Your *Clinics* subscription just got better!

You can now access the FULL TEXT of this publication online at no additional cost! Activate your online subscription today and receive...

- Full text of all issues from 2002 to the present
- Photographs, tables, illustrations, and references
- Comprehensive search capabilities
- Links to MEDLINE and Elsevier journals

Activate Your Online Access Today!

Plus, you can also sign up for E-alerts of upcoming issues or articles that interest you, and take advantage of exclusive access to bonus features!

To activate your individual online subscription:

1. Visit our website at **www.TheClinics.com**.

2. Click on "Register" at the top of the page, and follow the instructions.

3. To activate your account, you will need your subscriber account number, which you can find on your mailing label (note: the number of digits in your subscriber account number varies from six to ten digits). See the sample below where the subscriber account number has been circled.

This is your subscriber account number

```
************************************3-DIGIT 001
FEB00   J0167   C7   ( 123456-89 )  10/00   Q: 1

J.H. DOE, MD
531 MAIN ST
CENTER CITY, NY  10001-001
```

4. That's it! Your online access to the most trusted source for clinical reviews is now available.

theclinics.com

ELSEVIER

BRUCE H. THIERS, MD, Consulting Editor

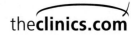

DERMATOLOGIC CLINICS

Dermatologic Therapy

DAVID I. McLEAN, MD
W. STUART MADDIN, MD
Guest Editors

April 2005 • Volume 23 • Number 2

SAUNDERS

An Imprint of Elsevier, Inc.
PHILADELPHIA   LONDON   TORONTO   MONTREAL   SYDNEY   TOKYO

W.B. SAUNDERS COMPANY
A Division of Elsevier Inc.

The Curtis Center • Independence Square West • Philadelphia, Pennsylvania 19106

http://www.theclinics.com

DERMATOLOGIC CLINICS
April 2005
Editor: Robert G. Gardler

Volume 23, Number 2
ISSN 0733-8635
ISBN 1-4160-2816-1

The ideas and opinions expressed in *Dermatologic Clinics* do not necessarily reflect those of the Publisher. The Publisher does not assume any responsibility for any injury and/or damage to persons or property arising out of or related to any use of the material contained in this periodical. The reader is advised to check the appropriate medical literature and the product information currently provided by the manufacturer of each drug to be administered to verify the dosage, the method and duration of administration, or contraindications. It is the responsibility of the treating physician or other health care professional, relying on independent experience and knowledge of the patient, to determine drug dosages and the best treatment for the patient. Mention of any product in this issue should not be construed as endorsement by the contributors, editors, or the Publisher of the product or manufacturers' claims.

Dermatologic Clinics (ISSN 0733-8635) is published quarterly by Elsevier Inc. Corporate and editorial offices: Elsevier, 170 S Independence Mall W 300 E, Philadelphia, PA 19106-3399. Accounting and circulation offices: 6277 Sea Harbor Drive, Orlando, FL 32887-4800. Periodicals postage paid at Orlando, FL 32862, and additional mailing offices. Subscription prices are USD 205 per year for US individuals, USD 314 per year for US institutions, USD 236 per year for Canadian individuals, USD 368 per year for Canadian institutions, USD 260 per year for international individuals, USD 368 per year for international institutions, USD 103 per year for US students, and USD 130 per year for international students. International air speed delivery is included in all *Clinics* subscription prices. All prices are subject to change without notice. POSTMASTER: Send address changes to *Dermatologic Clinics*, W.B. Saunders Company, Periodicals Fulfillment, Orlando, FL 32887-4800. **Customer Service: 1-800-654-2452 (US). From outside of the US, call 1-407-345-4000. E-mail: hhspcs@harcourt.com.**

Reprints. For copies of 100 or more, of articles in this publication, please contact the Commercial Reprints Department, Elsevier Inc., 360 Park Avenue South, New York, New York 10010-1710. Tel.: (212) 633-3813; Fax: (212) 462-1935; E-mail: reprints@elsevier.com.

The *Dermatologic Clinics* is covered in *Index Medicus, Current Contents/Clinical Medicine, Excerpta Medica, Chemical Abstracts,* and *ISI/BIOMED*.

Printed in the United States of America.

CONSULTING EDITOR

BRUCE H. THIERS, MD, Professor, Department of Dermatology, Medical University of South Carolina; Chief, Dermatology Service, Veterans Affairs Medical Center, Charleston, South Carolina

GUEST EDITORS

DAVID I. McLEAN, MD, Department of Dermatology, University of British Columbia, Vancouver, British Columbia, Canada

W. STUART MADDIN, MD, Department of Dermatology, University of British Columbia, Vancouver, British Columbia, Canada

CONTRIBUTORS

MEI CHEN, PhD, Professor, Medicine (Dermatology), University of Sourthern California Dermatology, Norris Cancer Center, Keck School of Medicine, University of Southern California, Los Angeles, California

BAHAR DASGEB, MD, Fellow in Dermatology, Department of Dermatology, Boston University School of Medicine, Boston, Massachusetts

WILLIAM H. EAGLSTEIN, MD, Department of Dermatology and Cutaneous Surgery, University of Miami School of Medicine, Miami, Florida

WARREN GARNER, MD, Associate Professor, Division of Plastic Surgery, Doheney Eye Institute, Keck School of Medicine, University of Southern California, Los Angeles, California

MARSHA L. GORDON, MD, Associate Clinical Professor, Department of Dermatology, Mount Sinai School of Medicine, New York, New York

ILTEFAT HAMZAVI, MD, Clinical Assistant Professor; and Director, Photomedicine and Laser Unit, Department of Dermatology, Wayne State University, Detroit, Michigan

VINCENT C. HO, MD, Professor, Division of Dermatology, Department of Medicine, Vancouver Hospital and Health Sciences Center and University of British Columbia, Vancouver, British Columbia, Canada

DAVID B. HUANG, MD, MPH, Infectious Disease Fellow, Division of Infectious Diseases, Department of Medicine, Baylor College of Medicine; University of Texas at Houston School of Public Health; and Division of Infectious Diseases, Department of Medicine, University of Texas Health Science Center at Houston, Houston, Texas

STEVEN P. LaROSA, MD, Staff, Department of Infectious Diseases, Cleveland Clinic Foundation, Cleveland, Ohio

MELISSA CHESLER LAZARUS, MD, Resident Physician, Department of Psychiatry and Behavioral Sciences, University of Miami School of Medicine, Miami, Florida

MARK LEBWOHL, MD, Chairman, Department of Dermatology, The Mount Sinai School of Medicine, New York, New York

WEI LI, PhD, Professor, Medicine (Dermatology), University of Sourthern California Dermatology, Norris Cancer Center, Keck School of Medicine, University of Southern California, Los Angeles, California

YONG LI, MD, Research Associate, Division of Dermatology, University of Sourthern California Dermatology, Norris Cancer Center, Keck School of Medicine, University of Southern California, Los Angeles, California

HARVEY LUI, MD, FRCPC, Division of Dermatology, Vancouver General Hospital, University of British Columbia, Vancouver, British Columbia, Canada

KAREN MALLIN, PsyD, Clinical Psychologist/Instructor, Department of Psychiatry and Behavioral Sciences; and Department of Dermatology and Cutaneous Surgery, University of Miami School of Medicine, Miami, Florida

MONA Z. MOFID, MD, Assistant Professor, Department of Dermatology, Johns Hopkins University School of Medicine, Baltimore, Maryland

CHRISTIAN A. MURRAY, BSc, MD, FRCPC, Clinical Assistant Professor, Division of Dermatology, Department of Medicine, Sunnybrook and Women's College Health Sciences Centre, University of Toronto, Toronto, Ontario, Canada

JEAN-PAUL ORTONNE, MD, Professor and Chairman, Service de Dermatologie, Hôpital l'Archet 2, Nice, France

RAVINDRAN A. PADMANABHAN, MD, MRCP, Fellow, Department of Infectious Diseases, Cleveland Clinic Foundation, Cleveland, Ohio

KATIE R. PANG, MD, Dermatology Resident, Department of Dermatology, Wayne State University School of Medicine, Detroit, Michigan

THIERRY PASSERON, MD, Clinical Assistant, Service de Dermatologie, Hôpital l'Archet 2, Nice, France

TANIA PHILLIPS, MD, Professor, Department of Dermatology, Boston University School of Medicine, Boston, Massachusetts

ELIZABETH K. ROSS, MD, Division of Dermatology, University of British Columbia and Vancouver Coastal Health Research Institute, Vancouver, British Columbia, Canada

DANIEL N. SAUDER, MD, Professor and Chairman, Department of Dermatology, Johns Hopkins University School of Medicine, Baltimore, Maryland

JERRY SHAPIRO, MD, FRCPC, Division of Dermatology, University of British Columbia and Vancouver Coastal Health Research Institute, Vancouver, British Columbia, Canada

NEIL H. SHEAR, MD, FRCPC, Helen and Paul Phalen Professor and Chief, Division of Dermatology, Department of Medicine, Sunnybrook and Women's College Health Sciences Centre, University of Toronto, Toronto, Canada

ARTHUR J. SOBER, MD, Department of Dermatology; and Melanoma Center, Massachusetts General Hospital, Boston, Massachusetts

DANA KAZLOW STERN, MD, Fellow, Department of Dermatology, The Mount Sinai School of Medicine, New York, New York

TORY SULLIVAN, MD, Assistant Voluntary Professor, Department of Dermatology and Cutaneous Surgery, University of Miami School of Medicine, Miami, Florida

KENNETH J. TOMECKI, MD, Staff, Department of Dermatology, Cleveland Clinic Foundation, Cleveland, Ohio

JACKIE M. TRIPP, MD, Chief Resident, Division of Dermatology, Department of Medicine, Vancouver Hospital and Health Sciences Center and University of British Columbia, Vancouver, British Columbia, Canada

HENSIN TSAO, MD, PhD, Department of Dermatology; Melanoma Center; and Wellman Center for Photomedicine, Massachusetts General Hospital, Harvard Medical School, Boston, Massachusetts

STEPHEN K. TYRING, MD, PhD, MBA, Medical Director, Center for Clinical Studies; and Professor, Department of Dermatology, University of Texas Health Science Center at Houston, Houston, Texas

LAURENCE WARSHAWSKI, BSc, MD, FRCPC, Clinical Professor, Division of Dermatology, Department of Medicine, University of British Columbia, Vancouver, British Columbia, Canada

GAVIN A.E. WONG, MBChB, MRCP(UK), Clinical Fellow, Division of Dermatology, Department of Medicine, Sunnybrook and Women's College Health Sciences Centre, University of Toronto, Toronto, Canada

DAVID T. WOODLEY, MD, Professor and Chief, University of Sourthern California Dermatology, Norris Cancer Center, Keck School of Medicine, University of Southern California, Los Angeles, California

JASHIN J. WU, MD, Clinical Research Fellow, Department of Dermatology, University of California at Irvine, Irvine, California

DAVID ZLOTY, BSc, MD, FRCPC, Clinical Assistant Professor, Division of Dermatology, Department of Medicine, University of British Columbia, Vancouver, British Columbia, Canada

FORTHCOMING ISSUES

July 2005

Advanced Cosmetic Surgery
Neil Sadick, MD, *Guest Editor*

October 2005

Psychocutaneous Diseases
Madhulika A. Gupta, MD, *Guest Editor*

January 2006

Sunscreens
Zoe D. Draelos, MD, *Guest Editor*

RECENT ISSUES

January 2005

Advanced Surgical Reconstructive Techniques
Marc D. Brown, MD, *Guest Editor*

October 2004

Psoriasis
Alan Menter, MD, and
Jennifer Cather, MD, *Guest Editors*

July 2004

Bioterrorism
Boni E. Elewski, MD, *Guest Editor*

THE CLINICS ARE NOW AVAILABLE ONLINE!

Access your subscription at:
http://www.theclinics.com

CONTENTS

Preface   xi
David I. McLean and W. Stuart Maddin

Treating Children Is Different   171
Karen Mallin and Melissa Chesler Lazarus

This article discusses how treating children is different from treating adults and shows areas where physicians can enhance their practice of medicine by addressing these developmental factors in their dermatology clinic.

Wound-Healing Perspectives   181
Wei Li, Bahar Dasgeb, Tania Phillips, Yong Li, Mei Chen, Warren Garner, and David T. Woodley

Wound-healing in the skin is a complex orchestration of cellular processes, which has been perfected throughout the eons of phylogeny. It has so many coordinated biologic processes invoked both simultaneously and in a regulated orderly fashion that it has been likened to a recapitulation of gestation. Part of the problem with studying wound healing is in analyzing the processes independently and then seeing how they fit together and influence each other. This article discusses selected and recent scientific observations that have given insight into the biology of human skin wound healing. The article then discusses selected clinical advances that are based less on evidence-based observation and more on what works in practice and promotes wound healing.

Cyanoacrylates for Skin Closure   193
William H. Eaglstein and Tory Sullivan

Cyanoacrylates (CAs) were not widely adopted for medical use until recently because of lingering concerns regarding the initial tissue toxicities of the short-chain CAs. The medium-chain CAs, primarily butyl-cyanoacrylate, have been widely used in Europe and Canada for several decades and have gone a long way in dispelling any lingering concerns about tissue toxicity. The newer, longer chain CA, octyl-2-cyanoacrylate (2-OCA), now has been approved for multiple uses in the United States and has achieved widespread acceptance by the medical and lay communities. The current authors believe that this is probably only the beginning of the use of 2-OCA and other CAs in cutaneous medicine. This article discusses the use of CAs in their original cutaneous use as glues for the repair of lacerations and incisions and in their more recent use as dressings for the treatment of abrasions and wounds.

Using Light in Dermatology: An Update on Lasers, Ultraviolet Phototherapy, and Photodynamic Therapy   199

Iltefat Hamzavi and Harvey Lui

Indications for light-based treatments, such as lasers, UV phototherapy, and photodynamic therapy, are rapidly increasing within the arena of skin disorders. Physicians can remain current in their understanding of these modalities if they understand a few basic principles outlined in this article. Once these concepts are understood, all the rapid advances can be kept in perspective and physicians can apply the most appropriate technology to the care of their patients while informing them about the limitations of overmarketed but poorly proved strategies.

Melanin Pigmentary Disorders: Treatment Update   209

Jean-Paul Ortonne and Thierry Passeron

Most of the melanin pigmentary disorders are cosmetically important and have a strong impact on the quality of life of affected individuals. This article examines recent advances in the treatment of melanin pigmentary disorder including hypermelanosis and hypomelanosis. The development of laser technologies has completed the use of the increasing number of bleaching agents in treating hyperpigmented lesions. The treatment of hypomelanotic disorders is still often disappointing, but new therapeutic options provide encouraging results.

Management of Hair Loss   227

Elizabeth K. Ross and Jerry Shapiro

The management of patients with hair loss requires a customized plan. Diagnosis, prognosis, psychosocial impact, treatment options, and patient preference are key determinants. This article discusses current agents for the treatment of three commonly encountered nonscarring alopecias: male- and female-pattern hair loss, telogen effluvium, and alopecia areata. Algorithmic approaches to management are provided.

Topical Immunotherapy: What's New   245

Daniel N. Sauder and Mona Z. Mofid

Further understanding of the pathogenesis of dermatologic conditions at a molecular level has led to targeted therapies. The topical immune response modifiers have contributed significantly to the treatment of cutaneous diseases. New topical remedies, particularly the Toll-like receptor agonists and calcineurin inhibitors, have added to the clinical armamentarium and have further advanced clinicians' ability to treat a wide variety of benign, premalignant, and malignant conditions. Furthermore, these agents have contributed to the understanding of the disease process. The next decade will witness even greater advances in targeted immunotherapies for dermatologic disease.

The Use of Systemic Immune Moderators in Dermatology: An Update   259

Dana Kazlow Stern, Jackie M. Tripp, Vincent C. Ho, and Mark Lebwohl

In addition to corticosteroids, dermatologists have access to an array of immunomodulatory therapies. Azathioprine, cyclophosphamide, methotrexate, cyclosporine, and mycophenolate mofetil are the systemic immunosuppressive agents most commonly used by dermatologists. In addition, new developments in biotechnology have spurred the development of immunobiologic agents that are able to target the immunologic process of many inflammatory disorders at specific points along the inflammatory cascade.

Alefacept, efalizumab, etanercept, and infliximab are the immunobiologic agents that are currently the most well known and most commonly used by dermatologists. This article reviews the pharmacology, mechanism of action, side effects, and clinical applications of these therapies.

What's New in Antibiotics? 301
Ravindran A. Padmanabhan, Steven P. LaRosa, and Kenneth J. Tomecki

Antibiotics are important agents in dermatologic practice. New drugs have expanded the therapeutic approach to uncomplicated skin infections and complicated infections involving deeper soft tissue or infections that require surgical intervention. This article reviews new antibiotics of dermatologic importance, including daptomycin (cyclic lipopeptide), linezolid (oxazolidinone), quinupristin-dalfopristin (streptogramins), moxifloxacin and gatifloxacin (fluoroquinolones), and dalbavancin and oritavancin, which are presently under investigation.

Advances in Antiviral Therapy 313
Jashin J. Wu, Katie R. Pang, David B. Huang, and Stephen K. Tyring

Infections with five of the herpesviruses (herpes simplex virus 1 [HSV-1], HSV-2, varicella zoster virus, Epstein-Barr virus, and cytomegalovirus) are treated with topical or systemic antiviral therapies. There are more than 100 genotypes of human papillomaviruses (HPVs), which may manifest as warts, skin cancers, cervical cancer, anogenital cancers, and upper digestive tract cancers. Molluscum contagiosum (MC) is a common, benign viral infection of the skin. Immunomodulating agents, such as imiquimod, act on HPV and MC indirectly by inducing host immune responses, such as cytokines and cell-mediated immunity, and thereby reduce recurrences. There are multiple vaccines available for certain viral diseases and others in development for HSV-2 and HPV.

Melanoma Treatment Update 323
Hensin Tsao and Arthur J. Sober

Except for high-dose interferon as adjuvant therapy in stage III disease, little success has emerged over the last 20 years for metastatic melanoma. Recent advances in melanoma biology suggest that disarming oncogenic mechanisms in melanoma may be an attractive approach to therapy. For instance, sustained expression of Bcl2 has been associated with an increased resistance to apoptosis, and recently, anti-sense–mediated reduction of Bcl2 levels was shown to chemosensitize patients to dacarbazine, dimethyl triazino imidazole carboxamide, or DTIC. Likewise, the identification of activating mutations in the RAS signaling pathway, including the *NRAS* and *BRAF* genes, opens up new therapeutic options for RAS and RAF inhibitors. A more thorough understanding of melanoma biology and tumor immunology will undoubtedly yield new promise for patients with advanced disease.

Adverse Drug Interactions and Reactions in Dermatology: Current Issues of Clinical Relevance 335
Gavin A.E. Wong and Neil H. Shear

This article highlights several adverse drug interactions and reactions relevant to current dermatologic practice. Absorption interactions between drugs and compounds containing polyvalent cations, potential interactions between herbal and conventional medicines, the meaning of *sulfa allergy*, and adverse cutaneous reactions caused by epidermal growth factor receptor inhibitors are discussed.

The Evolution of Soft Tissue Fillers in Clinical Practice   **343**
Christian A. Murray, David Zloty, and Laurence Warshawski

To remain experts in skin care and treatment, every dermatologist must be aware of the evolving role of soft tissue fillers in dermatology. Patients with facial scarring, lipodystrophy, contour abnormalities, and age- and sun-induced rhytids can be successfully treated. A literature review, industry recommendations, and the authors' experience serve to highlight fillers most appropriate for each patient's complaint. Newer agents, including the hyaluronic acids and human collagens, and long-lasting materials, such as polymethlymethracrylate and calcium hydroxlyapatite, are reviewed. This discussion of the specific risks, indications, and technical pearls for the various fillers will allow clinicians to accurately advise or treat patients.

Current Therapy

A Conservative Approach to the Nonsurgical Rejuvenation of the Face   **365**
Marsha L. Gordon

With ever-increasing frequency, dermatology patients are requesting information and treatments that improve the appearance of their skin. Corresponding to this trend, there is an ever-increasing number of products and procedures available that claim to aid in this pursuit. Finding a suitable regimen is a challenge for patients and physicians alike. Many different approaches may be helpful. This article outlines one general approach to choosing effective and safe treatments and procedures.

Index   **373**

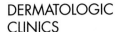
ELSEVIER
SAUNDERS

Dermatol Clin 23 (2005) xi – xii

Preface

Dermatologic Therapy

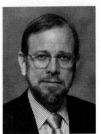 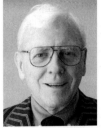

David I. McLean, MD   W. Stuart Maddin, MD
Guest Editors

The trend in medical care is toward personalized and predictive therapeutics. Individual variation in responsiveness and toxicity is increasingly recognized by the pharmaceutical industry and serious attempts have been made to tailor treatment to subsets of patients who are more likely to respond. Many of the thorough reviews in this issue of the *Dermatologic Clinics* reflect this new knowledge. We are on the edge of a revolution in health care.

We expect that many of the new treatments—as outlined in the review by Lebwohl and colleagues of system immunosuppressives, for example—will be increasingly used in a cost-effective manner. If nonresponders or poor responders can be weeded out before therapy, even otherwise expensive therapy can be used in a cost-effective manner.

The arrival of topical immune response modifiers in the 1990s ushered in a new era: that of a topical therapeutic approach in the treatment of diseases such as warts, and more recently, actinic keratosis and superficial basal cell carcinoma. The authoritative information regarding the use of this interferon-inducing agent has been prepared by Dr. Sauder, a pioneer in the field.

The update on the treatment of melanoma prepared by Drs. Tsao and Sober provides a clinical overview of the limited choices available along with practical therapeutic suggestions. Melanoma remains a fruitful area for potential research gains.

The advances in antiviral drugs include both preventative strategies and current treatment protocols. Tyring and colleagues have provided a thorough and current review of this rapidly changing field.

The increasing concern about the appropriate use of antibiotics is critically reviewed and is accompanied by practical recommendations. As with antivirals, antibiotic use in clinical practice is a rapidly evolving therapeutic area important to every clinician, and Tomecki has provided clear guidance to we practitioners.

Dr. Woodley covers wound healing, including basic mechanisms and how they affect wound management. We have learned much in the past decade, and it is important to bring that updated knowledge into our practices.

Providing a simple and cosmetically acceptable method for wound closure has long been a target. The use of tissue glue in the form of cyanoacrylates is reviewed by Dr. Eaglstein. Such tissue glue has the potential to reduce "railroad tracks" in surgical scars and allow for a better edge attachment of grafts. It is also an ideal treatment for painful fissures of the palm and soles.

Drs. Ross and Shapiro have provided a series of management approaches that give answers to clinicians who are called upon to treat diseases causing hair loss. The treatment algorithm outlines are of considerable clinical use.

Pigmentary disorders and their successful treatment play an expanding role in most clinical medical practices. Dr. Jean Paul Ortonne outlines a practical series of therapeutic approaches that meet this need.

Our concerns with drug reactions and interactions have not diminished. The introduction of new chemical entities presents new challenges. Dr. Shear, in his coverage, has been successful in laying down tenets that, if followed, will reduce risks to patients.

Quite often dermatologists and rheumatologists are called upon to treat the same diseases. Dr. Jan Dutz, with his unique background as both a dermatologist and a rheumatologist, has successfully bridged the disease overlap and the therapeutic approaches used by both.

The need for dermatologists to be aware of the changes taking place in phototherapy, photodynamic therapy, and lasers is highlighted in the section produced by Dr. Lui. All of us are aware that these modalities have revolutionized the practice of dermatology, and Dr. Lui has provided clinically relevant recommendations that should accompany their use.

Drs. Murray, Zloty, and Warshawski have in their review covered surgical injectables, which include a variety of new fillers that emphasize the ease of use and increased durability, as well as enhanced safety. Working in Canada, they have had extensive experience in using fillers just now becoming available in the United States, and they are willing to share that experience with us.

Lastly, not all dermatologists feel comfortable in dealing with children and their skin conditions. Drs. Mallin and Lazarus have succinctly outlined a series of easy-to-follow recommendations that will make dermatologists more confident when treating children with skin problems. Children really are different, and the effective treatment of children demands a thoughtful approach that takes these differences into consideration.

With this issue, we will have edited three issues of the *Dermatologic Clinics* targeting therapy, starting in 1993. We have seen dramatic improvements in therapy during this time, including new fields of major therapeutic options that were not even contemplated 12 years ago. For this issue, we have invited the current global leaders to introduce us to new options and to update us on improvements in the use of more familiar therapeutic interventions. We hope that you find this issue rewarding.

David I. McLean, MD
W. Stuart Maddin, MD
Department of Dermatology
University of British Columbia
855 West 10th Avenue
Vancouver, BC V5Z 4E8, Canada
E-mail address: dmclean@interchange.ubc.ca
(D.I. McLean)

ELSEVIER
SAUNDERS

Dermatol Clin 23 (2005) 171 – 180

Treating Children Is Different

Karen Mallin, PsyD[a,b,*], Melissa Chesler Lazarus, MD[b]

[a]Department of Psychiatry and Behavioral Sciences, University of Miami School of Medicine, 1600 NW 10th Avenue, R-250,
Miami, FL 33136, USA
[b]Department of Dermatology and Cutaneous Surgery, University of Miami School of Medicine, 1600 NW 10th Avenue,
Miami, FL 33136, USA

Dermatology has changed over the past several decades to a field that incorporates a more psychosocial approach to treatment. The current economic climate exerts pressure to keep costs to a minimum while increasing high-volume bottom lines. The challenge to physicians is deciding where to make sacrifices in their clinical practice to meet demands. Those working in pediatrics know that attending to several key developmental factors can make a significant difference in obtaining a thorough clinical history and physical examination, thus enhancing the ability to provide quality care. These factors include the following: decreasing stress in the child and his or her parent from the moment they enter the office, minimizing pain during procedures, and addressing issues that impede on adherence to the prescribed treatment regimen. This article discusses how treating children is different from treating adults and areas where physicians can enhance their practice of medicine by addressing these developmental factors in their dermatology clinic.

The office visit

The approach to the office visit is similar in many ways to that of a general pediatrician. It is important to create a comfortable environment for the child and the parent. A waiting room that is calm and invit-ing will help decrease the stress of waiting for both child and parent. Activities or a play area for pediatric patients and appropriate reading materials for both children and adults can help decrease initial anxiety associated with visiting the physician.

Parents often rush from home or work to see the physician. Therefore, it is important to help decrease parental stress on arrival before meeting with the physician. Children notice when their parents are under stress or nervous; this is called *social referencing*. The parent's behavior provides clues to the child that something is about to occur. Although the parent may be anxious for other reasons (eg, later needing to pick up another child after school on time), the child in the waiting room may feel that the parent is anxious about the dermatology visit. This perception may elevate the child's own anxiety about the visit. Therefore, it is important to see patients in a timely manner, especially when dealing with energetic children. If it is not possible to see the patient on time, parents should be informed of the situation and an explanation provided.

Children have specific developmental needs at each age period. Dermatologists who masterfully combine the science of observation and interpretation of developmental needs with the art of how to sequence and pace information while distracting the patient during a clinical examination will best meet the patient and families overall affective, cognitive, and physical development [1].

Infants

Examining infants who are younger than 1 year is generally easier than examining older infants and

---

* Corresponding author. Department of Psychiatry and Behavioral Sciences, University of Miami School of Medicine, 1600 NW 10th Avenue, R-250, Miami, FL 33136.
 E-mail address: kmallin@med.miami.edu (K. Mallin).

toddlers. It is important for the physician to carefully acquaint his- or herself to the child patient and the parent. Infants younger than 6 months have virtually no fear of physicians because stranger anxiety does not typically develop until age 8 to 10 months. Separation anxiety begins around 6 months, however. It is therefore important to put the parent at ease by encouraging his or her close proximity to the infant to provide comfort. Infants should be seated on the parent's lap, on a chair, or the examining table. Separation and stranger anxiety usually peak at approximately the age of 18 months, making examination more difficult. Reminding the parent that this is a normal developmental milestone can remove the frustration and concern that the infant or toddler is exceptionally fearful. In extremely fearful children, however, better results occur if the physician begins the examination by sitting as far away as possible, avoids eye contact, speaks softly, and moves slowly, with gradual movement closer to the child [1].

Infants should remain swaddled until the physical examination. On the first visit, the child should be examined head to toe. Once the examination begins, the child should be completely undressed. The parent best facilitates this process. Parents should be reassured that most infants cry when undressed in cold examining rooms. Often, a pacifier is useful to calm a crying child. The entire examination can occur on the parent's lap to facilitate the child's comfort and cooperation.

Toddlers and preschool-aged children

Before beginning the history and physical examination, it is important to engage the child by asking direct questions about their likes, games they play, siblings at home, school, best friends, and "what they do for fun." It is important to note these responses on the progress note so that the patient feels validated when he or she returns to the clinic because the physician remembered personal details.

Given the wide range of activity levels and cooperation in this age group, this is often the most difficult group to examine. Initiating play and incorporating this into the physical examination can be useful with these patients. The use of a parent's lap as an examining table can be useful in this age group as well. The physician should begin the history and physical examination seated at or below the level of the child to align with the child and to appear less "gigantic." The physician should also be aware not to sit or stand in a position that blocks the door, allowing the patient to visualize the door during the entire examination.

This technique allows the child to feel more control over his or her environment.

Young children between the ages of 2 years and 6 years often engage in imaginative play. Some may believe the physician in a white coat is a dangerous figure. Some physicians do not wear white coats when examining children for this reason. Language development is growing rapidly yet is still simplistic and concrete. Wording that does not carry multiple meanings, which could scare them, should be chosen. The same principle holds true for materials used in the clinic. Although liquid nitrogen splashed on the floor may be exciting for much older children, this common practice may confirm in young children's minds that the physician has magical powers capable of making things disappear into thin air, including them.

School-aged children

All of the rules for toddlers and preschool-aged children previously discussed apply to school-aged children, except that children will sit alone on the table for the physical examination. Physicians can address patients directly for history, with assistance from parents when the patient is unclear of the answer or seems shy and inhibited. School-aged children are able to tell where their skin problem is located, how it feels, and what makes it better or worse. Obtaining a personal history directly from the child is important to engage the child and make them feel more involved in the medical visit. School-aged children are capable of understanding what is going on during the visit. Therefore, it is important to explain everything that will happen, when it will happen, and what it will feel like. Involving the patient in the clinic visit helps to reduce fears that he or she may have before seeing the physician.

Adolescents

Adolescents are developing and exercising increasing independence as they mature. Speaking directly to them to obtain the history, instead of to parents in the room, reinforces that independence. Beginning the history with asking personal information about the patient, such as school, work, sports, or other activities, typically produces more information and builds rapport. This method also often helps to gain insight into the patient's life and actively engages the patient. At times, it may be necessary to obtain the history without the parents present to obtain a more accurate history. Simply explain to parents that with all teenage patients, having the parent step out of the room for part of the history is customary. Reinforce and emphasize to the teenager that discussions are confidential, and that unless the patient reveals information that could be life threatening to him/her, or others, the contents of the discussion will not be shared with others. Issues relating to confidentiality are discussed later.

It is important to remember that in this developmental age group, inherent concerns about modesty and body image exist. Providing appropriate gowns, drapes, and privacy for the physical examination is essential. Adolescents, in general, are able to cooperate with the physical examination and should be examined in a manner similar to adults.

Before treating adolescent patients for a condition, such as acne, ascertain whether the patient is concerned about the dermatologic problem or if the parent is more worried. Most treatment failures are because of overzealous parents and unconcerned adolescents. A teenager indifferent about a skin problem will not be motivated to treat it.

Dealing with pain and intrusive procedures

Originally, the belief was that infants and toddlers were incapable of feeling pain [2]. One of the first physicians to recognize that pediatric patients experienced pain during injections was MacKenzie [3], who first published a method of alleviating the pain of injections in 1954. She reported a technique that provided localized analgesia by freezing a 1:1000 solution of Zephiran (benzalkonium chloride) in ice cubes. The frozen solution was rubbed on the patients' skin before injections, providing temporary pain relief.

Since that time, an increased interest in the management of pain in the pediatric population has sparked extensive research. Researchers have shown that even very-low-birth-weight premature infants experience pain [4]. In dermatology, it is often necessary to perform potentially painful procedures on pediatric patients. Local anesthesia, injections, biopsies, and cryotherapy are the most frequently performed procedures that illicit pain and prompt anxiety in the patient, the parent, and the physician. There are many pharmacologic and nonpharmacologic approaches to dealing with pain and intrusive procedures. These techniques can help minimize the discomfort experienced by the pediatric patient, and thereby that of the parent and physician.

Nonpharmacologic approaches

Minimizing the trauma of painful procedures requires an understanding of pediatric developmental stages. Generalizations can be made about children in each developmental stage, which can help dermatologists develop different approaches to performing these procedures. For simplicity, pediatric patients are divided into three groups: (1) infants, (2) toddlers and preschool-aged children, and (3) school-aged children and adolescents.

Infants

When treating infants, it is important to note that the level of anxiety experienced by the infant is often a reflection of parental fears. Research has identified that infants can recognize when their parents are nervous and react to these emotions [5]. Attending to the parents' comfort level and understanding of procedures can secondarily decrease anxiety in the infant. Babies younger than 6 months will rarely demonstrate distress if the parent is not in the room. Although their presence is beneficial, parents should not be made to feel guilty if they choose to leave the room during painful procedures. Effective modalities to decrease pain in this age group include the following: those of external comfort, such as swaddling and providing a pacifier; offering a distracting activity, such as bubbles; or having the parent hold and soothe the infant immediately after the procedure [6]. A pacifier soaked in a sucrose solution has shown effectiveness in decreasing the pain of procedures in the newborn period, although the most effective dose of sucrose has not been determined [7].

Because babies begin to develop stranger anxiety at the age of approximately 8 months, it is important to decrease this anxiety by encouraging the parent to be present with the child during the procedure. Research has shown across all age groups that the presence of parents during a painful procedure has beneficial effects on children and their parents [8]. Often, procedures can be performed on a parent's lap, if the parent agrees. Do not use parents to restrain a child during a painful procedure, however.

Toddlers and preschool-aged children

In this developmental age group, physicians can use the toddler's parental attachment as an ally. Ask parents to sit on the examining table with the child for painful procedures. Because children are trusting and curious at this age, it is important not to lie to children about pain. Honesty is the best policy; therefore, it is often helpful to describe to the child exactly what the procedure will feel like. Explaining to toddlers what will happen and what their role is, in simple language they can understand, is extremely useful to instill cooperation. Whenever giving an injection, avoid the word "shot" if possible. Substitute words such as "sting" or "pinch" instead. A scalpel, if seen by the patient, should be called "a green stick" because often children have heard the word "scalpel" on television associated with surgery. Distraction in this age group is an extremely effective method of pain reduction. Blowing bubbles or a pinwheel, counting, and reading a pop-up book are useful distractions. Patients in this age group also benefit from engaging in constant conversation.

It is best to have all of the materials prepared for procedures, such as a biopsy, before entering the room. It is often helpful to keep the scary items, such as needles, hidden until needed. Before beginning the procedure, children should be informed what their job is in the process. They need to hold very still and not kick; they can hold someone's hand, count backward to zero, yell, or cry. If patients need restraining, the parent should never be used to help restrain the child. Toddlers and early school-aged children should be constantly encouraged on their efforts during the procedure and commended for behaving very well, even if they are not. Reward good behavior with a tangible gift, such as a sticker.

School-aged children and adolescents

As noted previously, children in this age group also benefit from distraction techniques. Handheld video games, music on a walkman, or a television set in the room are better distractions for these patients. The previously described rules of yelling, but not moving, apply to this age group as well. Again, honesty is the best policy, and clear explanations of what the patient will experience are essential. Helping the patient retain control, by giving the choice of biopsy site for example, may be helpful in eliciting cooperation from school-aged children and adolescents. Children in this age group should be able to cooperate without restraint.

Pharmacologic approaches

Topical anesthetics

Since MacKenzie [3] reported the use of benzalkonium chloride (Zephiran), many new topical formulations and techniques have been used to decrease the pain of the needle stick. Local cooling is used

extensively and is relatively inexpensive. Skin cooling can be achieved by using ice or frozen gel packs. In addition, volatile liquid sprays (vapocoolant sprays), such as ethylchloride or fluorimethane (Gebauer), have been reported to be effective [9]. A study of 4- to 6-year-old children reported that when combined with distraction, vapocoolant spray is equally effective as an eutectic mixture of local anesthetics (EMLA) cream in reducing vaccination pain, and both are superior to distraction alone [10]. Vapocoolants may be applied directly from the container in a fine spray, or may be used to saturate a cotton ball that is applied to the skin for 15 seconds [11]. The liquid evaporates and provides pain relief for 1 to 2 minutes.

EMLA, which is an eutectic mixture of 2.5% prilocaine and 2.5% lidocaine, is reported to induce anesthesia to a depth of 3 to 5 mm on intact skin [12]. EMLA cream, available by prescription, must be applied under occlusion at least 1 hour before procedures and 2 hours before intramuscular injections to have an analgesic effect. Topical lidocaine (4% and 5% L-M-X, previously known as Ela-Max) is another over-the-counter topical anesthetic that can be used with and without occlusion, and should be applied 30 minutes before injection. Eichenfield et al [13] found that a 30-minute application of Ela-Max without occlusion is as safe and as effective for ameliorating pain associated with venipuncture as a 60-minute application of the prescription product EMLA, which requires occlusion.

Other topical agents, such as 4% tetracaine gel and betacaine-LA ointment (formerly eutectic-LA), have been shown to reduce pain but not as effectively as L-M-X or EMLA [14]. The use of lidocaine iontophoresis, which allows for the active transdermal delivery of lidocaine under the influence of a low-level electric current, has been reported to be effective for pain management of venipuncture [15]. Currently, however, few studies have been conducted to determine its utility in dermatology. Additional new topical treatments include amethocaine, which is not yet approved by the US Food and Drug Administration, and the S-caine patch.

Lidocaine

The use of lidocaine is necessary for many dermatologic procedures. The injection of lidocaine can potentially be very painful. Many techniques can be used to decrease the pain of injection, however. As discussed earlier, there are many effective topical methods to decrease the pain of the "prick" caused by the needle in local anesthesia. Other ways to decrease the pain of injection is to use a 30-gauge needle, puncture the skin rapidly at a 90° angle, and inject the medication slowly to minimize tissue distortion [16]. Punching or rubbing the skin in the area of injection before, and during injection, can also decrease pain by activating p-fibers in the skin and causing their depletion [17].

Altering the properties of injectable medications can also decrease the pain associated with injection. The pain of lidocaine infiltration can be decreased by warming the drug to body temperature or, at the minimum, room temperature before injection [18]. Buffering the anesthetic solution with sodium bicarbonate (1 mEq of sodium bicarbonate to 9 mL lidocaine) to raise the pH closer to a neutral pH decreases the burning associated with lidocaine [19].

Conscious sedation

Conscious sedation is an often-underused modality because of the fear of respiratory suppression in pediatric patients. Although beyond the scope of this article, enlisting a pediatric anesthesiologist, or becoming proficient in pediatric support, allows the incorporation of this useful pain control modality.

Adherence to dermatologic treatment programs

There is nothing more frustrating in dermatology and medicine in general than dealing with a patient, or family, who does not adhere to the prescribed treatment regimen. Studies in the pediatric literature report that significant percentages of children and adolescents do not adhere to treatment regimens in acute to chronic illnesses, making this an important issue in the daily practice of dermatology [20–22]. Estimates of overall adherence range between 10% to 60% in pediatric practice, although for some treatments, nonadherence has been reported as high as 70% [23–27]. Research exploring factors contributing to treatment adherence has increased over the past 30 years in response to these striking statistics. Despite these reports, a paucity of research on adherence exists in dermatology, with even fewer studies examining methods for improving treatment adherence [28,29]. As advances in science and technology are made, especially with the approval of biologic agents and topical immune modulators, concerns about treatment adherence increases, because many of these agents require more complex treatment regimens. Current research on treatment adherence in dermatology has identified approaches to improve the overall health status of children and adolescents affected by their skin disease.

Understanding treatment adherence from multiple perspectives

The literature often uses the terms *adherence* and *compliance* interchangeably [30]. One definition of compliance used most often in the medical literature states that compliance is the degree to which a person's behavior coincides with medical or health advice [31]. This definition places power with the physician for deciding what treatment is best and states that the patient needs to acquiesce and comply fully with directions, regardless of the effectiveness of the medical recommendations, their cost, their level of inconvenience, their discomfort, the developmental level of the child, or the impact on quality of life on the patient and family. This authoritarian medical view represents much of the older research on compliance, which describes reasons for noncompliance as caused by patient ignorance, disobedience, or forgetfulness, or as a reaction to the disease treatments [32].

Over the last 25 years, health care practices in dermatology have changed to incorporate the patient's and family's perspective on medical treatment decisions. Rather than identifying patients as adherent or not, adherence is operationalized on a continuum where various health care behaviors are rated by dividing the number of adherence behaviors completed by the number prescribed. Nonadherence therefore represents reasoned decision making rather than deviance. The strength of this approach to adherence in pediatric dermatology is that it can be used in the following ways: to measure different aspects of the treatment regimen over time, to highlight the complexity of health care behaviors for a particular skin disease, to allow a comparison of rates across different behaviors, and to compare with other research studies of adherence and with different dermatologic diseases [33].

Multidimensional factors associated with adherence

Treatment adherence is a multidimensional concept impacted by multiple factors and systems that affect children's health behaviors [27,34]. These include developmental factors, age factors, cognitive factors, social and emotional factors, and psychologic factors, and the role of the family and the physician. Understanding how these various factors can play a part in impeding medical outcome, and assessing which are present in patients, can guide the dermatologist to making adjustments in treatment recommendations necessary to ameliorate outcomes.

Developmental factors

A developmental perspective is an important factor, often overlooked although pediatric dermatologists are constantly evaluating the cognitive, motor, social, emotional, and physiologic functioning of the child. The developmental status of the child dictates how the skin disease is managed, how much responsibility is given and who is primarily responsible for following through with the treatment regimen, and barriers that may interfere with adequate health care delivery. These factors affect the course and management of skin disease and change as a child develops. This situation indicates that each component of treatment be evaluated individually and that adherence should be assessed over time.

Age factors

Age is an important factor identified in research on adherence with different medical populations [35]. For example, younger children have more difficulty participating in medical procedures, often showing more distress and uncooperative behaviors. Adolescents are expected to have more skills and knowledge regarding their skin disease than younger children, and yet they tend to be less adherent to prescribed therapy regimens than younger children [36]. Suggested reasons for nonadherence in adolescents are as follows: the level of parental support; peer pressure to conform; other factors, such as the impact of treatment regimens on major lifestyle requirements; cosmetic side effects; or treatments that interfere in social interactions. Furthermore, other research has found that, depending on the severity or chronicity of the disease, these factors may actually encourage better adherence because the adolescent is more aware of the need for treatment.

Cognitive factors

According to Piagetian theory, a child's view of health and illness changes over time as his or her cognitive abilities shift from a toddler or preschool-age child's preoperational thinking to more formal operational thinking found in adolescence. Preschoolers frequently regard illness causation with magical thinking as discussed earlier, often believing that their own negative behaviors or some other temporal event caused the skin disease to occur. When certain painful or aversive treatments are required, such as steroid injections for alopecia areata, the child may become overly distressed because he or she believes this treatment may be a punishment for previous misbehavior. Preparing young children for unpleasant procedures and clarifying the purpose of the treatment by reframing it in a way that makes sense to the young child can have a lasting impact on more chronic diseases and long-term therapies as they develop.

Early school-age children have the ability to understand that some external factors may play a role in disease processes, such as cold weather aggravation of eczema or the spread of germs or viruses by scratching as in molluscum contagiosum or verruca vulgaris. The cognitive stage of preoperational thinking is one made up of rigid rules that dictate behavior and outcome. They believe that strict adherence to these rules will provide relief or recovery from their skin disease, thinking that is very conducive to medical compliance. This factor most likely explains why many younger children are more adherent to their treatments than adolescents.

Once children reach adolescence, they are able to think abstractly, taking into account both internal and external factors that play a role in illness recovery and the complexities of health and disease. They continue to consider the immediate needs and desires of wanting to alleviate their skin disease, especially if it is visible to others. It is not until an individual reaches late adolescence or young adulthood that the implications of health behavior and adherence to treatment regimens is understood to impact future consequences of illness (eg, picking at acne pimples now likely creates permanent scarring later).

Social and emotional factors

Children's social and emotional development progresses through various stages much like their cognitive development. Infants begin this process by moving from a state of total physical dependence on the primary caregiver, to establishing relational attachments to parents. This relationship continues through the early preschool years. Once a child enters the school system, other relationships and peer friendships develop, taking on a new importance. Fitting into the crowd and feeling accepted plays a key role in certain health behaviors. Peer acceptance, independence, and autonomy also become major forces in the later school-age years through the adolescent period. These often-opposing developmental needs (autonomy versus affiliation) can interfere with an adolescent's motivation to adhere to dermatologic treatment regimens, often for reasons of not wanting to appear remarkably different from his or her peers. It is common for adolescents to use camouflage cosmetics, or clothing, to hide skin disease, such as vitiligo, psoriasis, or acne. They may refuse to apply creams or lotions to affected areas if the treatment is noticeable to others because of its appearance or smell. They may even engage in behaviors that might exacerbate their skin disease, such as contact with certain substances or environmental triggers, especially if their peer group is unaware of their specific needs, or because they fear peer rejection if they do not acquiesce.

Psychologic factors

Personality, temperament, and psychologic factors also play a role in adherence behaviors in children, depending on the emotional functioning, behavioral style, attitudes and beliefs about the skin disease, and the recommended treatment. Psychologic factors affecting children include whether they are experiencing distress or using avoidant coping behaviors. Dermatologists treating children and adolescents need to assess and address the psychosocial and psychologic factors that create barriers to treatment adherence. These factors include issues of self-esteem, coping with peer pressure, and dealing with social demands. Research has linked positive emotional functioning with good treatment adherence, especially for children with more chronic diseases [37]. Self-esteem that is more positive, flexible and adaptive coping styles, and lower levels of maladaptive coping have been associated with better adherence to medical regimens. The establishment of a trusting and collaborative relationship with a pediatric patient is reinforced when a dermatologist asks questions that help illuminate how the child's skin disease affects various aspects of his or her life. This approach builds a stronger collaborative working relationship with the family as well, and reinforces adherence behaviors to the prescribed treatment regimen. By evaluating the cognitive, motor, social, emotional, and physiologic functioning of the child or adolescent, the physician is able to identify the specific factors that play a role in adherence or nonadherence behaviors, allowing for flexibility in the treatment regimen and removing the blame from the individual.

The role of the family

Dealing with children is different from dealing with adults in that the physician works directly with the patient and all family members. Family members often take on the major responsibility for helping the child follow through on his or her treatment regimens; this situation is especially true for younger children [38]. Depending on how complex or cumbersome the regimen, these factors may restrict or interfere with the daily routines and functions of the family. Family factors may include financial constraints, the lack of social support, limited problem-solving abilities, a lack of family cohesion, and poor communication skills. How accepting family members are of the skin disease, how well they cope with and adjust to the needs of the child, and how restrictive their attitudes are toward parenting play a role in whether the child will remain adherent or believe in the treatment recommended [35].

It is often mistaken that adherence behaviors are synonymous with health outcome. Nonadherence and nonresponse to a treatment regimen are two distinct issues [39]. Even when complete adherence occurs, there is no guarantee of symptom relief or illness recovery. This situation directly influences motivation to follow through with the prescribed regimen. Dermatologists and family members may also believe that maintaining good health or preventing future complications should provide sufficient motivation to ensure treatment adherence in children. This perception rarely takes into consideration developmental issues and child concerns about feeling different. To facilitate long-term treatment adherence, external positive reinforcers may need to be used to maintain a child's adherence behaviors [40].

Parental involvement in the treatment of pediatric dermatology patients requires that the physician assess active knowledge of the skin disease and the parent's skill in managing the tasks to provide the care required. With advances in treatments for challenging skin conditions, such as psoriasis, epidermolysis bullosa, and ichthyosis, increasing behavioral demands burden children and their families. These demands may involve multiple daily procedures, careful dosing, and increased time demands. Basic understanding of the skin disease may or may not be as related to adherence as active knowledge of the illness process and the ability to accurately execute tasks, making adjustments when problems arise. This situation is especially true for episodic diseases, such as atopic dermatitis, where parents need to quickly problem-solve and alter regimens during the first signs of disease flare for successful treatment management. Unique to working in pediatrics is that knowledge and problem-solving skills change over time as a function of developmental progress. As children age, so do their cognitive abilities and the level of responsibility to manage more of their own disease therapy. Dermatologists also need to take these factors into account when designing a treatment protocol, which should include an educational component [31].

Family variables, such as socioeconomic status, family cohesiveness, and family constellation factors, play a role in how to manage skin disease. Parental and social supports are instrumental in successful adaptation to chronic skin conditions and disease management. In many cases, a child's skin disease can disrupt family routine and lifestyle, and, depending on the demands placed on the family, the family can harbor resentment and frustration. The role of family support is critical for pediatric health care, especially when the family situation is less than optimal. Research has reported that family conflict and stress often coincide with poor treatment management. Although it is assumed that there is a bidirectional influence of family functioning and adherence to treatment, these factors play an important role in clinical application when well documented.

The role of the physician

Physicians aspiring to improve medical adherence need to consider the family's parenting style and adopt a family systems perspective when developing their interventions with pediatric dermatology patients. This perspective takes into account that each family member's physical, social, and emotional functioning is profoundly interdependent with that of other family members; changes in one part of the system reverberate in other parts.

Illness and treatment factors influencing adherence include the following: the complexity of the treatment regimen, the duration of the skin disease, and whether the skin disease is acute or chronic. Dermatology treatment regimens for acne involve multiple complex behaviors requiring several different strategies for assessing adherence. For example, an adolescent may consistently adhere to washing his or her face with a mild soap and waiting 30 minutes before applying Tazarac (tazarotene) cream before bedtime. He or she may not be adherent to taking oral antibiotic medication several times a day, however. Thus, adherence to one aspect of a regimen does not necessarily imply adherence to others.

At times, a child's self-care behaviors do not match the prescribed medical recommendations. Usually when this occurs, what appears as nonadherence to a treatment regimen can be explained by either lack of understanding or lack of knowledge about the treatment. This situation can also occur

from the incomplete specification by the physician about expectations in desired health care behavior.

Adherence is a very difficult construct to assess and measure reliably [25,41]. Various methods used to assess treatment adherence are better than others. Several measures include the following: treatment outcome/health status; drug assays or biochemical markers of medication; self-reports; ratings by health care professionals; child or parent behavioral observations; monitoring devices, such as Medication Event Monitoring Systems; pill counts; and interview and 24-hour recall [33,42–44]. Measures appropriate for short-term treatment regimens may not be practical for chronic diseases, such as atopic dermatitis, with complex regimens [24]. Each method has assets and limitations. The use of multiple procedures works best to improve adherence. Various techniques have been used successfully to increase treatment adherence. They include simplifying treatment demands on the patient and family as much as possible. In addition, specifying the particular behaviors expected of the patient helps to clarify health behavior expectations. Adherence is enhanced when physicians attempt to incorporate the treatment regimen into the patient's lifestyle [33]. The referral of patients to a pediatric psychologist, who can use interventions including education, cognitive/behavioral approaches, and self-regulatory skills training to enhance adherence, has been shown to be effective [33]. In addition, the availability of adequate health care, a positive relationship with the health care system, and trust in the physician treating the child play a role in satisfaction with care and willingness to follow through. Demographic variables, such as race, gender, religion, and educational level of the parent, have not been good predictors of adherence in pediatric populations [45]. Factors involving the physician include poor communication skills and having conflicting goals for managing disease than those desired by the patient or family.

In summary, to understand and predict adherence behavior in pediatric patients, it is important to consider that it is a multidimensional concept impacted by multiple factors and systems. Health behavior and health status are dynamically interrelated. Gathering a child's and family's history of adherence efforts, and the effects of additional health care behaviors on health status, may determine subsequent disease management. If a child or adolescent has presented with a suboptimal response to medical treatment, anticipated compliance may be problematic. As previously discussed, however, suboptimal response to treatment also can be impacted by a multitude of developmental factors, family dynamics, prior medical history, response to pain, and fear of medical procedures. The intricacy of different disease requirements, coupled with the diverse challenges faced by children and their families at different developmental stages, may prevent establishing models of health care behavior, making this one of the many unique challenges for those working in pediatrics versus adult dermatology. Using the techniques discussed previously will maximize health outcomes in young patients and bring the art and science of dermatology to the forefront. Most important, dermatologists working with children consider these factors every time they step into the room as they begin their assessment, which is why treating children is different.

References

[1] Algranati PS. Effect of developmental status on the approach to physical examination. Pediatr Clin North Am 1998;45(1):1–23.

[2] McGee JP, Stapleton FB. Painless injections in pediatric practice. J Pediatr 2004;144(4):436.

[3] MacKenzie EP. Painless injections in pediatric practice. J Pediatr 1954;44:421.

[4] Johnston CC, Stevens BJ, Yang F, Horton L. Differential response to pain by very premature neonates. Pain 1995;61(3):471–9.

[5] Landolf-Fritsche B, Powers SW, Sturges JW. Differences between high and low coping children and between parent and staff behaviors during painful medial procedure. J Pediatr Psychol 1991;16:795–809.

[6] Campos RG. Soothing pain-elicited distress in infants with swaddling and pacifiers. Child Dev 1989;60: 781–92.

[7] Stevens B, Ohlsson A. Sucrose for analgesia in newborn infants undergoing painful procedures. Cochrane Database Syst Rev 2000;2:CD001069.

[8] Bauchner H, Waring C, Vinci R. Parental presence during procedures in an emergency room: results from 50 observations. Pediatrics 1991;87:544–88.

[9] Ebner CA. Cold therapy and its effects on procedural pain in children. Issues Compr Pediatr Nurs 1996;19: 197–208.

[10] Reis EC, Holubkov R. Vapocoolant spray is equally effective as EMLA cream in reducing immunization pain in school-aged children. Pediatrics 1997;100:e5.

[11] Reis EC, Jacobson RM, Tarbell S, Weniger BG. Taking the sting out of shots: control of vaccination-associated pain and adverse reactions. Pediatr Ann 1998;27(6): 375–86.

[12] Gajraj NM, Pennant JH, Watcha MF. Eutectic mixture of local anesthetics (EMLA) cream. Anesth Analg 1994;78:574–83.

[13] Eichenfield LF, Funk A, Fallon-Friedlander S, Cunningham BB. A clinical study to evaluate the efficacy of ELA-Max (now known as L.M.X.4™) (4% lipo-

somal lidocaine) as compared with eutectic mixture of local anesthetics cream for pain reduction of venipuncture in children. Pediatrics 2002;109(6): 1093–9.

[14] Friedman PM, Fogelman JP, Nouri K, Levine VJ, Ashinoff R. Comparative study of the efficacy of four topical anesthetics. Dermatol Surg 1999;25(12): 950–4.

[15] Rose JB, Galinkin JL, Jantzen EC, Chiavacci RM. A study of lidocaine iontophoresis for pediatric venipuncture. Anesth Analg 2002;94(4):867–71.

[16] Wagner AM. Pain control in the pediatric patient. Dermatol Clin 1998;16(3):609–17.

[17] Barnhill BJ, Holbert MD, Jackson NM, Erickson RS. Using pressure to decrease the pain of intramuscular injections. J Pain Symptom Manage 1996;12:52–8.

[18] Davidson JAH, Boom SJ. Warming lidocaine to reduce pain associated with injection. BMJ 1992;305:617–8.

[19] Bartfield JM, Gennis P, Barbera J, et al. Buffered versus plain lidocaine as a local anesthetic for simple laceration repair. Ann Emerg Med 1990;19:1387–90.

[20] Cork MJ, Britton J, Butler L, Young S, Murphy R, Keohane SG. Comparison of parent knowledge, therapy utilization and severity of atopic eczema before and after explanation and demonstration of topical therapies by a specialist dermatology nurse. Br J Dermatol 2003;149(3):582–9.

[21] D'Alessandro DM, Kingsley P, Johnson-West J. The readability of pediatric patient education materials on the World Wide Web. Arch Pediatr Adolesc Med 2001;155(7):807–12.

[22] Koo J. How do you foster medication adherence for better acne vulgaris management? Skin Med 2003;2(4):229–33.

[23] Dunbar-Jacob J, Dunning EJ, Dwyer K. Compliance research in pediatric and adolescent populations: two decades of research. In: Krasnegor NP, Epstein LH, Johnson SB, Yaffe SJ, editors. Developmental aspects of health compliance behavior. Hillsdale, NJ: Erlbaum; 1993. p. 29–51.

[24] Fischer G. Compliance problems in paediatric atopic eczema. Australas J Dermatol 1996;37:510–3.

[25] LaGreca AM, Schuman WB. Adherence to prescribed medical regimens. In: Roberts MC, editor. Handbook of pediatric psychology. 2nd edition. New York: Guilford Press; 1995. p. 55–83.

[26] Renzi C, Picardi A, Abeni D, et al. Association of dissatisfaction with care and psychiatric morbidity with poor treatment compliance. Arch Dermatol 2002; 138:337–42.

[27] Sherbourne CD, Hays RD, Ordway L, DiMatteo MR, Kravitz RL. Antecedents of adherence to medical recommendations: results from the Medical Outcomes Study. J Behav Med 1992;15(5):447–68.

[28] Roter DL, Hall JA, Merisca R, Nordstrom B, Cretin D, Svarstad B. Effectiveness of interventions to improve patient compliance: a meta-analysis. Med Care 1998; 36(8):1138–61.

[29] Renzi C, Abeni D, Picardi A, et al. Factors associated

with patient satisfaction with care among dermatological outpatients. Br J Dermatol 2001;145(4):617–23.

[30] Rapoff MA. Adherence to pediatric medical regimens. Boston: Klewer Academic; 1999.

[31] Haynes RB, McDonald HP, Garg AX. Helping patients follow prescribed treatment. JAMA 2002; 288(22):2880–3.

[32] Witkowski JA. Compliance: the Dermatologic Patient. Int J Dermatol 1988;27(9):608–11.

[33] Meichenbaum D, Turk DC. Facilitating treatment adherence: a practitioner's guidebook. New York: Plenum Press; 1987. p. 11–75.

[34] Fielding D, Duff A. Compliance with treatment protocols: interventions for children with chronic illness. Arch Dis Child 1999;80:196–200.

[35] Manne SL, Jacobsen PB, Gorfinkle K, Gerstein F, Redd WH. Treatment adherence difficulties among children with cancer: the role of parenting style. J Pediatr Psychol 1993;18(1):47–62.

[36] Friedman IM, Litt IF. Promoting adolescents' compliance with therapeutic regimens. Pediatr Clin North Am 1986;33(4):955–73.

[37] Reid GJ, Dubow EF, Carey TC, Dura JS. Contribution of coping to medical adjustment and treatment responsibility among children and adolescents with diabetes. J Dev Behav Pediatr 1994;15:327–35.

[38] LaGreca AM. Issues in adherence with pediatric regimens. J Pediatr Psychol 1990;15:285–308.

[39] Koehler AM, Maibach HI. Electronic monitoring in medication adherence measurement. Implications for dermatology. Am J Clin Dermatol 2001;2(1):7–12.

[40] Varni JW, Babani L. Long-term adherence to health care regimens in pediatric chronic disorders. In: Krasnegor NA, Arasteh JD, Cataldo MF, editors. Child health behavior: a behavioral pediatrics perspective. New York: Wiley; 1986. p. 502–20.

[41] Cluss PA, Epstein LH. The measurement of medical compliance in the treatment of disease. In: Karoly P, editor. Measurement strategies in health psychology. New York: Wiley; 1985. p. 403–32.

[42] Balkrishnan R, Carroll CL, Camacho FT, Feldman SR. Electronic monitoring of medication adherence in skin disease: results of a pilot study. J Am Acad Dermatol 2003;49(4):651–4.

[43] Christophersen ER. Pediatric compliance: a guide for the primary care physician. New York: Plenum Press; 1994.

[44] Parrish JM. Parent compliance with medical and behavioral recommendations. In: Krasnegor NA, Arasteh JD, Cataldo MF, editors. Child health behavior: a behavioral pediatrics perspective. New York: Wiley; 1986. p. 453–501.

[45] Lemanek KL, Kamps J, Chung NB. Empirically supported treatments in pediatric psychology: regimen adherence. J Pediatr Psychol 2001;26(5):253–75.

ELSEVIER
SAUNDERS

Dermatol Clin 23 (2005) 181 – 192

DERMATOLOGIC
CLINICS

Wound-Healing Perspectives

Wei Li, PhD[a], Bahar Dasgeb, MD[b], Tania Phillips, MD[b], Yong Li, MD[a],
Mei Chen, PhD[a], Warren Garner, MD[c], David T. Woodley, MD[a],*

[a]University of Southern California Dermatology, Norris Cancer Center, Keck School of Medicine,
University of Southern California, 1441 Eastlake Avenue, Los Angeles, CA 90033, USA
[b]Department of Dermatology, Boston University School of Medicine, 609 Albany Street, Boston, MA 02118, USA
[c]Division of Plastic Surgery, Doheney Eye Institute, Keck School of Medicine, University of Southern California, 3rd Floor,
1500 San Pablo Avenue, Los Angeles, CA 90033, USA

Wound healing in the skin is a complex orchestration of cellular processes, which have been perfected throughout the eons of phylogeny. This process has so many coordinated biologic processes invoked both simultaneously and in a regulated orderly fashion that it has been likened to a recapitulation of gestation. Part of the problem with studying wound healing is dissecting out the processes independently and then seeing how they fit together and influence each other. This article discusses selected, recent scientific observations that have given insight into the biology of human skin wound healing. The article then turns to selected clinical advances that are based less on evidence-based observation and more on what has been found to work and to promote wound healing in practice.

Selected scientific observations

What are the intrinsic prohealing elements in skin?

The first phase of wound healing includes the following processes: clotting of the blood, aggregation of platelets, release of platelet contents, the transformation of plasma into serum, and inflammation [1]. Wound healing of skin involves so many

processes that it is difficult to determine the origins of biologic elements within a complex wound. To get around this problem, investigators have attempted to isolate processes in vitro and dissect what a given cell or tissue can contribute. Falanga et al have been working with a commercially available, three-dimensional skin substitute, Apligraf (Organogenesis, Canton, Massachusetts). This construct consists of a collagen lattice gel containing human dermal fibroblasts overlaid with human keratinocytes. After appropriate culture, including time for keratinocyte expansion and a period of air-fluid culture to stratify and mature the differentiation of the keratinocytes, the construct consists of a bilayer of a neodermis covered with a stratified epithelium of human keratinocytes. This skin equivalent construct can then be used for grafting onto human skin wounds. The construct does not engraft permanently on the human recipient because it is made of allogeneic cells. Nevertheless, its presence in human wounds for a period of time is believed to promote wound healing by the provision of growth factors, cytokine release, structural support, and a moist wound environment [2]. The skin equivalent in culture does not have all of the inflammatory or clotting elements involved in an acute human skin wound, such as platelets or inflammatory cells; therefore, the skin equivalent provides an opportunity to see what the intrinsic cells of the construct can contribute to the wound by wounding the construct in vitro.

The skin equivalent can be wounded in vitro by meshing the construct as a surgeon would do for the

* Corresponding author.
  E-mail address: dwoodley@hsc.usc.edu
(D.T. Woodley).

preparation of split-thickness skin for mesh grafts on burn wounds or by creating a scalpel incision wound into the construct. It was found that the skin equivalent stimulated by wounding produced an ordered and reproducible cytokine profile reminiscent of that seen in human skin wounds. Interleukin 1β (IL-1β) was expressed 12 hours after wounding, whereas IL-1α and transforming growth factor α (TGF-α) expression peaked at 24 hours. Other cytokines were expressed as well but later in the sequence, including TGF-β and insulinlike growth factor 2 at 48 hours and platelet-derived growth factor BB (PDGF-BB) at 72 hours. The specificity of this cytokine staged progression was suggested not only by the reproducibility of the timing but because certain cytokines did not change at all during the postwound period of observation. This model makes it clear that two predominant cells intrinsic to the skin, namely keratinocytes and dermal fibroblasts, are capable of contributing growth factors and cytokines believed to be essential to wound healing. Furthermore, the expression of the keratinocyte- and fibroblast-derived cytokines was associated with a functional component within the skin equivalent: the transformation of the keratinocytes from a differentiation or proliferative mode into a mode of cell migration.

Associated with the ordered cytokine progression, there was decreased keratinocyte proliferation and a coordinate increase in keratinocyte motility and re-epithelialization. Sarret et al [3] showed that the proliferative potential of human keratinocytes could be driven essentially to zero by the presence of TGF-β, and yet the keratinocytes were readily capable of cell migration on promigratory extracellular matrices (ECMs), such as type I collagen and fibronectin. This finding suggests that keratinocytes can either be in a proliferative mode or a migratory mode but cannot do both biologic functions at the same time. The TGF-β expression within the skin equivalent likely contributes to the keratinocyte hypoproliferative and promigratory mode associated with re-epithelialization of the incision or mesh wound. Epidermal growth factor (EGF), TGF-α, and IL-1α promote human keratinocyte migration if the cells are apposed to a promotility matrix [4–6]. These selected cytokines and growth factors are expressed strongly in the postwound period of the skin equivalent at a time when the keratinocytes in the construct are involved in re-epithelialization.

This model increases the understanding of the healing of skin wounds because it dissects the wound-healing process such that the immune system, bone marrow, and inflammatory cells have been nullified because they are absent from Apligraf. These obser-

vations dissect out what the intrinsic contributions of the skin are to many important elements in wound healing. In addition, these observations are in accordance with the current authors' clinical impressions of skin wound healing. Clinically, the authors know that when patients have had chemotherapy and bone marrow ablation for stem cell or bone marrow transplantation, these procedures are not associated with delayed healing of skin wounds in any significant or consistent manner.

Serum versus plasma

A simplistic view of the influences on cells in a wound could be that there are essentially two elements: small soluble factors, such as cytokines and growth factors, or large connective tissue macromolecules, such as ECM components. The nutrients supplied to keratinocytes, fibroblasts, melanocytes, Merkel cells, Langerhans' cells, and endothelial cells in unwounded healthy skin come from a filtrate of plasma. The proteins within the plasma of the circulation must pass through a basement membrane zone (BMZ) that surrounds each dermal blood vessel. These proteins are then available to bathe and influence the biology of dermal fibroblasts. The same proteins may diffuse from the dermis, cross the dermal-epidermal junction where another basement membrane zone lies, and enter the epidermis where they may influence the biology of epidermal cells.

Little is known about which plasma proteins selectively diffuse through the vascular basement membranes and influence the dermal cells versus which plasma proteins selectively diffuse through the basement membrane zone at the dermal-epidermal junction and influence the epidermal cells. This question is interesting because the vascular BMZ and the BMZ of the dermal-epidermal junction have both common and different elements. Common elements include type IV collagen, laminin-1, and heparin sulfate proteoglycans. The BMZ at the dermal-epidermal junction, however, also contains type VII collagen, type XVII collagen, and anchoring filament proteins, such as laminin-5. During wounding, the blood vessels are cut, clotting mechanisms are invoked, platelets aggregate, releasing their contents, and the plasma is converted into serum. The skin cells in a wound, therefore, for the first time are confronted with serum rather than plasma. In most in vitro keratinocyte cultures and keratinocyte motility assays, bovine pituitary extract (BPE) is present as a source of growth factors because of a long tradition of culturing human keratinocytes in low-calcium, serum-free conditions as established by Boyce and Ham [7]. In this keratinocyte culture medium, the medium is supplemented with BPE, transferrin, hydrocortisone, and EGF. Nevertheless, little is known about the contents of BPE except that it contains keratinocyte growth factor 2 (fibroblast growth factor 10) and basic fibroblast growth factor. Henry et al [8] studied standard keratinocyte migration assays but used human serum, human plasma, or BPE as a source of growth factors for keratinocytes migrating on promigratory matrices, such as collagen I, collagen IV, and fibronectin. The investigators found that human serum augmented human keratinocyte migration on these matrices, whereas plasma was incapable of promoting cellular motility. They found that serum has at least two cellular mechanisms by which it promotes keratinocyte motility: first, serum promotes the keratinocyte-derived expression of metalloproteinases; second, serum promotes the p38 mitogen-activated protein kinase–signaling pathway. Both metalloproteinase expression and the p38 signaling pathway are believed to be essential for human keratinocyte motility. These laboratory findings are significant because they make sense with what physicians know about real human skin wounds. These findings also raise the next important question: what is it in human serum that augments ECM-driven human keratinocyte migration in the wound?

Human keratinocytes must migrate from the cut edges of the wound and from the cut epidermal appendages to re-epithelialize, resurface, and close human skin wounds. Therefore, these cells are transformed from cells destined to a tightly regulated program of terminal differentiation into dead *Stratum corneum* cells, the most external layer of skin that provides humans with a critical permeability barrier. In addition to keratinocytes being transformed into a migratory cell type, within the dermis and wound bed, fibroblasts also must be stimulated to migrate. Fibroblasts in the unwounded dermis juxtaposed to the clot and wound bed must migrate into the wound bed and begin to contribute cytokines and growth factors, release metalloproteinases to help clear the wound debris, and begin to lay down essential ECM macromolecules to form the neodermis, which will then undergo a long process of remodeling. The wound bed is swamped by serum, and dermal fibroblasts experience serum rather than plasma in the wound setting for the first time. Fibroblasts, like keratinocytes, become migratory in the setting of a cutaneous wound. Recently, Li et al [9] showed that the element within human serum that enhances dermal fibroblast motility is PDGF-BB. PDGF-BB can completely replace serum in terms of promoting human dermal fibroblast migration on a type I collagen matrix. Likewise, the promotility activity in human serum for dermal fibroblasts is completely blocked by the presence of functional antibodies to PDGF-BB in the migration assays. Therefore, the element within human serum responsible for human dermal fibroblast migration has been identified. In contrast, the factor (or factors) in human serum that promotes human keratinocyte migration remains unknown.

The role of soluble growth factors and extracellular matrix in skin motility

The scientific literature on human keratinocyte and human fibroblast migration could be understood to suggest that small soluble growth factors or cytokines alone can induce cell migration. This is a false impression. The current authors do not believe that any soluble cytokine or growth factor alone can make fibroblasts or keratinocytes migrate on the bottom of a Petri dish (tissue culture polystyrene plastic) or a Petri dish coated with albumin, laminin-1, processed laminin-5, or any substratum that allows cell attachment but is not intrinsically promotile. For example, keratinocytes can be initiated to migrate significantly by apposition to promotile matrices, such as collagen I and fibronectin, even in the absence of added growth factors. The addition of promotility soluble factors, such as serum, EGF, or IL-1α, enhances the matrix-initiated cell motility and gives the cells polarity and direction [4,5]. If the cells themselves contribute small soluble factors as autocrines, these factors are unable to optimize the matrix-initiated motility or give the cells directionality. In a real skin wound, the cells are influenced by both contact with ECMs in the wound bed and by soluble growth factors within the microenvironment of the wound, including those in serum. Nevertheless, it is significant that ECM provides the stimulus and activates the necessary signaling pathways by way of integrin receptors to initiate the cell motility of skin cells. It is likely that the presence of growth factors and cytokines then initiate other signaling pathways by way of the activation of their tyrosine kinase receptors. The exact mechanisms are still not well defined. Nevertheless, it is believed that the matrix-initiating and the growth factor–enhancing signals likely cross-talk in an orchestrated manner to optimize cell migration. Li et al [9,10] have shown that the signals from matrix that initiate keratinocyte and fibroblast motility and the signals from growth factors that enhance and optimize matrix-initiated motility use common and disparate signaling pathways within the cytosol of the cell.

Oxygen tension and wound healing

It is believed that low oxygen tension in the long run inhibits wound closure. Although there are few controlled blinded studies, hyperbaric oxygen chambers have been used to help heal chronic wounds, particularly when it is believed that arterial disease hampers the delivery of oxygen to the wound tissue. Nevertheless, during an acute wound, the periwound tissues experience sudden and extreme hypoxia. Many signaling pathways in cells are activated by nonspecific stress signals that in turn activate survival genes. Keratinocytes next to the wound and fibroblasts around the wound dermal defect likely experience acute hypoxia because all of the blood vessels are rapidly clotted to prevent the patient from exsanguinating. Red blood cells and hemoglobin therefore are not getting to these tissues. It is conceivable that this situation creates stress signals that, at least in the short run, promote the transformation of keratinocytes and fibroblasts into migratory cells and cells that help initiate the healing of the wound. For example, TGF-β produced by dermal fibroblasts increases the ECM by causing the same cells to synthesize more matrix macromolecules, such as collagens, and synthesize and secrete fewer matrix-degrading enzymes, such as collagenases (matrix metalloproteinases). Falanga et al [11] have shown that hypoxia up-regulates the synthesis of TGF-β1 by human dermal fibroblasts. Therefore, this important wound-healing growth factor would be available within the wound to stimulate cells to make more ECM and fill in the rent in the skin. In addition, a hypoxic environment promotes the growth potential of fibroblasts and helps them avoid senescence [12]. In keratinocytes, it has been shown that human keratinocytes migrate better on collagen I, collagen IV, and fibronectin under hypoxic conditions compared with normoxia. This superior migration under hypoxia is associated with an up-regulation in proteins that build cell lamellipodia with increased keratinocyte expression of collagenases—both elements that promote cellular locomotion [13]. The current authors' view of these data is that hypoxia in acute wounds may serve as a stress signal to the wound cells which invokes a series of signaling pathways that transform the cells from maintenance, stationary skin cells into cells that are activated and migratory to begin healing the wound.

The origin of stem cells in healing skin wounds

Stem cells are slow-cycling cells that are considered the "mother cells" that give rise to a progeny of cells. Keratinocyte stem cells are located within the basal keratinocyte layer and within the bulge region of the pilosebaceous unit [14,15]. The general view of healing skin wounds has been that the healing is generated by local cells at the site of the wound. Nevertheless, this view may need to be modified. Investigators have taken bone marrow cells from one animal and, by transfection methods, induced the cells in culture to express green fluorescent protein (GFP). They then took these GFP-positive bone marrow cells and injected them into the circulation of mice of identical species. The investigators then wounded the mice and noted that many of the GFP-positive cells homed to the wound and were involved in the wound-healing process [16]. Similarly, patients with nonhealing wounds have had their wounds treated with autologous bone marrow cells—either by direct inoculation of the wound with bone marrow aspirates or with bone marrow cells after culturing. Although the number of patients was small and the results uncontrolled, wounds that had not healed for more than 1 year healed by these maneuvers [17]. These observations, although preliminary, are encouraging. They potentially open a new way of looking at the wound-healing process and at strategies for healing large nonhealing wounds.

Clinical advances in wound healing

Likely because of natural selection, living creatures are adept at healing cutaneous wounds. Although many components of the wound-healing cascade have been characterized, the use of exogenously administered cytokines and growth factors to wounds with the hope of improving wound healing has not been consistently successful. Recombinant EGF has been shown to speed the healing of skin graft donor sites (ie, acute healing wounds) [18]. Further, human recombinant PDGF was found to increase the efficiency of healing when healing is impaired, such as in diabetic foot ulcers or pressure ulcers [19]. Many other proteins have been tested, however, and have not been found to significantly alter wound healing. Further, when the mediators affect healing in clinical studies or experimental models, the gain in wound-healing time is minimal. Because these mediators are expensive, the cost–benefit ratio is not favorable. In short, it has been difficult for biotechnological advances to improve on the designs of nature.

Another factor that confounds true data-driven conclusions about the healing of human skin wounds is the paucity of controlled studies. The use of historical controls is fraught with errors. In therapy for acute and chronic wounds, there is more tradition and art than much evidence-based support for a given therapy. Perhaps one of the most notable examples of this situation is the use of hydrogen peroxide as a recommended part of a patient's wound care regime. Hydrogen peroxide is not a particularly good antiseptic or debridement reagent. It likely gives the patient something to do, however, and usually is harmless when used on the head and neck. Nevertheless, it has been shown that hydrogen peroxide at concentrations used clinically likely inhibits the migration of human keratinocytes [20].

Autologous cultured keratinocytes for burn wounds

Since the development of techniques to culture epidermal keratinocytes, autologous, cultured, keratinocyte sheets have been used to heal burn wounds in children and adults [21,22]. These sheets have the theoretic advantage that a small skin biopsy could be used to introduce the keratinocytes into tissue culture and expanded over 2 to 4 weeks into large sheets of epidermis that could be transplanted back onto prepared wound sites on the patient. These sheets are currently commercially available (eg, Genzyme, Cambridge, Massachusetts). Despite clinical success and the survival of patients with burns over more than 90% of their body surface area, the technique has not been generally accepted. The technical demands of a meticulously prepared burn wound site, the delay of 2 to 4 weeks needed for the cultures to expand, and the lack of improved outcomes have limited the impact of this technique [23].

Cultured allogeneic keratinocyte sheets and "skin equivalents" for wounds

Allogeneic cultured keratinocyte grafts have been used to heal various chronic cutaneous wounds, including venous stasis ulcers, vasculitis ulcers, and even pyoderma gangrenosum [24]. Because the grafts come from the same species but not the same person, the grafts take for a brief time and do not persist. Nevertheless, their presence on the wound, even for a short period of time, has beneficial effects. The grafts provide protection to the wound from desiccation, reduce pain, condition the wound bed, and provide keratinocyte-derived growth factors, such as PDGF and EGF, which may help accelerate the wound-healing process.

Since the original studies using autologous or allogeneic cultured keratinocyte sheets to help heal skin wounds, there have been other technologies developed to cover the wound with a composite culture consisting of an epidermis and dermis, which is then transplanted onto the patient's wound. In some cases, these composite cultures provide the wound with a dermal equivalent and in some cases a "skin equivalent" is provided, which has an epidermal and a dermal component. Table 1 summarizes some of these approaches and products and compares their advantages and disadvantages with transplanted culture autologous or allogeneic keratinocyte sheets. To date, there have been no head-to-head comparison studies of these products in terms of ultimate efficacy and wound healing. In one multicenter study, however, the application of a culture-derived skin equivalent transplanted onto diabetic foot ulcers resulted in enhanced healing rates compared with state-of-the-art wound care [25].

The role of antibiotics in wounds

When wound healing is delayed or fails, local wound infection is usually a contributor. Many practitioners find that many chronic wounds heal simply by daily treatment with broad-spectrum topical antibiotics, such as Silvadene. These daily dressings have the disadvantage of requiring repeated, painful, and messy dressing changes. A recently developed alternative is the use of silver-releasing dressings. The best known and studied of these dressings, Acticoat, has a broad spectrum of activity against resistant grampositive and gram-negative pathogens and releases antibacterial levels of silver for 3 to 7 days, depending on the particular product [26]. This characteristic allows antibacterial treatment without the need for frequent dressings. Further, the silver seems to displace the zinc ions in matrix metalloproteinases linked to wound chronicity (Greg Schultz, PhD, personal communication, 2004). Because it is believed that certain metalloproteinases are overexpressed in the wound bed of a nonhealing wound, displacing the zinc cations around this enzyme may attenuate its activity.

Although appropriate antibacterial treatment can be essential for wound treatment, certain antibiotics applied topically to wounds can inhibit wound healing. Povodine iodine, for example, inhibits the wound from healing. Nevertheless, a newer formulation of iodine, cadexomer iodine, is a slow-release agent in which the iodine is released into the wound in small amounts from dextrin beads. In a recent study, Zhou et al [27] showed that this type of slow-release iodine preparation is not toxic to skin cells at the concentrations used clinically. Further, it does not

Table 1
Epidermal, dermal, and composite product comparison

Product	Description	Advantages	Disadvantages	Indications
Epidermal				
EpiDex, (IsoTis SA, Lausanne, Switzerland) [56,57]	Tissue-engineered, fully differentiated autologous epidermal equivalent derived from ORS keratinocytes of plucked anagen hair follicles	Easy application Outpatient procedure Rapidly growing stem cell Relieves pain As effective as skin graft [56]	Limited controlled studies	Recurrent venous or arterial ulcer Failed STSG
Allogeneic keratinocyte sheets, CEC [58]	Allogeneic keratinocyte culture derived from neonatal foreskin screened for HIV (PCR) and other viruses and bacteria	Rapid in vitro growth Immediate availability No need for biopsy Longer storage time (indefinite at −120°C and 6 mo at −20°C) Low-cost and effective in ulcers of different causes	Lack of dermal component Not commercially available Limited controlled trials	Burn, venous and diabetic ulcer, STSG donor site, epidermolysis bullosa, post Mohs, decubitus ulcer, laser and dermabrasion wounds
Autologous keratinocyte culture, Epicel [59]	Autologous skin keratinocyte cultures derived from biopsy specimens	Effective on ulcers of different causes	Biopsy needed Not immediately available	Burns Venous ulcer, vitiligo, mastoid vacity for chronic otorrhea, epidermolysis bullosa, pyoderma gangrenosum
Dermal				
Biodegradable mesh with allogenic fibroblast culture, Dermagraft [59,60]	Biodegradable mesh of PGA or PGL910 containing allogeneic fibroblasts	Immediate availability No need for biopsy Excellent cosmetic and functional result	Needs multiple applications Contraindicated in allergy to bovine protein	Burns Diabetic ulcer Full-thickness wounds

	Description	Advantages	Disadvantages	Indications
Allogeneic dermis				
Alloderm [61]	Human allograft skin treated with decellularization, matrix stabilization, and freeze drying	Immediate availability Allows ultrathin STSG with less scarring Immunologically inert	Allograft procurement, virus screening	Surgical wounds
Integra [61]	Bovine collagen and chondroitin sulfate over silastic	Bovine collagen and chondroitin sulfate over silastic	Susceptibility to infection, complete wound excision before application, expensive, contraindicated in allergy to bovine proteins	Excised burn wounds
Composite (epidermal and dermal)				
Living skin equivalent, Apligraf [62]	Bilayered construct of human keratinocytes and dermal fibroblast with bovine type 1 collagen. Matrix proteins and cytokines, lacks Langerhans' cells and melanocytes.	Immediate availability Easy handling Does not require subsequent skin graft	Contraindicated in hypersensitivity to bovine product Limited viability (5 d)	Venous ulcers Full-thickness diabetic ulcer
Skin equivalent, OrCell [63]	Bilayered cellular matrix with human keratinocytes and fibroblasts in separate layers on a bioabsorbable matrix made of bovine type 1 collagen	Immediate availability	Contraindicated in hypersensitivity to bovine proteins	Split-thickness donor sites in burn patients

Abbreviations: CEC, cryopreserved epithelial culture; PGA, polyglycolic acid; PGL910, polyglactin-910; STSG, split-thickness skin graft.

inhibit keratinocyte migration and does not depress the proliferative capacity of fibroblasts. This finding is consistent with clinical studies that indicate that cadexomer iodine is useful in venous stasis ulcers [28–30].

Clinical management of chronic wounds

Venous ulcers

The cornerstone of therapy for venous ulcers remains compression. It is generally agreed that venous ulcers heal more rapidly with compression than without, and that high compression is better than low compression [31]. In the United Kingdom, a multilayered elastic compression bandaging is the treatment of choice. In the United States, continental Europe, and Australia, short stretch bandages are used. In the United States, inelastic compression with the Unna or Duke boot tends to be favored. One method, popularized by Dr. Skip Burton of Duke University, is the so-called "Duke boot." This bandage consists of Duoderm applied to the non-healing leg ulcer. Then, a standard Unna boot zinc oxide bandage is applied from the foot to the knee. Last, 3- to 4-in Coban (3M, Minneapolis, Minnesota) is applied over the Unna boot with a compression gradient such that the maximal pressure is over the foot and ankle and there is progressively less pressure up to the knee. This appliance is then changed at weekly office visits. To date, there are no clear data as to which type of compression system is optimal.

For immobile patients, elastic bandages are recommended because inelastic bandages will fail to generate adequate compression if the calf muscle pump is weak or ineffective. For patients with a degree of arterial insufficiency, inelastic bandages that exert low pressure at rest are preferable (European Wound Management Association position document: Medical Education Partnership, Ltd., London, United Kingdom, 2003). Recurrence rates of venous ulcers are high (26%–28% in 12 mo). Surgery can be helpful in reducing recurrence rates, especially in patients who have superficial venous incompetence. A recent study comparing surgery and compression with compression alone in 500 patients who had venous ulcers showed that surgical correction of superficial venous reflux can reduce the 12-month ulcer recurrence rate. Overall 24-week healing rates were similar in the two treatment groups (65%), but the 12-month recurrence rates were significantly reduced in the compression and surgery group compared with

compression alone (12% versus 28%). Thus, most patients with chronic venous ulceration will benefit from the addition of simple venous surgery [32].

New technologies, such as skin substitutes, are approved by the US Food and Drug Administration (FDA) for venous ulcers but are expensive and should be reserved for hard-to-heal wounds. Poor prognostic indicators for venous ulcers include the following factors: large size, long duration, deep vein involvement, poor mobility, fibrin on the wound surface, an ankle–brachial index of less than 0.8, and a history of hip or knee replacement [33]. The rate of ulcer healing after initiation of compression therapy is also a predictor of healing: ulcers that heal slowly (<40% size reduction by 3 wk of compression therapy, or <0.05 cm/wk) are unlikely to heal and would likely benefit from intervention with advanced technologies [34].

Arterial ulcers

In patients who have arterial ulcers, the surgical re-establishment of an adequate vascular supply should be performed whenever possible. Medical management includes control of diabetes mellitus or hypertension, smoking cessation, and moderate exercise [35]. Cilostazol is a phosphodiastrase inhibitor that has antiaggregation effects on platelets, beneficial effects on serum lipids, and vasodilator effects. This drug has been approved by the FDA for the treatment of intermittent claudication.

In a double-blind, randomized, placebo-controlled trial to evaluate the relative efficacy and safety of Cilostazol versus pentoxifylline, 698 patients with moderate to severe claudication were randomly assigned to blinded treatment with either Cilostazol (100 mg, 2×/d), pentoxifylline (400 mg, 3×/d), or placebo. Cilostazol was significantly better than pentoxifylline or placebo for increased walking distance in patients who had intermittent claudication. It was, however, associated with a greater frequency of minor side effects, including headache, palpitations, and diarrhea. Pentoxifylline and placebo had similar effects [36]. Cilostazol is currently being evaluated in a multicenter trial for arterial ulcers.

Diabetic foot ulcers

Neuropathic diabetic foot ulcers are a leading cause of morbidity in patients who have diabetes. They develop in approximately 15% of patients who have diabetes, and 85% of lower limb amputations in patients who have diabetes are preceded by foot ulceration [37]. Ulceration is principally caused by neuropathy, but other causes include peripheral vascular disease, callus, edema, and deformity [38]. The management of diabetic neuropathic ulcers includes the following: treatment of infection, debridement of the wound, correction of any arterial disease, and removal of pressure from the ulcer. Glycemic control should be optimized, and patients should be advised to stop smoking [38]. Regular, sharp debridement of ulcers has been shown to promote healing [39]. The treatment of local edema with a pneumatic compression pump in addition to debridement has been shown to improve healing compared with debridement alone [40]. Pressure can be offloaded from the diabetic foot ulcer using various modalities, such as contact casting, boots, half shoes, sandals, or foam dressings [38]. Various dressings are available to provide a moist wound environment, but there are few randomized controlled trials to assess their efficacy. Dressings containing antibacterial agents, such as silver or iodine, in slow-release formulation may be helpful for superficially infected wounds.

Pexiganan is a 22-amino-acid antimicrobial peptide derived from magainin peptides isolated from the skin of the African clawed frog. It demonstrates antimicrobial activity against a broad range of organisms, including gram-positive aerobes and anaerobes, such as staphylococcus, streptococcus, enterococcus, corynebacterium, pseudomonas, acinetobacter, strenotrophomonas, bacteroides, and other species [41,42]. A randomized controlled trial of topical pexiganan compared with treatment with oral ofloxacin in patients who had mildly infected diabetic foot ulcers showed clinically equivalent response with equivalent healing rates [43].

For clinically infected wounds, culture-guided therapy with systemic antibiotics is required [38]. Linezolid (Zyvox) is the only oral antibiotic approved for the treatment of methicillin-resistant-*Staphylococcus aureus* infections and recently has been approved by the FDA to treat diabetic foot infections. In a randomized controlled trial, 371 patients who had diabetic foot infections were randomly assigned to receive Linezolid versus standard amino penicillin therapy of aminopenicillin/beta lactamase inhibitor with or without vancomycin. There was an 83% efficacy rate in the Linezolid arm versus a 73% rate in the control group [44].

Additional therapies may be helpful in the treatment of diabetic foot ulcers, which are slow to respond to traditional care. Recombinant PDGF has been approved by the FDA for the treatment of neuropathic foot ulcers in patients who have diabetes [45].

Two tissue-engineered skin products have been approved by the FDA for adjunctive treatment of diabetic foot ulcers. In a randomized trial of a bilayered skin constructs (Apligraf), higher healing rates, a lower incidence of osteomyelitis, and fewer lower limb amputations were found in the active treatment group compared with the control group [25,38]. A dermal equivalent (Dermagraft, Smith and Nephew, Cambridge, United Kingdom) also has been FDA-approved for the treatment of diabetic foot ulcers [46]. There have been no head-to-head comparisons of the efficacy of Apligraf versus Dermagraft.

Antimicrobial dressings

When chronic wounds fail to heal yet do not show clinical signs of systemic infection, there may be heavy bacterial contamination, principally located in the superficial zone of the wound. Topical antimicrobial agents can be used in this situation to reduce the wound bioburden and facilitate healing [47,48].

There has been a resurgence of interest in the use of topical antiseptics, such as iodine and silver, to control wound bioburden. These agents have a broad spectrum of antibacterial activity and are less likely to induce bacterial resistance than antibiotics [49,50].

New dressing formulations have been developed that allow the slow release of antibacterial agents, such as silver and iodine, in concentrations that are nontoxic to cells within the wound, yet have antibacterial activity. Silver has been used for centuries to prevent and treat various diseases. It was used in ancient Greece and Rome when silver coins were placed in jars of water to maintain the water's sterility. Silver ions can kill micro-organisms by blocking respiratory enzyme systems and seem to have no negative effects on human cells [51]. Silver has been shown to be effective in killing antibiotic-resistant bacteria, such as methicillin-resistant *S aureus* and vancomycin-resistant enterococcus [52].

In a study of patients with symmetric burn wounds randomized to treatment with a 0.5% silver nitrate solution versus a nanocrystalline silver dressing, burn wound sepsis and secondary bacteremias were reduced in the silver dressing group. In addition, dressing removal was less painful than with the silver nitrate solution [53]. Silver dressings may also alter the inflammatory environment of the chronic wound. Wounds treated with nanocrystalline silver dressings have decreased levels of matrix metalloproteinases, which are usually up-regulated in chronic wounds [54].

Cadexomer iodine is a three-dimensional starch lattice formed into spherical microbeads. Iodine is trapped within this lattice at 0.9% weight per volume. This product has a high absorptive capacity. It absorbs exudate from the wound and gradually releases iodine from the resulting gel. In a randomized controlled trial in 38 patients who had venous ulcers, topical cadexomer iodine reduced colonization with S aureus, beta hemolytic streptococcus, proteus, and klebsella ($P > 0.001$). There was a correlation between S aureus removal and the healing rate of the wounds [55].

These dressings are clinically promising, but larger randomized trials in different patient groups are required.

References

[1] Singer AJ, Clark RAF. Cutaneous wound healing. N Engl J Med 1999;341:738–46.
[2] Phillips TJ, Manzoor J, Rojas A, et al. The longevity of a bilayered skin substitute after application to venous ulcers. Arch Dermatol 2002;138:1079–81.
[3] Sarret Y, Woodley DT, Grigsby K, Wynn K, O'Keefe EJ. Human keratinocyte locomotion: the effect of selected cytokines. J Invest Dermatol 1992;98:12–6.
[4] Chen JD, Kim JP, Zhang K, et al. Epidermal growth factor (EGF) promotes human keratinocyte locomotion on collagen by increasing the alpha 2 integrin subunit. Exp Cell Res 1993;209:216–23.
[5] Chen JD, Lapiere J-C, Sauder DN, Peavey C, Woodley DT. Interleukin 1 alpha stimulates keratinocyte migration through an epidermal growth factor/transforming growth factor alpha-independent pathway. J Invest Dermatol 1995;104:729–33.
[6] Cha D, O'Brian P, O'Toole EA, Woodley DT, Hudson LG. Enhanced modulation of keratinocyte motility by transforming growth factor-alpha (TGF-alpha) relative to epidermal growth factor (EGF). J Invest Dermatol 1996;106:590–7.
[7] Boyce ST, Ham RG. Calcium-regulated differentiation normal human epidermal keratinocytes in chemically defined clonal culture and serum-free serial culture. J Invest Dermatol 1983;81(Suppl):33–40.
[8] Henry G, Li W, Garner W, Woodley DT. Migration of human keratinocytes in plasma and serum and wound re-epithelialization. Lancet 2003;361:574–6.
[9] Li W, Fan J, Chen M, et al. Mechanism of human dermal fibroblast migration driven by type I collagen and platelet-derived growth factor-BB. Mol Biol Cell 2004;15:294–309.
[10] Li W, Henry G, Fan J, et al. Signals that initiate, augment and provide directionality for human keratinocyte motility. J Invest Dermatol, in press.
[11] Falanga V, Qian SW, Danielpour D, et al. Hypoxia upregulates the synthesis of TGF-beta 1 by human dermal fibroblasts. J Invest Dermatol 1991;97:634–7.
[12] Falanga V, Kirsner RS. Low oxygen stimulates proliferation of fibroblasts seeded as single cells. J Cell Physiol 1993;154:506–10.
[13] O'Toole EA, Marinkovich MP, Peavy CL, et al. Hypoxia increases human keratinocyte motility on connective tissue. J Clin Invest 1997;100:2881–91.
[14] Cotsarelis G, Sun TT, Lavaker RM. Label-retaining cells reside in the bulge area of the pilosebaceous unit: implications for follicular stem cells, hair cycle and skin carcinogenesis. Cell 1990;61:1329–37.
[15] Taylor G, Lehrer MS, Jensen PJ, Sun TT, Lavker RM. Involvement of follicular stem cells in forming not only the follicle but also the epidermis. Cell 2000; 102:451–61.
[16] Badiavas EV, Abedi M, Butmarc J, Falanga V, Quesenberry P. Participation of bone marrow derived cells in cutaneous wound healing. J Cell Physiol 2003; 196:245–50.
[17] Badiavas EV, Falanga V. Treatment of chronic wounds with bone marrow-derived cells. Arch Dermatol 2003; 139:510–6.
[18] Brown GL, Nanny LF, Griffen J, et al. Enhancement of wound healing by topical treatment with epidermal growth factor. N Engl J Med 1989;321:76–9.
[19] Robson MC, Phillips LG, Thompson A, et al. Platelet-derived growth factor BB for the treatment of chronic pressure ulcers. Lancet 1992;339:23–5.
[20] O'Toole EA, Goel M, Woodley DT. Hydrogen peroxide inhibits human keratinocyte migration. Dermatol Surg 1996;22:525–9.
[21] Gallico GG, O'Connor NE. Cultured epithelium as a skin substitute. Clin Plast Surg 1985;12:149–57.
[22] Woodley DT, Peterson HD, Herzog SR, et al. Burn wounds resurfaced by cultured epidermal autografts show abnormal reconstitution of anchoring fibrils. JAMA 1988;259:2566–71.
[23] Paddle-Ledinek JE, Cruickshank DG, Masterton JP. Skin replacement by cultured keratinocyte grafts: an Australian experience. Burns 1997;23(3):204–11.
[24] Phillips T, Provan A, Colbert D, Easley KW. A randomized single-blind controlled study of cultured epidermal allografts in the treatment of split-thickness skin graft donor sites. Arch Dermatol 1993;129: 879–82.
[25] Veves A, Falanga V, Armstrong DG, Sabolinski ML. Apligraf Diabetic Foot Ulcer Study. Graftskin, a human skin equivalent, is effective in the management of noninfected neuropathic diabetic foot ulcers: a prospective randomized multicenter clinical trial. Diabetes Care 2001;24(2):290–5.
[26] Holder IA, Durkee P, Supp AP, Boyce ST. Assessment of a silver-coated barrier dressing for potential use with skin grafts on excised burns. Burns 2003;29: 445–8.
[27] Zhou LH, Nahm WK, Badiavas E, Yufit T, Falanga V. Slow release iodine preparation and wound healing: in vitro effects consistent with lack of in vivo toxicity

in human chronic wounds. Br J Dermatol 2002;146(3): 365–74.

[28] Ormiston MC, Seymour MT, Venn GE, et al. Controlled trial of Iodosorb in chronic venous ulcers. BMJ 1985;291:308–10.

[29] Holloway GA, Johansen KH, Barnes RW, et al. Multicenter trial of cadexomer iodine to treat venous stasis ulcers. West J Med 1989;151:35–8.

[30] Mober S, Hoffman L, Grennert ML, et al. A randomized trial of cadexomer iodine in decubitus ulcers. J Am Geriatr Soc 1983;31:462–5.

[31] Cullum N, Nelson EA, Fletcher AW, Sheldon TA. Cochrane database of systematic reviews. 2004.

[32] Barwell JR, Davies CE, Deacon J, et al. Comparison of surgery and compression with compression alone in chronic venous ulceration (ESCHAR study): randomized controlled trial. Lancet 2004;363:1854–9.

[33] Margolis DM, Berlin JA, Strom BL. Risk factors associated with the failure of venous leg ulcer to heal. Arch Dermatol 1999;135(8):920–6.

[34] Phillips TJ, Machado F, Trout R, et al. Prognostic indicators for venous ulcers: analysis of a randomized, double blind, placebo controlled study. J Am Acad Dermatol 2000;43:627–30.

[35] Bello YM, Phillips TJ. Recent advances in wound healing. JAMA 2000;283:716–8.

[36] Dawson DL, Cutler BS, Hiatt WR, et al. A comparison of Cilostazol and pentoxyfilline for treating intermittent claudication. Am J Med 2000;109:523–30.

[37] Palumbo PJ, Nelzen III LJ. Peripheral vascular disease and diabetes. In: Diabetes and America. Washington, DC: Government Printing Office; 1985 [NIH Publication #85-1468].

[38] Boulton AJN, Kirsner RS, Vileikyte L. Neuropathic diabetic foot ulcers. N Engl J Med 2004;351:48–55.

[39] Steed DL, Donohoe D, Webster MW, Lindsley L. Effect of extensive debridement and treatment on the healing of diabetic foot ulcers. J Am Coll Surg 1996; 183:61–4.

[40] Armstrong DG, Nguyen HC. Improvement in healing with aggressive edema reduction after debridement of foot infection in persons with diabetes. Arch Surg 2000:1351405–9.

[41] Ge Y, Macdonald DL, Holroyd KJ, Thornsberry C, Wexler H, Zasloff M. In vitro properties of pexiganan, an analog of magainin. Antimicrob Agents Chemother 1999;43:782–8.

[42] Ge Y, MacDonald D, Henry MM, et al. In vitro susceptibility to pexiganan of bacteria isolated from infected diabetic foot ulcers. Diagn Microbiol Infect Dis 1999;35(1):45–53.

[43] Lipsky BA, McDonald D, Litka PA. Treatment of infected diabetic foot ulcers, topical MSI-78 vs. oral ofloxacin. Diabetologica 1997;40:482–6.

[44] Lipsky BA, Itani K, Norden C. Treating foot infections in diabetic patients. A randomized, multicenter, open label trial of Linezolid versus ampicillin sulbactam/amoxicillin clavulanate. Clin Infect Dis 2004;38:17–24.

[45] Boulton MJ, Wieman TJ, Smiell JN, et al. Efficacy and safety of a topical gel formulation of recombinant human platelet derived growth factor BB (Bercaplamin) in patients with chronic neuropathic diabetic ulcers. A phase III randomized, placebo controlled, double blind study. Diabetes Care 1998;21:822–7.

[46] Marston WA, Hanst J, Norwood P, Pollack R. The efficacy and safety of Dermagraft in improving the healing of chronic diabetic foot ulcers: results of a prospective randomized trial. Diabetes Care 2003;26: 1701–5.

[47] Bowler PG, Duerden BI, Armstrong DG. Wound microbiology and associated approaches to wound management. Clin Microbiol Rev 2001;14:244–69.

[48] Robson MC. Wound infection: a failure of wound healing caused by an imbalance of bacteria. Surg Clin North Am 1997;77:637–50.

[49] White R, Cooper R, Kingsly A. Wound colonization and infection: the role of topical antimicrobials and guidelines in management. Br J Nurs 2001;10:563–78.

[50] Jones SA, Bowler PG, Walker M, Parsons D. Controlling wound bioburden with a novel silver containing hydrofiber dressing. Wound Repair Regen 2004;12: 288–94.

[51] Demling RH, Desan TL. The role of silver in wound healing. Wounds 2001;13:5–15.

[52] Wright JB, Lam K, Burrell RE. Silver coated wound dressings. Am J Infect Control 1998;26:572–7.

[53] Tredget E, Shankowsky HA, Groeneveld A, Burrell R. A matched pair randomized study evaluating the efficacy and safety of Acticoat silver-coated dressing for the treatment of burn wounds. J Burn Care Rehab 1998;19:532–7.

[54] Kirsner RS, Orsted H, Wright JB. Matrix metalloproteinases in normal and impaired wound healing: a potential of nanocrystalline silver. Wounds 2001;13:5–12.

[55] Skog E, Arnsjo B, Troeng T, et al. A randomized trial comparing Cadexomer iodine and standard treatment in the outpatient management of chronic venous ulcers. Br J Dermatol 1983;109:77–83.

[56] Touche AK, Skaria M, Bohlen L, et al. An autologous epidermal equivalent tissue-engineered from follicular outer root sheath keratinocytes is as effective as split-thickness skin autograft in recalcitrant vascular leg ulcer. Wound Repair Regen 2003;11:248–52.

[57] Limat A, French L, Blat L, Saurat J, Hunziker T, Soloman D. Organotypic cultures of autologous hair follicle keratinocytes for the treatment of recurrent leg ulcers. J Am Acad Dermaol 2003;48:207–14.

[58] Khachemount A, Bello Y, Phillips T. Factors that influence healing in chronic venous ulcers treated with cryopreserved human epidermal culture. Dermatol Surg 2002;28:274–6.

[59] Pollak R, Edingtin H, Jenson J, Kroeker R, Gentzkow G. A human dermal replacement for the treatment of diabetic foot ulcer. Wounds 1997;9:175–82.

[60] Hansborough J, Cooper M, Gohen R, et al. Evaluation of biodegradable matrix containing cultured human fibroblast as a dermal replacement beneath

meshed skin graft on athymic mice. Surgery 1992;111: 439–46.

[61] Kolenic SA, Leffell DJ. The use of cryopreserved human skin allografts in wound healing following Mohs surgery. Dermatol Surg 1995;21:615–20.

[62] Falanga V, Margolis D, Alvarez D, et al. Rapid healing of venous leg ulcers and lack of clinical rejection with an allogeneic cultured human skin equivalent. Arch Dermatol 1997;134:293–300.

[63] Lipkin S, Chaikof E, Isseroff Z, Silverstein P. Effectiveness of bilayered cellular matrix in healing of neuropathic diabetic foot ulcers: results of a multicenter pilot trial. Wounds 2003;15:230–6.

Cyanoacrylates for Skin Closure

William H. Eaglstein, MD*, Tory Sullivan, MD

*Department of Dermatology and Cutaneous Surgery, University of Miami School of Medicine, 1600 NW 10th Avenue,
RMSB 2023A, Miami, FL 33136, USA*

Cyanoacrylates (CAs), first produced in 1949 [1], are liquids that polymerize in the presence of moisture to form adhesives, glues, and films. The surgical use of these compounds was first proposed by Coover et al [2] in 1959. The short-chain cyanoacrylates (methyl, ethyl) [3,4] proved to be extremely toxic to tissue, however, preventing their widespread use as tissue glues. The short-chain CAs are used in nonmedical products, such as Krazy glue (Elmer's, Columbus, Ohio), and although they are not intended for medical use, dermatologists have been quoted in the popular press as recommending these glues for the treatment of fissures on fingers and toes [5]. Butyl cyanoacrylate (BCA), an intermediate-length CA, is not toxic when applied topically. Although it is not approved by the US Food and Drug Administration (FDA) for use in the United States, it has been used in Europe and Canada for middle ear procedures, to close cerebrospinal leaks, to repair incisions and lacerations, and to affix skin grafts [6–12]. Recently, a longer chain CA, octyl-2-cyanoacrylate (2-OCA), has been approved by the FDA and is now marketed (Dermabond topical skin adhesive) for closure of lacerations and incisions in place of sutures or staples. Even more recently, a 2-OCA formulated for greater flexibility, Liquid Bandage, has been approved for use in the over-the-counter market in the United States for the treatment of minor cuts and abrasions. This article discusses the use of CAs for their original cutaneous use as glues for the repair of lacerations and incisions and for their more recent use as films for use as dressings in the treatment of abrasions and wounds.

Butyl cyanoacrylate

BCA is an intermediate-length CA that was the first CA to be widely used for cutaneous wound closure. It has been available and widely used in Europe and Canada as Histoacryl Blue and Glustitch since as early as the 1970s. Although the short-chain CAs (methyl, ethyl) were toxic to tissue, BCA is generally considered to be nontoxic when applied topically. When used in an experimental model of incisional wound healing in hamsters, BCA resulted in less inflammation than 4.0 silk sutures on histologic assessment [7]. Furthermore, a randomized clinical trial involving 94 patients who had facial lacerations suitable for tissue adhesive closure and who underwent closure using either BCA or 2-OCA failed to reveal a difference in cosmetic result at 3 months as rated from photographs by a plastic surgeon using a visual analog scale [13]. Interpreting these data to imply that BCA has no tissue toxicity should be done with caution, however; care was taken to prevent the BCA from coming in contact with exposed wound tissue because of lingering concerns that BCA when trapped in the wound itself might cause a toxic reaction [14]. Because of these concerns, BCA has never been approved for use in the United States and has never been actively advocated for use on wounds as a film-forming or bandage-like agent.

Octyl cyanoacrylate

Octyl cyanoacrylates are CAs with a longer (8-carbon) side chain. This longer side chain gives

---

* Corresponding author.

2-OCA several potential advantages over CAs that have short or intermediate side chains. For example, 2-OCA is stronger and more flexible than BCA, with 4 times the three-dimensional breaking strength of this shorter chain CA [15]. Because of its improved strength and flexibility properties and because of reduced fears of tissue toxicity, 2-OCA is now widely used in the United States for wound closure, and it is currently one of the largest bandage brands as ranked by dollar sales in the United States.

Octyl cyanoacrylate and cosmetic outcome

Studies of 2-OCA have revealed that it is equivalent or superior to standard suturing of wounds as judged by several criteria. When evaluated prospectively for the treatment of cutaneous lacerations [16] and elective head and neck incisions [17], no differences in cosmetic outcome at 12 weeks were noted when compared with standard suture repair. In the same studies, patients rated 2-OCA closure as less painful than standard suture closure, and wound closure took significantly less time than with suture repair. A larger study of 814 patients who had a more diverse group of wounds (383 traumatic lacerations, 235 excisions of skin lesions or scar revisions, 208 minimally invasive surgeries, and 98 general surgical procedures) also showed the equivalence of closure with 2-OCA as compared with standard suture wound closure in terms of cosmesis at 3-month follow-up. Again, wound closure with 2-OCA was faster than with standard suture wound closure (2.9 min versus 5.2 min, $P < 0.001$), and at 1 week, infection rates were similar. There where were no differences in wound dehiscence rates in this study. Despite multiple studies that showed similar outcomes in 2-OCA–treated wounds and standard suture–treated wounds in both adults and pediatric patients in cosmetic appearance of the healed wound, there has been one study where 2-OCA–treated wounds had an inferior outcome [16–21]. In a study of 83 children who were seen in an emergency department with lacerations and randomized to receive either 2-OCA or non-absorbable sutures or staples, the children treated with 2-OCA ultimately had a slightly lower cosmesis score [22]. As in similar studies, however, treatment with 2-OCA resulted in a decreased repair time of 5.8 minutes with suture and staples to 2.9 minutes with 2-OCA, and a reduction was found in the parents' assessment of the pain felt by their children. Because this is the only study to show this outcome, it should be interpreted with caution, but physicians should consider whether 2-OCA is indicated for

lacerations in the pediatric population in cosmetically sensitive areas.

Octyl cyanoacrylate and infection

Because sutures inherently introduce foreign material into a wound, 2-OCA may have a natural comparative advantage in infection rates, especially with clean contaminated wounds. In addition, CAs have been reported to have inherent antimicrobial properties, especially against gram-positive organisms [23]. In a randomized, blinded study, incisions were made on guinea pigs and contaminated with *Staphylococcus aureus* [24]. The incisions were then randomly assigned to be closed with either 2-OCA or 5-0 polypropylene suture. At day 5, wounds were then examined histologically and determined to be infected if inflammatory cells with intracellular cocci were seen. On the same day, wounds were also examined for clinical evidence of infection and a quantitative bacteriologic analysis was performed. Of 20 wounds in the tissue adhesive group, 5 wounds were sterile on day 5, whereas all sutured wounds had positive cultures ($P < 0.05$). Fewer wounds in the tissue adhesive group were determined to be infected by histologic and clinical criteria. Generally, differences in infection rates in human trials between wounds closed with 2-OCA and standard suture wound closure techniques have not been statistically significant. Trials to date have frequently excluded patients with grossly contaminated wounds, however.

Octyl cyanoacrylate and cost

Despite the apparent evidence of equivalence or even advantage of 2-OCA for wound repair, its adoption over standard wound closure techniques has been relatively slow. This situation may be because of cost disadvantages to the treating physician or institutions. On a per-unit basis, 2-OCA (eg, Dermabond Ethicon Products, Somerville, New Jersey) is 10 times more expensive than a popular brand of black monofilament nylon sutures [25]. Despite this situation, the overall cost advantage to society and to patients probably lies with the CAs. When the three most commonly used methods for the repair of pediatric facial lacerations—nondissolving sutures, dissolving sutures, or a CA—were compared on an economic basis, which included factors such as equipment use, pharmaceutic use, health care worker time, and parental loss of income for follow-up visits, assuming an equal cosmetic outcome, there was a reduction in cost to the Canadian health care system from the use of CAs. The reduction in cost in

Canadian dollars per patient of switching from the standard nondissolving sutures to a CA was $49.60 and for switching to dissolving sutures was $37.90 [26]. In addition, when parents of treated patients were surveyed, they overwhelmingly (90% of parents) chose the use of the CA as their first choice for wound closure (10% chose dissolving sutures). Despite the preference of parents and reduced costs to the society, however, CAs will probably continue to be the last choice of health care providers as long as they are associated with increased direct cost to the providers.

Cyanoacrylates as wound dressings

As concerns about potential tissue toxicity abate and newer, more flexible 2-OCA formulations have become available, CAs have been used not only for the closure of wounds but also for the treatment of wounds and as a wound dressing. Many physicians remain skeptical about this use of 2-OCA out of concern of tissue toxicity in earlier CAs; however, animal studies have consistently failed to show any tissue toxicity from 2-OCA when applied directly to open tissue in wounds. In a guinea pig abrasion model of wounds, there were no differences in the mean wound-healing ratios on days 1, 7, or 14 for 2-OCA as compared with a control dressing (Biobrane), and histopathologic analysis on day 14 failed to find any differences between the treatments [27]. In a porcine model of acute partial-thickness wounds, 2-OCA did not produce tissue toxicity (Stephen C. Davis, William H. Eaglstein, MD, Alex L. Cazzaniga, and P.M. Metz, unpublished observations, 2000). Furthermore, faster healing was seen in the 2-OCA–treated wounds as compared with the wounds treated with commercial bandages. On day 5 post wounding, 67% of 2-OCA–treated wounds were completely healed as compared with 20% of Band-Aid–treated wounds. Other studies of 2-OCA for partial-thickness wounds in pigs confirm these results and suggest that 2-OCA compares favorably with other effective dressings. For example, 115 standardized partial-thickness wounds were created in a porcine wound-healing model and treated with 2-OCA, a hydrocolloid dressing, or gauze. Biopsy specimens were taken at days 4, 5, 6, and 21 post wounding. The percentage of re-epithelialization in wounds treated with the liquid occlusive and hydrocolloid dressings was significantly greater at days 4 and 5 compared with control wounds [28]. In addition, several benefits have been attributed to the treatment of

wounds with 2-OCA, including increased resistance to bacterial challenge of the wound and increased wound hemostasis [29]. In vitro testing of 2-OCA has confirmed that it forms an excellent barrier against several bacterial and fungal pathogens [30]. Similar results from the use of 2-OCA in burns have been observed. One author evaluated the use of 2-OCA second-degree burns as compared with treatment with a polyurethane film dressing (Tegaderm). Forty-four partial-thickness burns were created on the backs of pigs, and wounds were randomly treated with 2-OCA or the film dressing. Full-thickness biopsy specimens were taken on days 7, 10, and 14 and evaluated for infection and re-epithelialization. No statistically significant difference was seen in the rates of re-epithelialization and no wounds in either treatment group became infected [31]. Singer et al [32] compared the effects of treatment of partial-thickness burns in pigs with 2-OCA, silver sulfadiazine (SSD), polyurethane film (PU), and gauze on scarring after 3months. Forty partial-thickness burns were randomly assigned to be treated with 2-OCA, SSD, PU, or gauze. Digital images and biopsy specimens of the burns were obtained at 3 months. There were no statistical differences in the proportion of wounds with scarring among the groups (OCA = 10%, SSD = 22%, PU = 2%, gauze = 30%; $P = 0.89$) or in cosmetic scores among the groups ($P = 0.96$) as judged by blinded observers. The same authors also evaluated infection rates of contaminated second-degree burns in pigs treated similarly [33]. Eighty partial-thickness burns were created and contaminated with 0.1 mL of S $aureus$ 10(5) CFU/mL and then randomly treated with 2-OCA, SSD, PU, or gauze. The treatment of contaminated partial-thickness burns with 2-OCA resulted in fewer infections at 1 week compared with the other three treatments.

Results of the use of 2-OCA for the treatment of open wounds have been similar to those in animal models. The current authors recently compared a new, flexible formulation of 2-OCA (Liquid Bandage) to a commercially available over-the-counter bandage for the treatment of cuts and scrapes [34]. Because short-chain CAs are irritating and toxic to tissues and because Dermabond, which contains the same 2-OCA as Liquid Bandage, is approved only for application to the surfaces of wounds with approximated wound edges, the authors were particularly interested in evaluating the possibility that direct application of 2-OCA to open cuts and scrapes would be toxic or irritating to wounds. Eighty-two subjects in the study applied 2-OCA directly to their cuts or scrapes and none experienced pain, redness, warmth, or edema. In addition, neither infection nor delayed wound healing was seen in the 2-OCA–treated wounds.

Cyanoacrylates and wound hemostasis

The hemostatic activity of CAs has been reported in many studies [35–37]. In a porcine model of epistasis, one group of authors created 24 full-thickness wounds on the nasal septae of pigs with a 4-mm punch biopsy tool [38]. Wounds were randomized to either no treatment or to topical 2-OCA before and after heparinization of the animals. The authors reported that the time to complete hemostasis was significantly shorter in the wounds treated with 2-OCA versus control (mean difference, 150 s; $P < 0.001$). In porcine studies of partial-thickness wounds, 2-OCA has been an effective hemostatic agent [28,39]. In a human trial of 2-OCA for partial-thickness wounds, it was reported to stop bleeding or oozing immediately in 93% of wounds as compared with 46% of wounds treated with standard bandages. The ability to achieve rapid hemostasis is an attractive feature of the CAs.

Cyanoacrylates as drug delivery devices

CAs offer potential as a drug delivery device in which therapeutic agents can be directly incorporated into the CA itself and as a dressing, which can keep a therapeutic agent in place in a difficult anatomic location. For the former application, CAs have been used to create nanoparticles. These nanoparticles have then been incorporated in vehicles for topical application. BCA nanoparticles have been reported as drug carriers of 5-fluorouracil, paclitaxel, and indomethicin intended for use in topical treatment [40–42]. To the authors' knowledge, however, currently no therapeutic agents have been directly incorporated into a CA itself for cutaneous application. With regard to using 2-OCA as a device for maintaining an active agent in a difficult location, in one recent trial, 31 patients with recurrent aphthous lesions were treated with either an active agent or a placebo. Both the active agent and the placebo were maintained in place by coverage with a BCA [43]. Clearly, further research is needed in both possible uses.

Miscellaneous uses of cyanoacrylates

Another use for 2-OCA is for the treatment of wounds in the oral mucosa. Orabase (Colgate,

Conton, Massachusetts), a flexible form of 2-OCA, is specifically formulated for use in the oral mucosa [44]. It is a unique product in the over-the-counter market because, unlike other products, it is an occlusive dressing, not simply a topical anesthetic. To the current authors' knowledge, Orabase is the only over-the-counter product consumers can purchase that creates a mechanical barrier providing pain relief for oral ulcerations and abrasions. In two separate studies [45] of 200 patients with an aphthous ulcer, 2-OCA when used in the oral mucosa provided significant short- and long-term pain reduction as compared with placebo treatment.

Summary

Even though the first CAs were produced in 1949, they were not widely adopted for medical use until recently because of lingering concerns about the initial tissue toxicities of the short-chain CAs. Medium-chain CAs, primarily BCA, have been widely used in Europe and Canada for several decades and have gone a long way in dispelling any lingering concerns about tissue toxicity. The newer, longer chain CA, 2-OCA, now has been approved for multiple uses in the United States and has achieved widespread acceptance by the medical and lay communities. The current authors believe this development is probably only the beginning of the use of 2-OCA and other CAs in cutaneous medicine.

References

[1] Ardis AE. Cyanoacrylates. US patents 2467926 and 2467927. 1949.

[2] Coover HW, Joyner FB, Shearer NH, Wicker TH. Chemistry and performance of cyanoacrylate adhesives. J Soc Plast Eng 1959;15:413–7.

[3] Kline DG, Hayes GJ. An experimental evaluation of the effect of a plastic adhesive, methy-2-cyanoacrylate, on neural tissue. J Neurosurg 1963;20:647–54.

[4] Woodward SC, Hermann JB, Leonard F. Histotoxicity of cyanoacrylate tissue adhesive. Fed Proc 1964; 23:485.

[5] Johnson R. Of Krazy glue: a little dab will do for those unkind cuts. Wall Street Journal July 5, 2000:A-1.

[6] Quinn JV, Drzewiecki AE, Li MM, et al. A randomized, controlled trial comparing a tissue adhesive with suturing in the repair of pediatric facial lacerations. Ann Emerg Med 1993;22:1130–5.

[7] Galil KA, Schofield I, Wright GZ. Effect of n-2butyl cyanoacrylate (histoacryl blue) on the healing of skin wounds. J Can Dent Assoc 1984;50:565–9.

[8] Keng TM, Bucknall TE. A clinical trial of histoacryl

in skin closure of groin wound. Med J Malaysia 1989; 44:122–8.

[9] Mizrahi S, Bickel A, Ben-Layish E. Use of tissue adhesives in the repair of lacerations in children. J Pediatr Surg 1988;23:312–3.

[10] Applebaum JS, Zalut T, Applebaum D. The use of tissue adhesion for traumatic laceration repair in the emergency department. Ann Emerg Med 1993;22: 1190–2.

[11] Kamer FM, Joseph JH. Histoacryl: its use in aeshetic facial plastic surgery. Arch Otolaryngol Head Neck Surg 1989;115:193–7.

[12] Halopuro S, Rintala A, Salo H, Ritsila V. Tissue adhesive versus sutures in closure of incision wounds. Ann Chir Gynaecol 1976;65:308–12.

[13] Osmond MH, Quinn JV, Sutcliffe T, et al. A randomized, clinical trial comparing butylcyanoacrylate with octylcyanoacrylate in the management of selected pediatric facial lacerations. Acad Emerg Med 1999;6(3): 171–7.

[14] Gosain AK, Lyon VB. Plastic Surgery Educational Foundation DATA Committee. The current status of tissue glues: part II. For adhesion of soft tissues. Plast Reconstr Surg 2002;110(6):1581–4.

[15] Perry LC. An evaluation of acute incisional strength with Traumaseal surgical tissue adhesive wound closure. Leonia, NJ: Dimensional Analysis Systems; 1995. Taken from: Gosain AK, Lyon VB, Plastic Surgery Educational Foundation DATA Committee. The current status of tissue glues: part II. For adhesion of soft tissues. Plast Reconstr Surg 2002;110(6):1581–4.

[16] Quinn J, Wells G, Sutcliffe T, et al. A randomized trial comparing octylcyanoacrylate tissue adhesive and sutures in the management of lacerations. JAMA 1997;277(19):1527–30.

[17] Maw JL, Quinn JV, Wells GA, et al. A prospective comparison of octylcyanoacrylate tissue adhesive and suture for the closure of head and neck incisions. J Otolaryngol 1997;26(1):26–30.

[18] Singer AJ, Hollander JE, Valentine SM. Prospective, randomized, controlled trial of tissue adhesive (2-octylcyanoacrylate) vs standard wound closure techniques for laceration repair. Stony Brook Octylcyanoacrylate Study Group. Acad Emerg Med 1998;5(2):94–9.

[19] Holger JS, Wandersee SC, Hale DB. Cosmetic outcomes of facial lacerations repaired with tissue-adhesive, absorbable, and nonabsorbable sutures. Am J Emerg Med 2004;22(4):254–7.

[20] Quinn JV, Drzewiecki A, Li MM, et al. A randomized, controlled trial comparing a tissue adhesive with suturing in the repair of pediatric facial lacerations. Ann Emerg Med 1993;22(7):1130–5.

[21] Ong CC, Jacobsen AS, Joseph VT. Comparing wound closure using tissue glue versus subcuticular suture for pediatric surgical incisions: a prospective, randomised trial. Pediatr Surg Int 2002;18(5–6):553–5.

[22] Bruns TB, Robinson BS, Smith RJ. A new tissue adhesive for laceration repair in children. J Pediatr 1998;132(6):1067–70.

[23] Quinn JV, Osmond MH, Yurack JA, Moir PJ. N-2-butylcyanoacrylate: risk of bacterial contamination with an appraisal of its antimicrobial effects. J Emerg Med 1995;13(4):581–5.

[24] Quinn J, Maw J, Ramotar K. Octylcyanoacrylate tissue adhesive versus suture wound repair in a contaminated wound model. Surgery 1997;122(1):69–72.

[25] Care express products. Available at: http://www.care express.com. Accessed August 2, 2004.

[26] Osmond MH, Klassen TP, Quinn JV. Economic comparison of a tissue adhesive and suturing in the repair of pediatric facial lacerations. J Pediatr 1995; 126(6):892–5.

[27] Quinn J, Lowe L, Mertz M. The effect of a new tissue-adhesive wound dressing on the healing of traumatic abrasions. Dermatology 2000;201(4):343–6.

[28] Singer AJ, Nable M, Cameau P, et al. Evaluation of a new liquid occlusive dressing for excisional wounds. Wound Repair Regen 2003;11(3):181–7.

[29] Mertz PM, Davis SC, Cazzaniga AL, et al. Barrier and antibacterial properties of 2-octyl cyanoacrylate-derived wound treatment films. J Cutan Med Surg 2003;7(1):1–6.

[30] Narang U, Mainwaring L, Spath G, Barefoot J. In-vitro analysis for microbial barrier properties of 2-octyl cyanoacrylate-derived wound treatment films. J Cutan Med Surg 2003;7(1):13–9.

[31] Singer AJ, Mohammad M, Thode Jr HC, McClain SA. Octylcyanoacrylate versus polyurethane for treatment of burns in swine: a randomized trial. Burns 2000; 26(4):388–92.

[32] Singer A, Thode Jr H, McClain S. The effects of octyl-cyanoacrylate on scarring after burns. Acad Emerg Med 2001;8(2):107–11.

[33] Singer AJ, Mohammad M, Tortora G, et al. Octylcyanoacrylate for the treatment of contaminated partial-thickness burns in swine: a randomized controlled experiment. Acad Emerg Med 2000;7(3):222–7.

[34] Eaglstein WH, Sullivan TP, Giordano PA, Miskin BM. A liquid adhesive bandage for the treatment of minor cuts and abrasions. Dermatol Surg 2002;28(3):263–7.

[35] Al-Belasy FA, Amer MZ. Hemostatic effect of n-butyl-2-cyanoacrylate (histoacryl) glue in warfarin-treated patients undergoing oral surgery. J Oral Maxillofac Surg 2003;61(12):1405–9.

[36] Greenwald BD, Caldwell SH, Hespenheide EE, et al. N-2-butyl-cyanoacrylate for bleeding gastric varices: a United States pilot study and cost analysis. Am J Gastroenterol 2003;98(9):1982–8.

[37] Losanoff JE, Richman BW, Jones JW. Cyanoacrylate adhesive in management of severe presacral bleeding. Dis Colon Rectum 2002;45(8):1118–9.

[38] Singer AJ, McClain SA, Katz A. A porcine epistaxis model: hemostatic effects of octylcyanoacrylate. Otolaryngol Head Neck Surg 2004;130(5):553–7.

[39] Davis SC, Eaglstein WH, Cazzaniga AL, Mertz PM. An octyl-2-cyanoacrylate formulation speeds healing of partial-thickness wounds. Dermatol Surg 2001; 27(9):783–8.

[40] Simeonova M, Velichkova R, Ivanova G, et al. Poly(butylcyanoacrylate) nanoparticles for topical delivery of 5-fluorouracil. Int J Pharm 2003;263(1–2): 133–40.

[41] Mitra A, Lin S. Effect of surfactant on fabrication and characterization of paclitaxel-loaded polybutylcyanoacrylate nanoparticulate delivery systems. J Pharm Pharmacol 2003;55(7):895–902.

[42] Miyazaki S, Takahashi A, Kubo W, et al. Poly n-butylcyanoacrylate (PNBCA) nanocapsules as a carrier for NSAIDs: in vitro release and in vivo skin penetration. J Pharm Pharm Sci 2003;6(2):238–45.

[43] Ylikontiola L, Sorsa T, Hayrinen-Immonen R, Salo T. Doxymycine-cyanoacrylate treatment of recurrent aphthous ulcers. Oral Surg Oral Med Oral Pathol Oral Radiol Endod 1997;83(3):329–33.

[44] Narang U. Cyanoacrylate medical adhesives—a new era Colgate ORABASE Soothe. N. seal liquid protectant for canker sore relief. Compend Contin Educ Dent Suppl 2001;(32):7–11.

[45] Kutcher MJ, Ludlow JB, Samuelson AD, et al. Evaluation of a bioadhesive device for the management of aphthous ulcers. J Am Dent Assoc 2001; 132(3):368–76.

ELSEVIER
SAUNDERS

DERMATOLOGIC
CLINICS

Dermatol Clin 23 (2005) 199–207

Using Light in Dermatology: An Update on Lasers, Ultraviolet Phototherapy, and Photodynamic Therapy

Iltefat Hamzavi, MD[a],*, Harvey Lui, MD, FRCPC[b]

[a]Department of Dermatology, Wayne State University, 4201 St. Antoine, Suite 5F, Detroit, MI 48201, USA
[b]Division of Dermatology, Vancouver Coastal Health Research Institute, University of British Columbia, Vancouver, BC, Canada

It was just over a century ago that Niels Finsen was awarded the 1903 Nobel Prize in Medicine for establishing the scientific basis for using light to treat skin disease [1]. Despite the medical use of light in dermatology throughout the twentieth century, the fundamental mechanisms of action for its therapeutic effects have been systematically explored and clinically exploited only in the last couple of decades. This article highlights some of the most important advances in therapeutic photomedicine over the last decade with a focus on lasers, intense pulsed light (IPL), ultraviolet light (UV) phototherapy, and photodynamic therapy (PDT). Although these treatment modalities have each evolved quite independently of the others, there has been a convergence of interests among clinical practitioners and investigators who use light to treat diseased skin. For example, two very different photonic approaches have been introduced into clinical practice based on the concept that selective wavelengths within the UV light B (UVB) region are more effective for treating psoriasis: narrowband fluorescent lamps and pulsed excimer lasers. What unifies these two examples, and any other dermatologic light sources, is the fact that in essence all they really do is deliver external energy to the skin for therapeutic purposes. Regardless of the device or dermatologic indication, specific biophysical laws govern how all light affects the skin.

The key to developing and refining any type of light-based therapy is to understand how to deliver this energy to cutaneous structures efficiently and effectively in a highly targeted fashion so as to limit collateral light-induced damage to normal tissue. Treating the skin with light can be considered in two stages: understanding how selectively to deliver photons to specific structural targets in the skin (ie, tissue optics), and understanding the biologic processes that occur after a skin target absorbs light photons (ie, photobiologic reactions). Most refinements to phototherapeutic devices exploit either one or both of these two aspects, and the advances highlighted in this article are discussed using this mechanistic perspective.

Understanding tissue optics and photobiologic reactions

A detailed explanation of tissue optics and photobiologic reactions is beyond the scope of this article, but certain basic biophysical principles warrant a brief summary. The interaction of light with tissue is governed by three basic processes that can occur when a photon of light reaches the skin: (1) reflection, (2) scattering, and (3) absorption. Light that is reflected from the skin and perceived by the

---

* Corresponding author. Department of Dermatology, Henry Ford Hospital, 2799 West Grand Boulevard, Detroit, MI 48202.
E-mail address: ihamzavi@med.wayne.edu (I. Hamzavi).

human visual system provides the means for diagnosing skin disease, but reflected light does not itself result in any direct therapeutic effect. In the absence of an absorption event (see later), the forward propagation of light deeper within the skin is influenced by the degree to which its direction of travel has been scattered by tissue structures. Tissue scattering of UV, visible, and near infrared light is wavelength-dependent, and in general longer wavelength light penetrates the skin more deeply. Targets that are deeper in the skin require the use of devices that can deliver longer wavelength light.

Absorption is an important biophysical event that involves the transfer of energy from light to tissue. Without photon absorption, energy is not taken up by the skin and no biologic or therapeutic effect occurs. The absorption of photons by specific molecules within the skin also influences light penetration because any photon that is absorbed is no longer capable of propagating through the skin, because that particular photon no longer exists. Like scattering, absorption is wavelength-dependent, but in a somewhat more complicated manner because it depends on the absorption profile or "spectrum" of the light-absorbing molecule, which in this context is usually referred to as the "chromophore." With the possible exception of UVB phototherapy the specific chromophores for most light-based therapies are precisely known and include hemoglobin; melanin; water; exogenous dyes (ie, tattoo pigment); and photosensitizing drugs (ie, psoralens and PDT photosensitizers). It is ironic that although UVB light is the oldest and most widely used form of phototherapy, the precise chromophore and subsequent biologic tissue reactions for this modality remain unclear at this time.

In summary, both scattering and absorption determine the depth to which light penetrates the skin, but only absorption can lead to photobiologic and phototherapeutic effects. All phototherapeutic applications must by definition be mediated by chromophores present in the skin. For a given photon to have a clinical effect it must actually reach the target structure within the skin and then be absorbed by a specific chromophore within that target. Whether or not these events occur and the degree to which they occur is dependent on the wavelength of light used, the structure of the skin, the presence and location of chromophores, and the preferential ability of diseased tissue to absorb light more efficiently than normal unaffected skin. In clinical parlance, there is often an undue preoccupation with the technical specifications for a given light device rather than a well-grounded understanding of the desired underlying photobiologic and phototherapeutic end points. The reality is that for any clinical indication a multiplicity of possible photonic devices are often available. This simply reflects the fact that from the point of view of the tissue and its chromophores, the exact source of the photons (eg, laser versus IPL versus light-emitting diode versus fluorescent lamp) matters far less than whether the photons are of the appropriate wavelength and delivered to the target in sufficient quantity to cause irreversible tissue changes. As with any therapeutic modality, the ultimate arbiters for the bewildering array of competing light-based therapies and devices are well-designed and rigorously executed controlled clinical studies.

Once the photon is absorbed by the chromophore, the source's light energy is transferred to the skin either to generate heat or drive photochemical reactions. The former scenario encompasses most lasers and IPLs in dermatology, all of which in essence involve the selective and irreversible alteration of tissue using heat [2]. In contrast, UV phototherapy and PDT do not primarily involve the use of light to generate heat, but rather rely on photon absorption to energize photochemistry. In the case of UV therapy it is now generally accepted that the therapeutically useful photochemical reactions culminate in cutaneous immunosuppression, although the exact sequence of reactions is less clear. In PDT the first two photochemical reactions are very clearly defined. The energy of the excited chromophore is first transferred to molecular oxygen to form singlet oxygen, which then reacts with a diverse range of biomolecules. The everexpanding indications for PDT partly mirrors the multiple ways by which singlet oxygen generated by light can affect the skin.

Using lasers and intense pulsed light to heat the skin

Because most lasers in dermatology are used precisely to heat the skin, the advances for these applications are related to increasing the selectivity of these devices by fine tuning the wavelength and pulse duration (ie, the time over which the laser energy is delivered) [3], and simultaneously cooling the skin during light exposure. These modifications have increased the safety and efficacy for photothermal lasers in dermatology, particularly for targeting larger or deeper skin structures, such as larger blood vessels and hair follicles. Another driving force in the evolution of lasers and IPL has been the need to minimize downtime from postprocedure purpura and elaborate wound care protocols.

Extending the therapeutic range of vascular lasers

Although the principle for treating vascular lesions, such as port wine stains, with yellow 577- or 585-nm light was originally based on hemoglobin's absorption spectrum, red to infrared light seems to target blood vessels better that are situated more deeply. In addition, vascular laser pulse durations have been extended from the submicrosecond to millisecond domain for two reasons. A longer duration of exposure heats a greater tissue volume, which is necessary for larger-caliber vessels. Second, longer pulses conduct heat more gradually within blood vessels resulting in a lesser tendency to immediate purpura, which although temporary, patients find very disfiguring. The long-pulsed neodymium:yttrium–aluminum–garnet (Nd:YAG) and later-model pulsed dye lasers both expand the range of blood vessels that can be treated by incorporating these parameter changes. The longer penetration of the long-pulsed 1064-nm Nd:YAG laser facilitates its use for leg veins including blue veins up to 3 mm in diameter [4]. Not unexpectedly, these lasers are often less effective for finer red telangiectasias presumably because of a mismatch between the vessel's thermal relaxation time and the laser's pulsewidth [3]. Despite these advances, lasers have not yet supplanted conventional sclerotherapy for managing leg veins [5]. The deeper penetration of the recently developed 595-nm, long-pulse (up to 40 milliseconds) dye laser allows the operator to obtain clearance for some port wine stains that is equivalent to the original 585 nm, 450-μs pulsed dye laser results with fewer side effects, such as prolonged purpura and crusting [6]. It may also be helpful for red telangiectasias on the legs [7].

Cooling the skin to protect the epidermis and superficial dermis

Although the judicious selection of wavelength, pulse duration, and fluence allows lasers and IPL sources to generate heat at specific targets within the skin, collateral heat damage can still be sustained by surrounding structures, particularly the epidermis, which contains melanin, a broad-spectrum chromophore. Unwanted epidermal thermal damage becomes even more problematic when treating darker skin types or when using higher fluences as may be the case when treating deeper targets, such as hair follicles. Cooling the skin surface during laser exposures serves to protect the epidermis and superficial dermis from unintended photothermal effects. Skin cooling techniques include chilled probes held in contact with

the skin, timed cryogen sprays directed to the skin surface, and forced cold air fans directed at the treatment site. All forms of cooling aim to prevent the superficial layers of the skin from reaching the threshold temperature for thermal damage during laser exposure, and they all differ in terms of reliability and the cost of consumables, such as cryogen. An additional benefit of skin cooling beyond the reduction of superficial crusting and dyschromia [8] is intraoperative pain relief.

Intense pulsed light

IPL sources are now very popular in medicine and have been heavily marketed to the public, dermatologists, other physicians, and nonmedical practitioners. IPL devices are not lasers, but like most cutaneous lasers, produce their desired effect by generating heat. The core technology is relatively simple and involves the use of polychromatic broadband flashlamps equipped with optical filters that allow preselected visible to infrared wavebands (500–1200 nm) to reach the skin [9]. Because multiple wavelengths are delivered, several different chromophores including hemoglobin, melanin, and perhaps even water, can be targeted with the same light exposure. Photorejuvenation is a somewhat broad imprecisely defined concept whose aim is to improve the appearance of the skin by eliminating lentigines and dyspigmentation, telangiectasia, and fine wrinkles. Lasers and IPLs can achieve these effects to some extent, but the main purported advantage with IPLs is that these features can be treated simultaneously with one device [10], whereas with lasers several different devices may be required. There are few controlled clinical trials to confirm these claims for IPL, but nevertheless the systems have become quite popular [11]. In practical terms, multiple IPL treatment sessions are often required, and because of the complexity of selecting the appropriate wavelength cutoff filter, fluence, and pulse duration there is a risk for developing side effects secondary to nonspecific thermal damage. These side effects include crusting, pigmentary changes, and paradoxical increases in hair growth [12]. Another potential area of concern with IPL relates in part to the multiplicity of repeat treatments that are often advocated for both the initial treatment and subsequent maintenance sessions. Because IPL includes infrared radiation, it may be theoretically possible to sustain deleterious cutaneous effects from chronic infrared exposure. The versatility and effective marketing of these devices is a driving force behind their popularity but it remains to be seen if well-designed trials can confirm their efficacy.

From laser resurfacing to nonablative dermal remodeling

Within the span of less than a decade the use of carbon dioxide lasers (λ = 10,600 nm) for ablating rhytides and superficial scarring peaked and then abruptly declined. The controlled ablation of superficial skin layers with the carbon dioxide laser by tissue water as the chromophore improves the skin's texture and appearance, but carries with it significant risks for dyspigmentation and scarring, especially when performed by less experienced operators [13,14]. Ablative skin resurfacing is still relatively safe and effective in skilled hands when used for treating fine to medium rhytides and elastosis, and may be the gold standard for facial rejuvenation. This procedure is demanding on patients and practitioners, however, because success also requires meticulous and elaborate postoperative wound care and a willingness to accept weeks to months of facial erythema that can often be very conspicuous. More often than not, patients opt for less invasive procedures even if the improvement is less dramatic, and this preference has been fulfilled by the introduction of devices and techniques that replicate the clinical effects of the carbon dioxide laser while minimizing patient inconvenience and downtime.

The erbium (Er):YAG was initially believed to provide a wider safety margin for resurfacing as compared with the carbon dioxide laser because its shorter wavelength (2940 nm) and pulse width resulted in a more attenuated optical path length within tissue. The Er:YAG laser does indeed cause a narrower zone of ablation and residual tissue necrosis, but the tissue effects are probably too shallow to achieve the desired clinical effect. Intraoperatively, Er:YAG-based resurfacing is time consuming because more laser passes are required to ablate a given thickness of tissue. Furthermore, hemostasis is problematic because of this laser's inability coagulatively to seal off blood vessels, which is directly related to its attenuated tissue penetration. In terms of clinical results a controlled study showed that although the Er:YAG laser reduced healing times and side effects it did not produce the same degree of improvement in rhytides as the carbon dioxide laser [15].

To treat abnormal skin texture induced by photoaging effectively, photons must be delivered to the level of the dermis where collagen and elastin reside. Hence, the use of infrared wavelengths, such as with the carbon dioxide and Er:YAG lasers. Because the side effects associated with these two lasers are primarily the result of ablating and wounding the epidermis and superficial dermis, nonablative or subsurface dermal remodeling has been proposed as a preferred technique. Two methods are currently being used to spare the skin's surface when delivering infrared laser energy to the skin: using alternate infrared wavelengths and concurrent skin cooling during treatment. Lasers at 1320 nm Nd:YAG and 1450 nm (diode) seem to penetrate to the level of the dermis without affecting the skin surface, particularly when used in combination with dynamic skin cooling [16]. Commercial Food and Drug Administration (FDA) approval for these devices has established a foothold for nonablative resurfacing in the treatment of acne scars and rhytides [13,16]. Nonablative techniques require multiple treatments, however, and although histologic effects can be demonstrated, a corresponding clinical response may often be hard to discern [13].

Removing hair with light

The use of lasers and IPL systems for hair removal has expanded tremendously over the past decade. In fact, in many jurisdictions most treatments are now no longer performed through physician offices. The main advance in this application is the use of longer wavelengths and pulse durations to minimize side effects in darker-skinned patients [17].

The addition of radiofrequency pulses is suggested to remove blonde and gray hairs but there is scant published information to support that claim [11]. As hair removal technology has become more widespread unexpected side effects have been noted, such as the paradoxical stimulation of hair growth. This has been reported with IPL [12] and the long-pulsed alexandrite laser [18]. A striking reticulate erythema ab igne–type reaction has also been reported as being caused by infrared diode laser hair removal [19].

A need for well-designed trials

The widespread use of lasers and IPL has not necessarily been paralleled by an abundance of adequately powered controlled clinical trials with objective and reproducible end points that are assessed in a blinded fashion. This is partly related to the North American regulatory system for photonic devices, which is very different from the pharmaceutical approval process. Medical devices, such as light sources, can be approved primarily on the basis of technical equivalence to existing technologies without the need for multicenter, controlled trials. In many instances, controlled trials have not been able to confirm a significant advantage for lasers in the treatment of acne [20], warts [21], asymptomatic hemangiomas [22], scars [23,24], leg veins [5], and periorbital wrinkles [25]. Although promising "proof of concept" studies, clinical experience, marketing, and patient demand may indicate that a laser can be used for a given indication, good-quality controlled studies [26] are best for determining whether that laser should in fact be used.

Ultraviolet light as an immunomodulator

Recent advances in UV phototherapy include a better mechanistic understanding of its biologic effects, more rational dosimetry approaches, and the deployment of several novel UV sources. The basic science for UV phototherapy is characterized best for psoriasis, wherein the induction of T-cell apoptosis has been demonstrated for broadband [27] and narrowband UVB [28] and psoralen plus UV light A (UVA) [29]. Myriad other cutaneous immunologic reactions also occur with UV, but the T-cell−depleting effects are likely pivotal for clearing inflammatory dermatoses and cutaneous T-cell lymphoma. These cytolytic effects on activated immune cells may also explain why UV therapy can be considered a remittive form of psoriasis treatment. The fundamental shift in concept of UV phototherapy as a means of inducing localized cutaneous immunosuppression has provided a far more logical rationale for its general efficacy in a broad range of dermatoses.

In conventional UV phototherapy both diseased and normal skin are simultaneously exposed to light. Although the primary goal of treating inflammatory dermatoses, such as psoriasis, is to clear skin lesions using light, the current approach to UV dosimetry is limited by the need to avoid burning the unaffected skin. Very-high-dose UV exposures (as high as several multiples of the baseline minimal erythema [UVB [30]] or phototoxic [psoralen plus UVA [31]] dose) can indeed clear psoriasis fairly efficiently, but using such fluences on a whole-body basis at the outset of therapy causes severe burning of unaffected skin. With repetitive exposures, normal human skin gradually photoadapts or acquires tolerance to UV light, and the rate at which this develops in normal skin has been established empirically through clinical practice. The concept of UV [32] tolerance guides any course of phototherapy, and detailed insights into its biologic basis and kinetics are still under active systematic study [32].

Narrow-band ultraviolet light B

Although action spectrum studies of psoriasis from 1981 showed a clear therapeutic benefit for longer versus shorter wavelength UVB [33], the technology for exploiting this advantage became widely available only over the last decade. The development of the Tl-01 narrowband fluorescent UVB (NB-UVB) lamp by Philips Electronics (Utrecht, The Netherlands) probably represents the most significant advance in how phototherapy is now delivered. NB-UVB is the first widely available light source that confirmed the benefit of using selective wavelengths of UVB. The increasing popularity of NB-UVB contrasts with the abrupt decline in the use of systemic psoralen plus UVA, which clearly accelerates photoaging and causes skin cancer [34]. NB-UVB has been shown to be as effective as psoralen plus UVA without as many short-term side effects [35]. In hairless mice exposed to UVB, NB-UVB was shown to be more carcinogenic than broadband UVB [36], but NB-UVB has not been associated with an increased risk of skin cancer when used therapeutically [37]. The latter study evaluated patients who had received a relatively low cumulative NB-UVB number of exposures (mean of 44 treatments), and it is premature to conclude that NB-UVB will not be carcinogenic when used for phototherapy in humans.

Beyond psoriasis, NB-UVB has also been shown to be effective in controlled studies for the treatment of vitiligo, although the response is incomplete [38]. Using quantitative scales to measure depigmentation, Hamzavi et al [38] reported that narrowband phototherapy, even after 6 months of treatment, only repigments the skin by approximately 42%. Targeted phototherapy using the 308-nm excimer laser also treats vitiligo. It may work faster than whole-body NB-UVB but no head-to-head studies are available [39]. According to the British Photodermatology Group, there is good evidence to support the use of NB-UVB for chronic atopic dermatitis, and fair evidence for cutaneous T-cell lymphoma [40].

Novel ultraviolet light sources

Unlike selective photothermolysis with lasers, which is critically dependent on the rate and number (ie, irradiance and fluence, respectively) of photons delivered to the skin, the effects of UV phototherapy are primarily determined by the total number of photons that reach the skin. Depending on the specific light source, psoriasis can be cleared with UV light exposures ranging from several minutes (conventional fluorescent or incandescent lamps) to fractions of a second (lasers and IPL). UV lasers and IPL sources aim to clear psoriasis more efficiently than conventional broadband UVB in three ways. First, these sources emit relatively longer wavelength UVB; second, they can be targeted to expose only the affected areas while sparing normal skin, thereby allowing much higher fluences to be used safely; and finally, they operate at much higher irradiances so that exposure times are much shorter than with fluorescent lamps. There are now at least three commercial devices that can provide targeted phototherapy: (1) the 308-nm excimer laser, (2) broadband IPL, and (3) the broadband mercury lamp with dual UVB and UVA output. There are a few published controlled clinical studies to show that psoriasis responds to the excimer laser, whereas systematic studies for the other two systems are ongoing [30,41,42]. The disadvantages to targeted phototherapy are the higher cost and the relatively time-consuming aspect of covering broad plaques on the body with a series of relatively small spot-size exposures. Parenthetically, non-UV lasers have been used successfully for psoriasis [43,44], but these techniques have not been widely adapted in dermatology, presumably because of practical limitations.

As with UVB, UVA is also heterogeneous with respect to the clinical effects of specific wavelengths. For example, devices that deliver high-intensity UVA-1 light (ie, 340–400 nm) are effective for treating pruritic disorders, such as atopic dermatitis and mastocytosis [45]. The mechanism of action may hinge on the ability of this UVA waveband to reduce cellular IgE binding sites [46] and induce apoptosis by two different pathways while reducing IgE binding sites [47]. UVA-1 is also effective for sclerosing disorders [48]. Because of limited controlled and comparative data, long treatment times, and high costs, UVA-1 units have not been widely adapted in North America, with most units being installed at select university centers.

The arrival of photodynamic therapy

Following its approval by the FDA in 1999 for treating actinic keratoses, PDT was initially slow to catch on in dermatology, and this was largely caused by the low reimbursement for dermatologic PDT in the United States by third-party payers. The concept of PDT is a century old, and its dependence on oxygen-related photochemistry has been well known for most of that time. In clinical practice, the treatment involves the administration of a photosensitizer

followed by exposing the skin to light. The drug-activating photons can come from lasers or nonco-herent light sources. The photosensitizer, incubation period, and wavelength used to activate the photo-sensitizer allow the nonthermal selective destruction of neoplastic keratinocytes, sebaceous glands, and hair follicles to be fine-tuned. Indications for PDT can include oncologic uses and destruction of appendi-geal structures.

The efficacy of topical PDT using 20% amino-levulinic acid (ALA) and a blue light has been documented in the treatment of actinic keratosis [49]. The procedure as approved by the FDA is painful, however, and requires two visits on separate days [50]. A few studies where the incubation period was reduced to a few hours and a pulsed dye laser or IPL used to activate the photodynamic reactions [50,51] reduced the pain and overall patient treatment time. An experimental protocol used in mice showed that broad area application of the 20% ALA solution can treat subclinical neoplastic lesions, possibly preventing carcinogenesis [52]. In addition, the methylation of ALA to allow for deeper drug penetration has allowed for more effective treatment of superficial basal cell carcinomas in Europe [53]. This treatment was recently approved by the FDA for treatment of actinic keratosis when activated by a red light [54]. Systemic PDT has shown some promise using a systemic photosensitizer and a noncoherent red light diode array, but further confirmatory studies are needed [55].

The response of actinic keratoses to ALA PDT caused some investigators to evaluate the use of this treatment for the treatment of photoaging. Topical PDT has also been used to treat photoaging of the skin in a few case series with good results [51]. Studies on the long-term follow-up for this indication are lacking, although the procedure seems to be heavily promoted as an off-label cosmetic application.

The use of PDT to ablate appendigeal structures is an area of active investigation. There has been one case series on the use of topical 20% ALA to treat truncal acne with good results. Significant post-inflammatory pigmentation and pain, however, were reported [56]. Recently, this technique has been modified by decreasing the incubation period and activating the photosensitizer by a laser. This has been shown to be less painful and may induce a clinical remission of moderate acne [57]. To date, no controlled trials have been published.

Studies are ongoing but the evidence for the use of PDT for acne is limited. This would be a welcome addition to the few effective but safe treatment options for severe acne. The use of PDT for acne has increased significantly in the past year and it is likely that the use of PDT for acne has outpaced its FDA-approved use for actinic keratoses. This is as much a function of reimbursement as efficacy. The third-party payments for PDT for actinic keratosis in the United States have been poor as compared with lower-cost treatments, such as liquid nitrogen.

There are other forms of PDT that have entered the clinical arena for the treatment of acne. There are reports that certain wavelengths of light (blue and red) induce a PDT reaction in endogenous photosensitizers produced by *Propionibacterium acnes* bacteria resident in the skin. These treatments do not require an exogenous photosensitizer, such as ALA. Both lasers and noncoherent light sources have been reported to be effective [58]. The noncoherent light sources include red and blue wavelengths. They seem to reduce lesions initially with a gradual recurrence of the inflammatory papules and pustules over 3 to 12 months [11,59].

Summary

It is no longer possible to practice dermatology without drawing on the healing power of light. As compared with drugs, light therapy is in general vastly more versatile with an equal or better safety profile. The range of indications for using light in dermatology cuts across all areas including chronic inflammatory dermatoses, pigmentary disorders, cancer, infections, and cosmetic applications. Physicians can remain up-to-date in their understanding of current and evolving modalities by mastering the basic biophysical principles outlined in this article. Once these concepts are understood all the advances can be kept in perspective. Physicians can then apply the most appropriate technology to the care of their patients while informing patients and themselves about the potential limitations and pitfalls of over-marketed but inadequately proved strategies.

References

[1] Nobel Prize Organization. Niels Finsen. Available at: http://www.nobel.se/medicine/laureates/1903/press.html. Accessed August 17, 2004.

[2] Lui H. Advances in dermatologic lasers. Dermatol Clin 1998;16:261–8.

[3] Anderson RR, Parrish JA. Selective photothermolysis: precise microsurgery by selective absorption of pulsed radiation. Science 1983;220:524–7.

[4] Omura NE, Dover JS, Arndt KA, et al. Treatment of reticular leg veins with a 1064 nm long-pulsed Nd:YAG laser. J Am Acad Dermatol 2003;48:76–81.

[5] Lupton JR, Alster TS, Romero P. Clinical comparison of sclerotherapy versus long-pulsed Nd:YAG laser treatment for lower extremity telangiectases. Dermatol Surg 2002;28:694–7.

[6] Greve B, Raulin C. Prospective study of port wine stain treatment with dye laser: comparison of two wavelengths (585 nm vs. 595 nm) and two pulse durations (0.5 milliseconds vs. 20 milliseconds). Lasers Surg Med 2004;34:168–73.

[7] Sadick NS, Weiss RA, Goldman MP. Advances in laser surgery for leg veins: bimodal wavelength approach to lower extremity vessels, new cooling techniques, and longer pulse durations. Dermatol Surg 2002;28:16–20.

[8] Tunnell JW, Chang DW, Johnston C, et al. Effects of cryogen spray cooling and high radiant exposures on selective vascular injury during laser irradiation of human skin. Arch Dermatol 2003;139:743–50.

[9] Raulin C, Greve B, Grema H. IPL technology: a review. Lasers Surg Med 2003;32:78–87.

[10] Weiss RA, Weiss MA, Beasley KL. Rejuvenation of photoaged skin: 5 years results with intense pulsed light of the face, neck, and chest. Dermatol Surg 2002; 28:1115–9.

[11] Alam M, Dover JS, Arndt KA. Energy delivery devices for cutaneous remodeling: lasers, lights, and radio waves. Arch Dermatol 2003;139:1351–60.

[12] Moreno-Arias GA, Castelo-Branco C, Ferrando J. Side-effects after IPL photodepilation. Dermatol Surg 2002;28:1131–4.

[13] Leffell DJ. Clinical efficacy of devices for nonablative photorejuvenation. Arch Dermatol 2002;138: 1503–8.

[14] Rendon-Pellerano MI, Lentini J, Eaglstein WE, et al. Laser resurfacing: usual and unusual complications. Dermatol Surg 1999;25:360–6 [discussion: 366–7].

[15] Newman JB, Lord JL, Ash K, et al. Variable pulse erbium:YAG laser skin resurfacing of perioral rhytides and side-by-side comparison with carbon dioxide laser. Lasers Surg Med 2000;26:208–14.

[16] Tanzi EL, Alster TS. Comparison of a 1450-nm diode laser and a 1320-nm Nd:YAG laser in the treatment of atrophic facial scars: a prospective clinical and histologic study. Dermatol Surg 2004;30(2 Pt 1): 152–7.

[17] Ross EV, Cooke LM, Overstreet KA, et al. Treatment of pseudofolliculitis barbae in very dark skin with a long pulse Nd:YAG laser. J Natl Med Assoc 2002; 94:888–93.

[18] Alajlan A, Shapiro J, Rivers JK, et al. Paradoxical hypertrichosis after laser epilation. J Am Acad Dermatol, in press.

[19] Lapidoth M, Shafirstein G, Ben Amitai D, et al. Reticulate erythema following diode laser-assisted hair removal: a new side effect of a common procedure. J Am Acad Dermatol 2004;51:774–7.

[20] Orringer JS, Kang S, Hamilton T, et al. Treatment of acne vulgaris with a pulsed dye laser: a randomized controlled trial. JAMA 2004;291:2834–9.

[21] Robson KJ, Cunningham NM, Kruzan KL, et al. Pulsed-dye laser versus conventional therapy in the treatment of warts: a prospective randomized trial. J Am Acad Dermatol 2000;43(2 Pt 1):275–80.

[22] Batta K, Goodyear HM, Moss C, et al. Randomised controlled study of early pulsed dye laser treatment of uncomplicated childhood haemangiomas: results of a 1-year analysis. Lancet 2002;360:521–7.

[23] Manuskiatti W, Fitzpatrick RE. Treatment response of keloidal and hypertrophic sternotomy scars: comparison among intralesional corticosteroid, 5-fluorouracil, and 585-nm flashlamp-pumped pulsed-dye laser treatments. Arch Dermatol 2002;138:1149–55.

[24] Wittenberg GP, Fabian BG, Bogomilsky JL, et al. Prospective, single-blind, randomized, controlled study to assess the efficacy of the 585-nm flashlamp-pumped pulsed-dye laser and silicone gel sheeting in hypertrophic scar treatment. Arch Dermatol 1999;135:1049–55.

[25] Reynolds N, Thomas K, Baker L, et al. Pulsed dye laser and non-ablative wrinkle reduction. Lasers Surg Med 2004;34:109–13.

[26] Kopera D, Smolle J, Kaddu S, et al. Nonablative laser treatment of wrinkles: meeting the objective? Assessment by 25 dermatologists. Br J Dermatol 2004;150:936–9.

[27] Krueger JG, Wolfe JT, Nabeya RT, et al. Successful ultraviolet B treatment of psoriasis is accompanied by a reversal of keratinocyte pathology and by selective depletion of intraepidermal T cells. J Exp Med 1995;182:2057–68.

[28] Ozawa M, Ferenczi K, Kikuchi T, et al. 312-nanometer ultraviolet B light (narrow-band UVB) induces apoptosis of T cells within psoriatic lesions. J Exp Med 1999;189:711–8.

[29] Johnson R, Staiano-Coico L, Austin L, et al. PUVA treatment selectively induces a cell cycle block and subsequent apoptosis in human T-lymphocytes. Photochem Photobiol 1996;63:566–71.

[30] Trehan M, Taylor CR. High-dose 308-nm excimer laser for the treatment of psoriasis. J Am Acad Dermatol 2002;46:732–7.

[31] Taylor CR, Kwangsukstith C, Wimberly J, et al. Turbo-PUVA: dihydroxyacetone-enhanced photochemotherapy for psoriasis: a pilot study. Arch Dermatol 1999;135:540–4.

[32] Oh C, Hennessy A, Ha T, et al. The time course of photoadaptation and pigmentation studied using a novel method to distinguish pigmentation from erythema. J Invest Dermatol 2004;123:965–72.

[33] Parrish JA, Jaenicke KF. Action spectrum for phototherapy of psoriasis. J Invest Dermatol 1981;76:359–62.

[34] Stern RS, Nichols KT, Vakeva LH. Malignant melanoma in patients treated for psoriasis with methoxsalen (psoralen) and ultraviolet A radiation (PUVA). The PUVA Follow-Up Study. N Engl J Med 1997;336:1041–5.

[35] Snellman E, Klimenko T, Rantanen T. Randomized half-side comparison of narrowband UVB and trimethylpsoralen bath plus UVA treatments for psoriasis. Acta Derm Venereol 2004;84:132–7.

[36] Wulf HC, Hansen AB, Bech-Thomsen N. Differences in narrow-band ultraviolet B and broad-spectrum ultraviolet photocarcinogenesis in lightly pigmented hairless mice. Photodermatol Photoimmunol Photomed 1994;10:192–7.

[37] Weischer M, Blum A, Eberhard F, et al. No evidence for increased skin cancer risk in psoriasis patients treated with broadband or narrowband UVB phototherapy: a first retrospective study. Acta Derm Venereol 2004;84:370–4.

[38] Hamzavi I, Jain H, McLean D, et al. Parametric modeling of narrowband UV-B phototherapy for vitiligo using a novel quantitative tool: the Vitiligo Area Scoring Index. Arch Dermatol 2004;140:677–83.

[39] Baltas E, Csoma Z, Ignacz F, et al. Treatment of vitiligo with the 308-nm xenon chloride excimer laser. Arch Dermatol 2002;138:1619–20.

[40] Ibbotson SH, Bilsland D, Cox NH, et al. An update and guidance on narrowband ultraviolet B phototherapy: a British Photodermatology Group Workshop Report. Br J Dermatol 2004;151:283–97.

[41] Dierickx C. Optimalization of treatment of psoriasis with B clear system [abstract]. Lasers Surg Med 2003;32(Suppl 15):37.

[42] Hu J, Kaur M, Feldman S. Non-laser targeted UV treatment for localized psoriasis. Presented at the 62nd Annual Meeting of the American Academy of Dermatology, Poster 581, 2004; Washington DC, T500X Targeted phototherapy. Available at: http://www.daavlin.com/T500x.shtml. Accessed September 19, 2004.

[43] Zelickson BD, Mehregan DA, Wendelschfer-Crabb G, et al. Clinical and histologic evaluation of psoriatic plaques treated with a flashlamp pulsed dye laser. J Am Acad Dermatol 1996;35:64–8.

[44] Alora MB, Anderson RR, Quinn TR, et al. CO_2 laser resurfacing of psoriatic plaques: a pilot study. Lasers Surg Med 1998;22:165–70.

[45] Krutmann J, Diepgen TL, Luger TA, et al. High-dose UVA1 therapy for atopic dermatitis: results of a multicenter trial. J Am Acad Dermatol 1998;38:589–93.

[46] Grabbe J, Welker P, Humke S, et al. High-dose ultraviolet A1 (UVA1), but not UVA/UVB therapy, decreases IgE-binding cells in lesional skin of patients with atopic eczema. J Invest Dermatol 1996;107:419–22.

[47] Godar DE. UVA1 radiation triggers two different final apoptotic pathways. J Invest Dermatol 1999;112:3–12.

[48] Dawe RS. Ultraviolet A1 phototherapy. Br J Dermatol 2003;148:626–37.

[49] Jeffes EW, McCullough JL, Weinstein GD, et al. Photodynamic therapy of actinic keratoses with topical aminolevulinic acid hydrochloride and fluorescent blue light. J Am Acad Dermatol 2001;45:96–104.

[50] Alexiades-Armenakas MR, Geronemus RG. Laser-mediated photodynamic therapy of actinic keratoses. Arch Dermatol 2003;139:1313–20.

[51] Touma D, Yaar M, Whitehead S, et al. A trial of short incubation, broad-area photodynamic therapy for facial actinic keratoses and diffuse photodamage. Arch Dermatol 2004;140:33–40.

[52] Bissonette R, Bergeron A, Liu Y. Large surface photodynamic therapy with aminolevulinic acid: treatment of actinic keratoses and beyond. J Drugs Dermatol 2004;3(1 Suppl):S26–31.

[53] Rhodes LE, de Rie M, Enstrom Y, et al. Photodynamic therapy using topical methyl aminolevulinate vs surgery for nodular basal cell carcinoma: results of a multicenter randomized prospective trial. Arch Dermatol 2004;140:17–23.

[54] Photocure. FDA approval. Available at: http://www.photocure.com. Accessed August 29, 2004.

[55] Lui H, Hobbs L, Tope WD, et al. Photodynamic therapy of multiple nonmelanoma skin cancers with verteporfin and red light-emitting diodes: two-year results evaluating tumor response and cosmetic outcomes. Arch Dermatol 2004;140:26–32.

[56] Hongcharu W, Taylor CR, Chang Y, et al. Topical ALA-photodynamic therapy for the treatment of acne vulgaris. J Invest Dermatol 2000;115:183–92.

[57] Goldman MP, Boyce SM. A single-center study of aminolevulinic acid and 417 NM photodynamic therapy in the treatment of moderate to severe acne vulgaris. J Drugs Dermatol 2003;2:393–6.

[58] Tzung TY, Wu KH, Huang ML. Blue light phototherapy in the treatment of acne. Photodermatol Photoimmunol Photomed 2004;20:266–9.

[59] Papageorgiou P, Katsambas A, Chu A. Phototherapy with blue (415 nm) and red (660 nm) light in the treatment of acne vulgaris. Br J Dermatol 2000;142:973–8.

ELSEVIER
SAUNDERS

Dermatol Clin 23 (2005) 209–226

DERMATOLOGIC
CLINICS

Melanin Pigmentary Disorders: Treatment Update

Jean-Paul Ortonne, MD*, Thierry Passeron, MD

Service de Dermatologie, Hôpital l'Archet 2, BP 3079, Cedex 3, 06202 Nice, France

Three clinical alterations of skin color have been described: (1) a darkening, (2) a lightening, and (3) the occurrence of an unusual skin color [1]. This article focuses on melanin pigmentary disorders. Skin darkening may be the result of several different pathophysiologic processes including increased amounts of melanin and abnormal distribution of melanin.

An increased amount of melanin in the skin is called hypermelanosis or melanoderma. According to the skin color, two types of hypermelanosis occur: brown hypermelanosis, caused by excessive amounts of melanin within the epidermis, and ceruloderma (blue hypermelanosis resulting from large amounts of melanin in the dermis). Mixed hypermelanosis, characterized by an excess of melanin in both the epidermis and the dermis, may also occur. Brown hypomelanosis may result from increased melanin production by a quantitatively normal melanocyte density in the epidermis (melanotic hypermelanosis) or by an increased number of epidermal melanocytes (melanocytic hypermelanosis). Ceruloderma can result from three different mechanisms:

1. Abnormal transfer of melanin from epidermal cells to the dermis (pigmentary incontinence). In this situation, melanin granules accumulate within melanophages or may be free in the extracellular matrix of the dermis.
2. Production of melanin by ectopic dermal melanocytes.
3. Binding of melanin to exogenous pigments deposited in the dermis.

Skin lightening or whitening (leukoderma, hypopigmentation) is most commonly the result of decreased melanin content in the skin (hypomelanosis). Epidermal hypomelanosis may be the result of at least two different pathogenic mechanisms: partial or total absence of epidermal melanocytes (melanocytopenic hypomelanosis); or melanin synthesis, melanosome biogenesis, transport, and transfer despite a normal number of epidermal melanocytes (melanopenic hypomelanosis). Increase of epidermal turnover can also induce hypomelanosis. Hypomelanosis may affect hair color. Canities means a generalized loss of hair color, whereas poliosis refers to localized hypomelanosis involving a tuft of hair or a few hairs in the eyebrows or eyelashes.

Many treatment modalities including chemical agents and physical therapies are now available to treat hypermelanosis. New therapeutic strategies are presently developed to repigment hypomelanotic or amelanotic skin. This article examines the recent advances in the treatment of melanin pigmentary disorders including both hypermelanosis and hypomelanosis.

Wood's light examination: a key step in the diagnosis of melanin pigmentary disorders

This simple technique is performed in the dark. Wood's light emits wavelengths ranging from 320 to 400 nm with a peak emission at 365 nm. Ultraviolet light (UV) from the Wood's lamp penetrates predominantly in the stratum corneum and epidermis where melanin is distributed. When melanin is abundant, such as in black skin, most of the light is absorbed by melanin and only a small amount returns to the eye. The skin appears black. When melanin is decreased

---

* Corresponding author.
E-mail address: ortonne@unice.fr (J.-P. Ortonne).

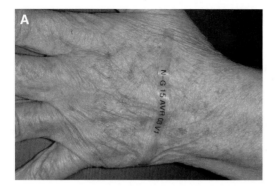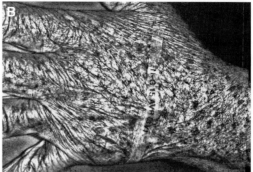

Fig. 1. (*A*) Actinic lentigo, normal light. (*B*) Actinic lentigo, UV plus polarized light.

in the epidermis, such as in light skin, more light goes back to the eye and the skin appears white. Only a small amount of UV light reaches the dermis. This dermal melanin does not affect the amount of light observed. Wood's light accentuates changes in epidermal melanin pigmentation. Furthermore, variations in dermal pigmentation are less visible under Wood's light than under visible light. The unique limitation of Wood's light is that it cannot be used reliably in skin types V and VI. Indeed, normally dark skin melanin pigmentation obscures the detection of dermal melanin.

Wood's light examination is very useful in two clinical situations. The first is to detect variations of epidermal pigmentation that are not apparent under visible light. It is sometimes difficult to detect hypomelanotic or amelanotic maculae in vitiligo patients with fair or pale skin. Indeed, the contrast between involved and noninvolved vitiligo skin in these patients is very faint. The greater the loss of epidermal melanin, the more marked the contrast on

Wood's light. This explains why vitiligo maculae that are completely devoid of melanin become obvious when examined under this technique. In contrast, lightly pigmented café-au-lait spots or ephelides becomes more visible when examined with Wood's light (Fig. 1). The second clinical situation is to determine the depth of melanin pigmentation in hypermelanotic skin (Fig. 2). In dermal melanosis, the contrast between involved and noninvolved skin is considerably decreased or even unapparent than under ambient visible light.

Treatment of hypomelanosis

Phototherapy

Phototherapy is considered one of the most effective therapies. Several strategies are used including UV light A (UVA) phototherapy; photochemotherapy (oral and topical), such as psoralen plus UVA

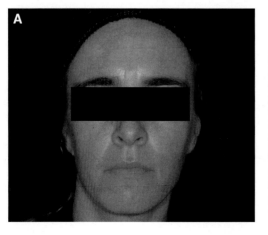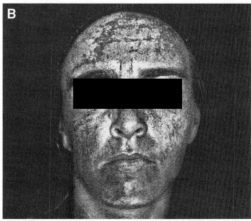

Fig. 2. (*A*) Melasma, normal light. (*B*) Melasma, UV plus polarized light.

(PUVA); PUVAsol; broadband and narrowband UV light B (UVB) phototherapy; 308-nm excimer laser; and combination phototherapy.

Ultraviolet light A phototherapy

Topical psoralen plus ultraviolet light A (paint) photochemotherapy. Most investigators agree that topical psoralen photochemotherapy should be restricted to vitiligo patients with an involvement of less than 20% of the body surface. This treatment can be used in children. Topical PUVA is difficult to perform because of the high risk of phototoxicity from the topical psoralen formulations. Advantages of topical PUVA, however, include lower cumulative UVA doses than oral PUVA and lack of ocular and systemic toxicity. Low concentrations of psoralens should be used. A 0.1% concentration of 8- methoxypsoralen (MOP) has the same effectiveness as higher concentrations (0.5% or 1%), but a lower risk of toxicity. The commercially available 1% 8-MOP lotion should be diluted 1:10 to 1:100. The patient should be exposed to UVA approximately 20 to 30 minutes after application of the topical preparation (preferentially cream or ointment to avoid *running* leading to streaks of hyperpigmentation) with a cotton-tipped applicator by a physician or a nurse to avoid a rim of hyperpigmentation around the lesions if the psoralen is applied on the surrounding normally pigmented skin. The initial dose should not exceed 0.25 J/cm^2. This treatment is performed once or twice a week, never on consecutive days, with increments of 0.12 to 0.25 J/cm^2 per week until mild erythema is achieved at the treated sites. Following treatment the area is washed, a broad-spectrum sunscreen is applied, and excessive sun exposure is avoided for at least 24 hours [2].

The mean clinical response is about 60% repigmentation, depending on the anatomic site. Because of the risk of severe blistering reactions, topical photochemotherapy should never be used with sunlight as a UVA source. A home topical PUVA protocol using very dilute 8-MOP (0.001%) has been proposed for the treatment of vitiligo. In a large cohort of patients (N = 125), only 3% had blistering reactions [3].

Oral psoralen plus UVA photochemotherapy. PUVA involves the use of psoralens followed by exposure to long-wavelength UVA irradiation. Oral PUVA is used most commonly in patients with extensive vitiligo. Other less common indications include pityriasis alba, postinflammatory hypopigmentation, and chemical leukoderma.

There are numerous psoralens occurring naturally in plant species. Of these, only a few are used therapeutically, including methoxsalen (8-MOP); 4,5′,8-trimethoxypsoralen; and recently bergapten (5-MOP), almost exclusively for vitiligo. Trioxsalen is no longer available and 5-MOP is pending approval in the United States.

By far the most commonly used oral psoralen is 8-MOP (0.4–0.6 mg/kg) and treatments are typically administered two times per week. For patients with vitiligo, the initial dose of UVA is usually 0.5 to 1 J/cm^2. This dose is gradually increased until minimal asymptomatic erythema of the involved skin occurs. 5-MOP has about the same response rate as 8-MOP in repigmenting vitiligo. The former seems to be more suitable for the treatment of vitiligo because of its lower incidence of adverse affects, in particular a reduced phototoxicity of depigmented skin and less nausea and vomiting.

The response rate of PUVA is variable, and complete repigmentation is achieved in only a few patients. Some degree of repigmentation is seen in about 60% to 80% of treated patients. A satisfactory cosmetic result is usually obtained in less than 20% of cases. According to a recent meta-analysis, the mean success rate in treating vitiligo for oral methoxsalen plus UVA was 51%. As with other forms of phototherapy and topical corticosteroids, the areas that respond most favorably are the face, the mid-extremities, and the trunk [4]. The total number of PUVA treatments required is between 50 and 300. Evidence of repigmentation is usually first seen after 1 to 4 months of treatment, but complete repigmentation usually requires 100 to 300 treatments. Repigmentation, as with narrowband UVB, usually appears in a perifollicular pattern or from the periphery of the lesions. The former represents the repopulation of the interfollicular epidermis from the follicular reservoir, and pigmented hairs are a better prognostic sign than depigmented hairs. General contraindications to oral PUVA include photosensitivity disorders, pregnancy and lactation, a history of skin cancer, arsenic exposure, cutaneous radiation therapy, cataract, and retinal disease. To date, only a few vitiligo patients with PUVA-induced cutaneous carcinomas have been reported. This may reflect a smaller cumulative UVA dose, but large follow-up studies have not yet been done in PUVA-treated vitiligo patients. Until more data are available, it seems wise to recommend a maximum cumulative PUVA dose and a maximum number of UVB treatments of 1000 J/cm^2 and 300 treatments, respectively, to vitiligo patients.

Rate of oral PUVA repigmentation varies depending on the anatomic site. Schematically, two groups

of lesions can be identified: the UV-responsive lesions that include the face and neck, the trunk, and
the proximal extremities; and the UV-resistant areas,
including the bony prominences, the distal digits,
and the lips. Children with vitiligo tend to respond
somewhat better to PUVA than adults. Darkly pigmented patients often achieve more repigmentation
with PUVA than patients with lighter skin, probably
because they tolerate higher UVA doses.

Retention of PUVA-induced repigmentation has
been observed in more than 90% of patients 14 to
15 years after discontinuation of treatment. Retention
of repigmentation seems to be more common in areas
with complete repigmentation.

Ultraviolet light B phototherapy
Broadband ultraviolet light B.   Very few studies
evaluating the potential of broadband UVB in the
treatment of vitiligo are available. One of them
reports that 75% repigmentation was achieved in
8 of 14 patients, mostly in patients with skin
phototype IV to VI [5]. This observation needs to
be confirmed by larger studies.

Psoralen plus ultraviolet light B.   A left-side comparative study suggests that PUVB is equally
effective as PUVA therapy [6] in the treatment of
vitiligo. Unfortunately, no comparative study of
PUVB versus UVB monotherapy is yet available. In
this trial, broadband UVB initial dose of 0.03 J/cm^2
was increased by 0.03 J/cm^2 every session. All the
patients were skin type III and IV.

Narrowband ultraviolet light B.   Narrowband fluorescent tubes (Philips TL01/Waldman) with an
emission spectrum of 311 nm are used for this
therapy. Narrowband UVB has been shown to be an
effective and well-tolerated therapeutic option for
vitiligo. The starting dose varies from 100 to
250 mJ/cm^2, with increments of 10% to 20% at each
subsequent exposure, and then held once a mild
erythema develops. Treatments are administered two
to three times per week, never on two consecutive
days. Several studies have demonstrated the effectiveness of narrowband UVB as monotherapy. About
60% of patients obtain greater than 75% of repigmentation. Short-term side effects include pruritus
and xerosis. Long-term side effects are unknown. The
advantages of narrowband UVB over oral PUVA
include shorter treatment times; no drug cost; and no
or fewer side effects, such as nausea or phototoxic
reactions. There is no need for posttreatment photoprotection. This treatment can be used in children,
pregnant or lactating women, and in individuals with

hepatic and kidney dysfunctions. Furthermore, there
is less contrast between depigmented and normally
pigmented skin, and possibly fewer long-term side
effects. Narrowband UVB therapy is becoming the
first choice of therapy for adults and for children
(over 6 years of age) with vitiligo [7,8].

Narrowband UVB has been used in combination
with pseudocatalase. No control study has been
performed, however, to validate the beneficial effect
of adjuncting pseudocatalase [9].

Focused microphototherapy.   In the last few years
new devices delivering UVB light have been developed for the treatment of localized vitiligo. Narrowband UVB microphototherapy uses a device that
delivers a focused beam with spectrum from 300 to
320 nm with a peak emission of 311 nm. Two studies
report excellent results [10,11], but comparative
studies versus Xecl excimer lasers (Excilite–DEKA
MELA, Florence, Italy) are still lacking. Monochromatic excimer light 308 nm can also be delivered by
lamps. A pilot study using such a device reports that
18 out of 37 vitiligo patients achieved 75% or more
repigmentation after 6 months of treatment. These
observations should be confirmed by a comparative
trial (excimer laser versus excimer lamp) in a larger
population [12].

Excimer laser.   The xenon chloride Xecl excimer
laser generates UVB radiation at a wavelength of
308 nm. Several reports have shown that this device is effective in the treatment of vitiligo. Patients
are treated twice or three times a week for 1 to
6 months depending on the series. Low fluencies
(50–200 mJ/cm^2) are used. In most studies, the
percentage of treated lesions achieving at least 75%
repigmentation is about 30% [13–17]. As for the
different phototherapies, the rate of repigmentation
varies depending on the anatomic sites. The rate of
repigmentation is very high on UVB-responsive
areas, such as the face, whereas the extremities and
bony prominences (well recognized UVB-resistant
areas) show a statistically significant inferior repigmentation rate [17]. Side effects are limited to mild
erythema and uncommon blistering. The major
advantage of the Xecl excimer laser is to confine
the treatment only to the vitiliginous lesions. The
Xecl excimer laser represents a useful tool for the
treatment of localized vitiligo. It gives the possibility
to choose only a limited number of lesions without
whole-body irradiation.

Therapy with the 308-nm excimer laser is also
safe and effective in pigment correction of hypopigmented scars and striae alba [18]. Mean final pigment

correction rates of approximately 60% to 70% by visual assessment and 100% by colorimetric analysis were observed after nine treatments administered biweekly. A maintenance treatment of several months is required to sustain the cosmetic benefit.

Other photochemotherapies

Khellin (topical or systemic) plus UVA or phenylalanine plus UVA have also been proposed for the treatment of vitiligo. There have been conflicting reports regarding these treatment strategies, and there is a concern about the hepatic toxicity of khellin. For these reasons, these modalities are not recommended for the treatment of vitiligo.

Immunomodulators

Several preliminary studies have reported the efficacy of immunomodulatory drugs, including levamisole, anapsos, isoprinosine, and suplatast, as repigmenting agents for the treatment of vitiligo. Unfortunately, none of these initial observations have been following by clinical studies demonstrating the efficacy of these compounds in the treatment of vitiligo. As a consequence, these agents have not been widely used by vitiligo patients. Recent advances in vitiligo research, however, provide information strengthening the autoimmune therapy of vitiligo. Corticosteroids and topical immunomodulators, such as tacrolimus, demonstrate some efficacy for the treatment of vitiligo.

Corticosteroids

Topical steroids are useful for the treatment of localized vitiligo. Marked or almost complete repigmentation can be obtained with potent corticosteroids (eg, betamethasone valerate, triamcinolone) and very potent corticosteroids (eg, clobetasol, fluticasone propionate). Corticosteroids of low potency, however, show no therapeutic effect at all. A recent meta-analysis concluded that medium-potency and superpotent topical steroids are effective treatment for localized vitiligo [4].

Steroid-induced repigmentation occurs within 1 to 4 months of treatment in a perifollicular pattern and from the margins of the lesions. Side effects include dermal atrophy, steroid-induced acne, rosacea, telangiectasia, ecchymoses, and striae. Furthermore, suppression of the hypothalamic-pituitary-adrenal axis may occur after prolonged applications on large areas. To minimize the incidence of these side effects, it is recommended to use topical steroids on limited skin areas; to avoid prolonged use on sensitive areas, such as the face and body folds; and to use them once or twice daily for only 6 to 8 weeks followed by a treatment-free interval of several weeks as mild steroid-induced skin atrophy is reversible. No repigmentation after 3 months of treatment should lead to discontinuation of treatment. The mechanism of steroid-induced repigmentation is unknown, although several hypothesis are proposed, such as suppression of immunity-driven melanocyte destruction and stimulation of melanocyte proliferation and migration.

Intralesional corticosteroids must be avoided. Systemic steroids (high-dose pulsed therapy, minipulsed regimen, or daily oral low-dose) have been claimed rapidly to arrest spreading vitiligo and induce repigmentation. In most of these studies, a response to systemic corticosteroid therapy has been limited to patients with rapidly progressive generalized vitiligo. Given the significant potential for serious side effects of systemic corticosteroid therapy, the role of these drugs in the treatment of vitiligo remains confidential. The authors do not recommend this therapy for vitiligo patients.

Tacrolimus

Preliminary observations suggest that tacrolimus may be an effective treatment for both localized and generalized vitiligo [19]. A 0.1% tacrolimus ointment is applied twice daily for about 3 months [20]. Unfortunately, these studies are open label involving a very small number of patients.

A more recent 2-month double-blind randomized trial compared 0.1% tacrolimus with 0.05% clobetasol propionate in children with vitiligo [21]. This study confirmed the initial observation that tacrolimus stimulates vitiligo repigmentation. Interestingly enough, the best results where observed on sun-exposed areas suggesting that UV may also be involved in tacrolimus-induced repigmentation of vitiligo. Further studies are required to establish the safety and efficacy of topical tacrolimus in the treatment of vitiligo. Recent personal observations suggest that tacrolimus monotherapy in the absence of UV has little or no repigmenting potential in vitiligo (N. Ostovari, MD, submitted for publication, 2004).

Combination phototherapies

The interest of the combination treatments was first clearly demonstrated with the association of UVA and topical steroid. A prospective, randomized, controlled, left-right comparison study has shown that combination of UVA and fluticasone propionate was much more effective than UVA or topical steroid alone [22]. Several studies support the hypothesis that topical calcipotriol combined with sun exposure or

PUVA potentiates repigmentation of vitiligo. Topical calcipotriol as monotherapy, however, had no effect on vitiligo. Furthermore, calcipotriol in combination with narrowband UVB had no enhancing effect on vitiligo repigmentation [23]. Tacrolimus ointment has recently shown some interesting results in the treatment of vitiligo [24]. Best results, however, were achieved in sun-exposed areas. Two recent studies have evaluated if the combination of 308-nm excimer laser and topical tacrolimus is synergistic. These series have compared the efficiency of 308-nm excimer combined with tacrolimus ointment with excimer laser monotherapy [25] or associated with placebo ointment [26]. In both cases, a total of 24 sessions were done and tacrolimus ointment was applied twice a day. The results were similar and show a greater efficiency with the combined treatment as compared with laser alone (Fig. 3). Tolerance was good and side-effects were limited to constant erythema, sticking, and rare bullous lesions. These encouraging results are corroborated by two other reports associating UVB light and topical tacrolimus [24,27]. The increased risk of skin cancers, however, promoted by the association of two immunosuppressive treatments, cannot be excluded. Until there is long-term follow-up, this association should be reserved to control studies.

Surgical therapy

This approach aims to reconstitute the epidermal (and perhaps follicular) compartment of the melanocyte population of the skin in patients with a total destruction of pigment cells and a lack of response to medical treatment [28,29]. This option can be used in patients with stable vitiligo unlikely to respond to medical therapies and in patients with persistent depigmentation caused by halo nevi, thermal burns, trauma, or piebaldism [30–32]. For vitiligo, the selection criteria for these autologous transplantation strategies are stable vitiligo; localized involvement; unsatisfactory response to medical therapy; absence of Koebner phenomenon; positive minigrafting test (implantation of 2- to 3-mm punch biopsies to evaluate the spread of pigmentation at the recipient site and the risk of koebnerization at the donor site) [33,34]; no tendency for scar or keloid formation; and age above 12 years.

Several methods are available including punch grafts; blister grafts; split-thickness grafts; and autologous transplantation of melanocyte suspensions, cultured melanocytes, or cultured epidermal grafts including melanocytes. Grafting of follicular melanocytes to repigment vitiligo leukotrichia has also been performed successfully [35].

Punch grafts

Punch grafting (1.2- to 3-mm punch biopsies) is the simplest technique: grafts are implanted into perforations prepared at the recipient sites by different techniques (biopsy punch, lasers). Minigrafting using small grafts (1.2 mm) is the best technique. Pigment spread leading to repigmentation can be stimulated by phototherapies. Repigmentation usually appears after 2 to 6 weeks following grafting and the maximum repigmentation is reached within 6 months. The potential side effects include spotted pigmentation, polka-dot appearance, color mismatch, a cobblestone effect, sinking pits, and scarring. Furthermore, this technique is time consuming.

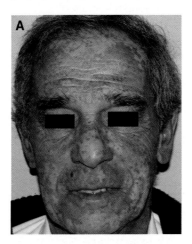 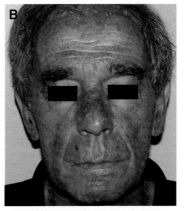

Fig. 3. Vitiligo patches on the face before (*A*) and after (*B*) 24 sessions of combination treatment with 308-nm excimer laser and topical tacrolimus.

Blister grafts

Autologous blisters can be induced by different ways, such as vacuum or liquid nitrogen. The mechanical split occurs at the dermoepidermal junction. The recipient site is prepared by dermabrasion; laser ablation (erbium:yttrium–aluminum–garnet [Er:YAG] or carbon dioxide laser); liquid nitrogen; PUVA-induced blisters; or dermatome. The graft (top of the blister) is applied and secured on the recipient site. Excellent cosmetic results ($\geq$ 95% repigmentation) are obtained in 50% to 88% of patients with segmental and localized vitiligo. The only adverse event is transient hyperpigmentation at both the donor and recipient sites. The advantages of this technique are the absence of scarring and the possibility of reusing the donor site. The repigmentation obtained by blister grafting is permanent.

Flip-top transplantation

The epidermis at the recipient site is used to form multiple hinged flaps, each covering an ultrathin 1.2-mm graft harvested from the donor site using a razor blade [36].

Split-thickness grafting

The graft is obtained by a standard or an electrical dermatome. The main advantage of this technique is to allow treatment of large areas. This approach, however, may be associated with esthetically unacceptable results at the donor site (dyspigmentation, scarring). Adverse events include milia-like cyst formation at the recipient site, partial loss of the grafts, hematoma formation, and thickening of the graft margins.

Transplantation of melanocyte suspensions

Noncultured keratinocyte-melanocyte suspensions can be obtained from a shave biopsy of the buttock or full-thickness biopsy of the scalp. Melanocytes obtained from the hair follicles and interfollicular epidermis and keratinocytes are placed into a suspension for direct application to the recipient site without expansion in culture [37].

Transplant of cultured epidermal cells

This technique initially used for the treatment of burn patients allows coverage of large areas. Applied on vitiligo lesions, it gives satisfactory results in 30% to 44% of patients. Improvement of melanocyte culture conditions and grafting devices has made possible the transplantation of autologous cultured melanocytes on large areas (up to 500 cm^2 during one session) of vitiligo-involved skin [38,39]. A 95% repigmentation is obtained in approximately 40% of the treated areas. All the techniques involving melanocytes culture and epidermal reconstruction require specialized laboratory expertise and are very expensive. For these reasons, they are not widely used [40–43].

Micropigmentation

The technique of permanent dermal micropigmentation using a nonallergenic iron oxide pigment can be used to camouflage recalcitrant areas of vitiligo. Micropigmentation may be useful to hide lesions of stable vitiligo in UV poorly responsive areas (eg, the lips, nipples, and distal fingers) [44]. Tattooing is also useful for posttraumatic amelanosis and for postcryotherapy leukoderma in which melanocytes have been destroyed. Side effects are rare, but can include bacterial infections, herpes simplex, warts, Koebner phenomenon, and keloids.

Depigmentation therapies

Patients who have widespread disease with only a few areas of normally pigmented skin on the face or other exposed areas can be treated with depigmenting agents. The patients must be chosen carefully; they must be adults who recognize that their appearance will be altered significantly and who understand that depigmentation also requires lifelong care of the skin (sunscreens, protective clothing, and so forth).

The guidelines for the using permanent depigmentation in vitiligo are as follows [45]:

1. Desire of permanent depigmentation
2. Age over 40
3. More than 50% of depigmentation of the sites to be treated
4. Willingness to accept the fact that repigmentation will no longer be possible.

A psychologic evaluation to the readiness of patients to undergo full skin bleaching is highly desirable. Previous studies have demonstrated such a procedure as valuable [46].

The most commonly used agent for further depigmenting vitiligo patients with an extensive involvement is monobenzylether of hydroquinone (MBEH) 20% applied twice daily to the affected areas for 9 to 12 months or more. MBEH is a potent irritant or allergenic compound. A patch-test to detect contact sensitivity to MBEH should be performed before starting therapy. It normally takes 1 to 3 months to initiate a response. Loss of pigment can also occur at distant sites of applications. Although depigmentation from MBEH is considered permanent, repigmentation following a sunburn or even intense sun exposure may occur. Monomethylether of hydroquinone, also named 4-hydroxyanisole or 4-methoxyphenol, in a 20% cream can be used as an alternative for MBEH. Side effects include contact dermatitis, pruritus, exogenous ochronosis, and leukomelanoderma en confetti. Depigmentation by Q-switched ruby laser therapy is reported to achieve faster depigmentation compared with depigmentation using a bleaching agent [47].

Others

Systemic antioxidant therapy

The rational for this approach rests on the hypothesis that vitiligo results from a deficiency of natural antioxidant mechanisms. Although to date not validated by a controlled clinical trial, selenium methionine, tocopherol, ascorbic acid, and ubiquinone are widely prescribed by dermatologists to arrest vitiligo spreading and to promote repigmentation.

Melagenina

Melagenina is a hydroalcoholic extract of the human placenta. An α-lipoprotein is said to be the active ingredient. Preliminary studies in Cuba claimed that 84% of vitiligo patients achieved total repigmentation. Experiments performed in other laboratories in the United States and other countries have not been able to confirm the animal and laboratory data claimed by the Cuban group. Several clinical trials have confirmed the lack of efficacy of melagenina.

Treatment of hypermelanosis

Depigmenting agents

Phenolic compounds
Hydroquinone. HQ is the most popular depigmenting agent [48]. Several studies have established the therapeutic effect of HQ in the treatment of hypermelanosis [49,50]. HQ is still the gold-standard of depigmenting agents. The effectiveness of HQ is related directly to the concentration of the preparations, the vehicle used, and the chemical composition of the final product. A 2% HQ was reported to improve hypermelanosis in 14% to 70% of the patients. HQ is most commonly used at a 4% concentration, however, by dermatologists. At this concentration HQ is very effective, but it can have a significant irritant effect. Concentrations as high as 6% to 10% are prescribed extemporaneously for

resistant cases, but may be a strong irritant effect. Because of the hazard of long-term treatments, the use of HQ in cosmetics has been banned by the European Committee (24th Dir. 2000/6/EC). Formulations are available only by prescription of physicians and dermatologists. A number of different vehicles can be used for HQ, but the most suitable for the formulation is a hydroalcoholic solution (equal parts of propylene glycol and absolute ethanol). A nitro-oxidant, such as ascorbic acid or sodium bisulphate, is regularly used to preserve the stability of the formulation.

The acute side effects of HQ include irritant and allergic contact dermatitis, nail discoloration, and postinflammatory hypermelanosis [51]. These adverse events are temporary and resolve after HQ discontinuation. Higher concentrations ($\geq 5\%$) may induce persistent hypomelanosis or amelanosis (leukoderma en confetti). Exogenous ochronosis is a very rare complication occurring in dark-skinned or black individuals after chronic use. This irreversible disorder presents in the form of reticulated, ripple like, sooty pigmentation affecting common sites of HQ applications (cheeks, forehead, periorbital areas). The lesions are typically localized on photoexposed areas (Fig. 4). Histologic examination of these lesions shows banana-shaped yellow-brown pigment granules in and around collagen bundles in conjunction with giant cells and melanophage-containing granulomas in the upper dermis.

The pathogenesis of HQ-induced ochronosis is unknown and no effective treatment is available. The mode of action of HQ is not fully understood. HQ seems to exert its effect mainly in melanocyte with active tyrosinase activity. Guidelines and radical oxy-

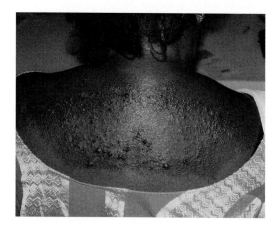

Fig. 4. Exogenous ochronosis induced by the prolonged used of hydroquinone. Note the photodistribution of the lesions.

gen species arising from the oxidation of HQ induce an oxidative damage of membrane lipids and proteins including tyrosinase, and depletion of glutathione contributes to the lightening action [52]. Other depigmenting pathways attributed to HQ include inhibition of tyrosinase through the covalent binding to histidine or interactions with copper at the active site of tyrosinase, inhibition of DNA and RNA synthesis, and alteration of melanosome formation and melanization extent.

Monobenzylether of hydroquinone. The clinical use of MBEH is restricted for generalized depigmentation in patients with extensive vitiligo. MBEH should never be used for the treatment of melasma or postinflammatory hypermelanosis. Indeed, MBEH can cause permanent depigmentation of the skin even at sites distant from those of application. MBEH-induced vitiligo depigmentation has been described in dark-skinned individuals. MBEH is metabolized to reactive free radicals inside the cells resulting in melanocyte destruction.

Monomethyl of hydroquinone. Monomethylether of hydroquinone is also called 4-hydroxyanisole (para-hydroxy-methoxy-benzene). This compound is oxidized by tyrosinase and exhibits strong melanocytotoxicity. Monomethylether of hydroquinone is used in France at 8% or 10% concentration for the treatment of various acquired hypermelanoses including melasma and postinflammatory hypermelanoses. Side effects include irritant and allergic contact dermatitis, postinflammatory hypermelanosis, and leukoderma en confetti at treated sites. Hypomelanosis at sites distant from the application areas has been reported.

Others

4-N-butylresorcinol. A lotion containing 0.3% 4-N-butylresorcinol has been demonstrated to improve melasma [53]. This product also decreases postinflammatory hyperpigmentation following laser therapy [54]. 4-N-butylresorcinol has an inhibitory effect on tyrosinase and tyrosinase-related protein.

4-Isopropylcatechol. 4-Isopropylcatechol (4-IPC) has been evaluated for the treatment of melasma. In a group of 54 melasma patients, two thirds of the patients showed significant improvement. Though 4-IPC is a potent depigmenting agent, it is no longer used because of its irritant potential [55].

Phenolic-thioether. N-acetyl-4-S-cystalminylphenol has been evaluated in a small number of patients

with melasma [56]. Marked improvement or complete clearing with minimal side effects were obtained in 75% of patients. These compounds are not widely used and large clinical trials to evaluate their safety and efficacy are not available.

Azelaic acid. Azelaic acid (AA) is a naturally occurring 9-carbon-dicarboxylic acid isolated from cultures of *Pityrosporum ovale*. AA is thought to play a key role in the pathogenesis of hypomelanotic tinea versicolor. AA has been used at concentrations of 15% to 20% for the treatment of melasma and postinflammatory hypermelanosis. The best results demonstrated that AA is more effective than 2% HQ and equivalent in efficacy with 4% HQ for the treatment of melasma in dark-skinned women [57]. Similar good results have never been obtained in European patients. AA is well tolerated. Adverse effects, such as pruritus, transient erythema, scaling, and irritation, are usually mild and disappear within a few weeks. Phototoxic and allergic reactions are rare.

AA may halt the progression of lentigo maligna and even induce its disappearance, suggesting that AA exerts an antiproliferative and cytotoxic effect mainly on hyperactive and abnormal melanocytes.

Kojic acid. Kojic acid is a fungal metabolic product used at 1% to 4% concentrations. In monotherapy, kojic acid shows a modest effectiveness. It is mainly used in combinations. It is a potent tyrosinase inhibitor and functions by chelating copper at the active site of the enzyme. Long-term side effects of kojic acid are not known. A high frequency of contact sensitivity has been reported [58]. The use of kojic acid in cosmetics has been banned in Japan.

Ascorbic acid. A stable ester of ascorbic acid (magnesium L-ascorbyl-2 phosphate) in a 10% cream base produced a significant lightening effect in patients with melasma after 3 months of twice daily application [59]. Ascorbic acid interferes with the different steps of melanogenesis by interacting with copper ions at the tyrosinase active site and reducing dopaquinone and by blocking dihydrochinindol-2-carboxyl acid oxidation. A randomized, double-blind, placebo-controlled trial of vitamin C iontophoresis in melasma has demonstrated that this strategy may be an effective treatment for melasma [60]. A double-blind, left-right randomized comparative study in melasma patients showed that 93% of good and excellent subjective results were observed on the 4% HQ side compared with 62.5% on the 5% ascorbic acid side. Colorimetric measures, however, showed no statistical differences. Side effects were more common with HQ (68.7%) than with ascorbic acid (6.2%) [61].

Retinoid monotherapy. Tretinoin (all-trans-retinoic acid) has been used in concentrations from 0.025% to 0.1% to treat a variety of pigmentary disorders, such as pigmented spots of photoaged skin, melasma, and postinflammatory hyperpigmentation in dark-skinned individuals [62–65]. Erythema and peeling in the area of application are adverse events of tretinoin 0.05% to 0.1%. Postinflammatory hyperpigmentation may also occur. Topical tretinoin seems to exert its action by enhancing keratinocyte proliferation and increasing epidermal cell turnover. Tretinoin, however, acting on retinoid-activating transcription factors interferes with melanogenesis. Tretinoin does not inhibit melanogenesis in skin equivalent or monolayer cultures of melanocytes, whereas it enhances the pigmentation of low-melanized melanoma cells and decreased that of highly pigmented normal melanocytes after UV irradiation [66].

Tazarotene, an acetylenic topical retinoid, improves the irregular hyperpigmentation associated with photoaging and lightening of the pigmented spots. Tazarotene 0.1% gel is associated with reduced mottling on the dorsal aspects of forearms. The Fontana stain showed a moderate to marked depigmenting effect with decreased pigmentation on the tazarotene-treated side. Melanin granules were sparser and less heavily pigmented, probably explaining the bleaching of hyperpigmented spots [67].

Adapalene gel 0.1% and 0.3%, a synthetic retinoid, improves solar lentigines and other features of photodamaged skin and is well tolerated [68].

Licorice extracts. Liquiritin, a flavonoid glycoside of licorice, has been found to induce a significant improvement of hypermelanosis in patients with bilateral epidermal melasma [69]. The mechanism proposed involved melanin dispersion and increased epidermal turnover. Glabridin, the main component of hydrophobic fraction of licorice extracts, decreases tyrosinase activity in melanoma cells. Furthermore, this compound inhibits UVB-induced skin pigmentation [70]. Although no clinical trials have evaluated its efficacy as a depigmenting agent, glabridin may be found in some cosmetics.

Thioctic acid (α-lipoic acid). This compound is a disulfide derivative of octanoic acid. It acts as ros scavenger and redox regulator but also inhibits tyrosinase activity probably by chelating the cooper ions and prevents UV-induced photoactive damage [71]. This product is commercially available.

Unsaturated fatty acids. Oleic acid (C18:1), linoleic acid (C18:2), and α-linolenic acid (C18:3) suppress pigmentation in vitro. Some of these compounds have in vivo a lightening effect in UVB-induced pigmentation without toxic effects on melanocytes [72]. Fatty acids have been shown recently to regulate pigmentation by proteosomal degradation [73]. Linoleic acid accelerates the degradation of tyrosinase, inhibiting melanogenesis. In contrast palmitic acid, a saturated fatty acid, retards the proteolysis of and accelerates melanogenesis.

Combination therapies. Widely used for the treatment of hypermelanosis, the purpose of these strategies is to augment the efficacy by associating active ingredients with different modes of action to obtain a synergic effect, to shorten the duration of therapy, and to reduce the risk of adverse effects. The most popular combination treatment for depigmenting skin is Kligman formula. This polytherapy includes 5% HQ, 0.1% tretinoin, and 0.1% dexamethasone in a hydrophilic ointment. Tretinoin functions as an enhancer of HQ penetration in the epidermis. Furthermore, tretinoin increases epidermal turnover, facilitating melanin dispersion within keratinocytes and also melanin removal from corneocyte shedding. Dexamethasone decreases the irritation and inflammation caused by HQ or tretinoin and the melanin synthesis by inhibiting metabolic activity. This formula demonstrated an efficacy in the treatment of melasma, ephelides, and postinflammatory hypermelanosis. Depigmentation occurs rapidly, beginning within 3 weeks after twice-daily application. Unfortunately, the efficacy of this formula depends on its stability. Extemporaneous formulation is useful, but bears a strong risk of instability. Recently, a stabilized formulation containing 4% HQ, 0.05% tretinoin, and 0.01% fluocinolone acetonide has been launched (Triluma). Two multicenter, randomized, double-blind, controlled trials demonstrated the safety and efficacy of this combination treatment in patients with moderate to severe melasma [74]. After 8 weeks of treatment, a 75% reduction of melasma was found in more than 70% of the patients. Furthermore, a superiority of the formulation over its three components (HQ, tretinoin, and fluocinolone acetonide) was demonstrated. There are already many variants of the extemporaneous Kligman formula. The suggestion that topical steroids are not necessary for achieving depigmentation led to a modification of this formula by removing topical steroids. Clinical trials demonstrated that 2% HQ combined with 0.05% to 1% tretinoin cream and lotions is also effective.

A solution containing monomethyl ether of 2% HQ and tretinoin 0.01% has been launched in North America for the treatment of actinic lentigo. This combination treatment has been shown to improve the appearance of these lesions in several controlled and noncontrolled studies [75,76].

A combination regimen of 20% AA with topical tretinoin 0.05% produces an earlier and more pronounced lightening pigmentation during the early phase of the treatment. An equivalent efficacy, however, of the combination 20% AA-topical tretinoin 0.05% versus AA monotherapy was obtained after 6 months of treatment [77]. The 20% AA has also been associated with 15% to 20% glycolic acid lotion. This combination regimen was as effective as 4% HQ cream for the treatment of facial hyperpigmentation in dark-skinned individuals [78].

Kojic acid has also been included in combination regimens. The 2% kojic acid in a gel containing 10% glycolic acid and 2% HQ improves epidermal melasma after 12 weeks of treatment. The 1-4 kojic acid combined with tretinoin, HQ, corticosteroid, or glycolic acid seems to act synergically [79].

The Westerhof formula, a combination of 4.7% N-acetylcysteine, 2% HQ, and 0.1% triamcinolone acetonide, has been shown to be effective in the treatment of melasma [80]. The mechanism of action of N-acetylcysteine is not fully characterized. N-acetylcysteine exerts an inhibitory effect on tyrosinase. It is likely the N-acetylcysteine stimulates pheomelanogenesis rather than eumelanogenesis, however, clinically producing lighter color.

Cosmetic use of bleaching products. The cosmetic use of bleaching products is a common practice in dark-skinned women from sub-Saharan Africa and a few other parts of the world. The products used include HQ; potent or superpotent topical glucocorticoids; mercury; salts; and caustic agents, such as liquid soaps, hydrogen peroxide, and salicylic preparations. Most users (> 90%) apply the products once or twice daily to the whole body, during months or years. Side effects, often very severe, include skin atrophy; delayed cicatrisation; infectious dermatoses (bacteria, mycoses, parasites); acne (Fig. 5); dyschromia with a typical pattern (Fig. 6); irritant and allergic contact dermatitis; prominent striae (Fig. 7); ochronosis (see Fig. 4); poikiloderma of the neck; and periauricular hyperchromia. Nephrotic syndrome can be observed after the use of mercurial derivatives. Finally, the daily use of potent topical steroids during years can lead to Cushing's syndrome (Fig. 8). This practice is a real health problem, not only in Africa,

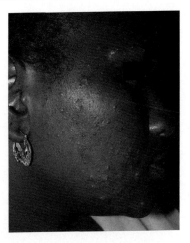

Fig. 5. Acne induced by the used of topical steroids.

but also in Northern countries receiving large immigrant communities. A careful dermatologic examination of patients is helpful to detect the skin symptoms resulting from this practice [81].

Chemical peels

Chemabrasion and peels using various chemicals is another treatment modality for removal of freckles, actinic lentigines, and other pigmented spots; melasma; and postinflammatory hypermelanosis. Deep peels are avoided in patients with hypermelanosis because of the high risk of postinflammatory hypermelanosis or hypomelanosis, scarring, and keloid formation. Superficial and medium-depth chemical peels have been used for the treatment of hypermelanosis, mainly in fair-skinned individuals.

Glycolic acid is an α-hydroxy acid that has an epidermal discohesive effect at low concentrations. Removal of corneocytes and epidermal upper layer keratinocytes by chemical peeling reduces the epidermal melanin content and improves hypermelanoses. Glycolic acid pills (50%–70%) are becoming increasingly popular in the treatment of melasma. They can be used safely in dark-skinned patients because of a low risk of hyperpigmentation [82].

A few studies have demonstrated the efficacy of chemical peels with other depigmenting agents in patients with hypermelanosis. Complete bleaching of diffuse melasma was observed in patients (30%) treated with glycolic acid 50% plus kojic acid 10%, and partial blanching in 60% of patients [79]. Serial glycolic acid peels (30%–40%) combined with a modified Kligman formula (2% HQ plus 0.05% tretinoin plus 1% hydrocortisone) provided an additional effect to the standard topical treatment in dark-

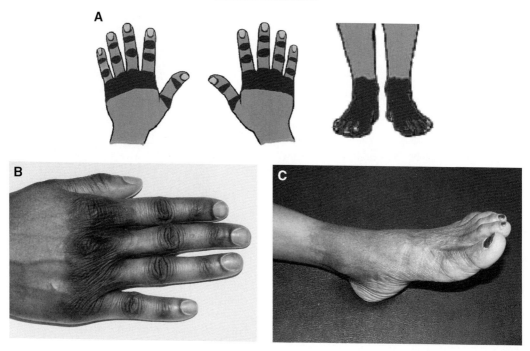

Fig. 6. (*A*) The feet and the joint hands are very difficult area to depigment. It results in a characteristic pattern of pigmentation that must make suspect the use of blanching creams. (*B*) Persistence of physiologic pigmentation on the joint hands and depigmentation of the rest of the skin leading to a characteristic pattern. (*C*) Pseudohyperpigmentation in *socks* caused by the depigmentation of the leg above.

skinned patients with melasma [83]. Another study suggested that daily application of 10% glycolic acid lotion and 2% HQ combined with 70% glycolic acid peels every 3 weeks showed some improvement of pigmented spots of photoaging in Asian women [84]. In contrast a split-face prospective study in 21 Hispanic women with melasma showed no differences in the bleaching effect of 4% HQ plus glycolic peels 20% to 30% versus HQ 4% alone.

Five peelings with salicylic acid 20% to 30% at 2-week intervals in dark-skinned patients (phototypes V to VI), after initial treatment with HQ 5% for 2 weeks, gave good results for melasma and other types of pigmentation [85]. The use of trichloroacetic

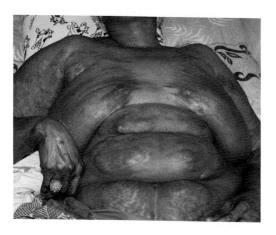

Fig. 7. Large stretch marks, skin atrophy, and erosions caused by a prolonged use of topical steroids.

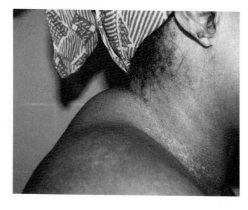

Fig. 8. Cushing syndrome with *buffalo neck* induced by the used of potent topical steroids on the entire body surface twice a day for more than 10 years.

20% to 35% followed by HQ hydroalcoholic 4% solution or tretinoin 0.05% plus hydrocortisone acetate 1% cream has produced excellent results for hypermelanosis in white patients with higher complexions [82].

Resorcinol is used as Jessner's solution (14 g resorcinol, 14 g salicylic acid, 14 g lactic acid 85%, and enough ethanol to make up 10 mL) or in Unna's paste (up to 10% resorcinol plus zinc oxide and ceisatile) and has been demonstrated to be effective in hypermelanosis with an acceptable rate of adverse effects. Peels that combine kojic acid, salicylic acid, α-hydroxy preparations with or without HQ, or resorcinol are commercially available [82]. Applied every 3 weeks they do not require neutralization.

Dermabrasion

Dermabrasion using rotary diamond fraises has been used for the treatment of melasma. Patients were followed for about 5 years [86]. According to the authors, most patients (97%) obtained a persistent clearance of melasma and only 12 out of 410 had a partial recurrence. Only two patients developed hypertrophic scars and one patient had permanent hypomelanosis.

Dermabrasion-induced postinflammatory hyperpigmentation, common in Asian and dark-skinned individuals, limits considerably the use of this strategy in these groups of patients. Even the more superficial microdermabrasion using a device emitting aluminum oxide crystals bears an important risk of postinflammatory dyspigmentation [87].

Liquid nitrogen cryotherapy

Melanocytes are particularly susceptible to freezing, and hence they should be avoided in dark-skinned people because of the risk of permanent depigmentation. The freezing agent must be applied gently to avoid blistering and skin necrosis. Cryotherapy with liquid nitrogen is commonly used successfully to treat individual pigmented lesions. Although satisfactory results are common, cryotherapy for benign epidermal lesion is problematic because of hypopigmentation, hyperpigmentation atrophy, scarring, or frequent recurrence. A randomized, controlled, prospective trial comparing liquid nitrogen cryotherapy with argon laser light delivered by a Dermascan shuttered delivery system and low-fluence carbon dioxide laser irradiation concluded that liquid nitrogen therapy was superior to the two lasers in the treatment of solar lentigines. More recently, a randomized, controlled, comparative study

with blinded observers has shown that the frequency-doubled Q-switched neodymium (Nd):YAG laser, the HGM K1 krypton laser, and the DioLite 532-nm diode-pumped vanadate laser were all superior to liquid nitrogen in the treatment of solar lentigines. Of the laser systems tested in this study, the frequency-doubled Q-switched Nd:YAG laser was the most effective [88].

Liquid nitrogen cryotherapy has also been used for the treatment of nevus of Ota, delayed nevus spilus, and blue nevus. The cryotreatment was performed using a liquid nitrogen cryogenic instrument with a removable disk-shaped copper tip called Cryo-mini. Liquid nitrogen has been proposed for the treatment of hypermelanoses (actinic lentigo and other pigmented spots of photodamaged skin, Ota's nevus) and hypomelanosis (idiopathic guttate hypomelanosis).

Laser surgery

Several types of lasers have been used to treat pigmented lesions. The four main short-pulsed pigment-selective lasers in clinical use nowadays are (1) the pigmented lesion dye laser (510 nm, 300 ns); (2) the Q-switched ruby laser (694 nm, 24–40 ns); (3) the Q-switched alexandrite laser (755 nm, 50–100 ns); and (4) the Q-switched Nd:YAG laser (1064 nm, 5–10 ns), which can be frequency-doubled to emit a green light at 532 nm of the same pulse duration. Intense pulsed light has also been demonstrated to improved solar lentigines [89]. These lasers have been used to treat epidermal hypermelanosis, such as ephelides, actinic lentigo, and café au lait spots [90,91]. For most dermatologists, laser therapy is of little use for treating melasma. Epidermal melasma responds well to laser therapy, but rapid recurrence occurs with both epidermal repigmentation and strong postinflammatory hyperpigmentation with an increased number of dermal melanophages [92]. This recurrence most likely results from the hyperactivation of melanocytes and for the laser-induced mediated inflammatory response that leads to additional postinflammatory hypermelanosis. Dermal and mixed-type melasma are resistant to laser therapy. To improve efficacy combination laser treatments are now promoted.

The combination of pulsed carbon dioxide laser to destroy melanocytes followed by Q-switched alexandrite laser to eliminate dermal melanin has been proposed for the treatment of dermal-type melasma [93]. Complete resolution of melasma was observed in all patients. The combination Er:YAG laser and glycolic acid peels has also been evaluated for the treatment of melasma [94]. Er:YAG laser resurfacing gives good improvement of hypermelanosis immediately after the treatment. The postinflammatory hypermelanosis that occurred 3 to 6 weeks after the laser treatment can be resolved with glycolic acid peels every 2 weeks. These observations suggest that combination laser therapy can be successful in clearing melasma. This has to be confirmed by controlled clinical trials.

Photoprotection

Photoprotection may be useful for patients with hypomelanotic disorders, such as vitiligo, to prevent sunburn of susceptible vitiligo skin or induction of Koebner phenomenon. Furthermore, sun exposure stimulates tanning of uninvolved skin and increases the contrast with lesional skin. Sun exposure can promote repigmentation of vitiligo, pityriasis alba, and postinflammatory hypomelanosis.

Sun avoidance is strongly recommended to prevent pigmented spots of photodamaged skin. Furthermore, sun exposure plays a key role in the pathogenesis of melasma. Sun block preparations containing zinc oxide or titanium dioxide are claimed to be more effective than other sunscreen preparations. The new broad-spectrum sunscreens providing both UVA and UVB protection are very efficient, however, provided they are reapplied every 2 or 3 hours. Use of sun-protective clothing, such as wide-brimmed hats, should also be recommended.

Camouflaging

The goal of camouflage is to normalize the appearance of a patient suffering from a disfigurement. This is usually done on lesions in the exposed areas, such as the face and the dorsal regions of the hands. Most pigmentary disorders are good candidates for this approach when they are resistant to the available medical and surgical treatments. Indeed, in these disorders only the skin color is altered, whereas the skin structure is usually normal. A recent study demonstrates that cosmetic camouflage advice improves quality of life in these patients [95]. Unlike traditional cosmetics, cover creams are used because of their unique properties. They are waterproof and opaque and offer wide varieties of cosmetic shades. Corrective cosmetics, such as Dermablend, Covermark, and Continuous Coverage, are available in various shades, allowing a perfect match to normal skin color in most patients. Synthetic melanin has

been incorporated into cover-ups that may be useful in patients with vitiligo [96].

The use of dihydroxyacetone 1,3-dihydroxydimethylcetone (DHA) to camouflage the depigmented lesions of patients with vitiligo vulgaris, segmental vitiligo, and piebaldism has been proposed recently [97]. DHA preparations color the stratum corneum brown because of its oxidative properties and provide temporary pigmentation resembling a UV-induced tan. In general, DHA pigmentation is not considered to be photoprotective. Recent investigations suggest that manipulation of the extent of hydration, pH, and availability of certain amino acids in the stratum corneum might produce DHA-induced pigmentation with greater photoprotection. For the camouflage of vitiligo lesions, DHA was stabilized at optimal levels. The 5% DHA was prepared with 10% ethanol and 1% sodium citrate buffer with 0.1% ethylenediaminetetraacetic acid at pH 4.5 at 4°C. After application with a sponge swab, the result appeared after a reaction time of approximately 6 hours. The pigmentation cannot be rubbed off on clothes or be removed by washing and remains for about 3 to 4 days. The color fades slowly with desquamation of skin. The main disadvantage is that it does not give a uniform color to the skin.

Betacarotene and canthaxanthin (phenoro-β-carotene, 10 mg, and canthaxanthin, 15 mg per capsule) oral preparations have been used to treat cosmetic defects in vitiligo. By darkening vitiliginous skin, they reduce the contrast between involved and normally pigmented skin. Good cosmetic results are seen in vitiligo patients with skin types I and II. In one study, 10% to 35% of patients gave very satisfactory responses, with the rest unsatisfactory. There is increased resistance to sun exposure in vitiligo. Because canthaxanthin is reported to produce retinopathy, proper ophthalmic consultations are mandatory.

Eye shadows, mascaras, and liners accentuate patients' eyes and draw attention to them to further distract from facial cosmetic defects, such as those seen in vitiligo around the eyes and in the nevus of Ota. Lipsticks can be used to cover vitiligo of lips.

Psychologic support

Vitiligo may cause a considerable level of distress because of its disfiguring nature and the quality of life of most patients is very severe. Vitiligo patients often experience indifference from doctors toward their skin problem and do not feel adequately supported by them. About 50% of vitiligo patients feel that they are not adequately informed about their disease and its treatment [98]. Only 36% of physicians encourage their patients to treat the disease, being pessimistic concerning expected treatment results [97].

Future strategies

A wide range of melanin pigmentary disorders are cosmetically important. They include both genetic and acquired hypomelanoses and hypermelanoses. Pigmentary abnormalities may have a strong impact on the quality of life of affected individuals, particularly when the lesions occur on exposed and visible skin areas. Many of these patients seek help from dermatologists. Among hypermelanosis, melasma, actinic lentigo, and postinflammatory hyperpigmentation are the top three reasons for dermatologic consultations. For hypomelanosis, vitiligo, pityriasis alba, postinflammatory hypomelanosis, and depigmented scars are the top four reasons.

An impressive number of molecules with well-established depigmenting properties that demonstrate in vitro systems (inhibition of mushroom tyrosinase, melanocytes and melanoma cells culture, skin equivalents) or sometimes in vivo (laboratory animals) have been identified. Unfortunately, many of them are toxic or do not penetrate in the skin because of their molecular size. After very promising preclinical studies, they end their therapeutic life after disappointing clinical trials. Readers should note an excellent review entitled "Chemical and instrumental approaches to treat hyperpigmentation," in which one finds information about potential molecules for skin depigmentation. These candidate molecules can even be classified based on their mode of action [52].

The main problem for achieving efficient depigmentation is to reach the appropriate targets. During the last two decades, pigment research has provided an incredible number of genes and related proteins involved in the regulation of skin pigmentation acting either within melanocytes or in other cells in the close vicinity of melanocytes. Present knowledge tells that the real machinery that controls melanin production is on the melanocyte surface or even inside the melanocyte in the cytoplasm, more precisely in a small organelle, the melanosome. There is a long way to penetrate into the melanosome starting from the skin surface after crossing obstacles, such as the stratum corneum, the different epidermal layers, the melanocyte cell membrane, and then the melanosome membrane. Failure of the many molecules characterized in vitro as good inhibitors of melanogenesis results from the poor bioavailability in the size where they should be to decrease melanin production.

A gene gun technique has been used to transfect and decolor pigmented rat skin with human agouti signaling protein cDNA [99]. This demonstration suggests that local cutaneous transfer of human cDNA plasmids using gene gun technology can effectively alter rat skin color without pleiotropic effect. The future will tell if such an approach can be applied to abnormal human skin color.

Summary

Through their aesthetical impact, pigmentary disorders are a frequent therapeutic demand in dermatology. Although therapeutic options are numerous, satisfactory cosmetic results are often difficult to obtain. The development of laser technologies has allowed improved treatment of some hyperpigmented lesions, such as solar lentigines. Other hypermelanosis, such as melasma, remains very difficult to treat. A paradox persists with the increased number of depigmenting agents effective in vitro that cannot produce really satisfactory clinical results. In addition, the treatment of hypopigmented disorders remains also very difficult. New therapeutic options, however, such as topical immunosuppressive drugs or new UV devices, have recently provided encouraging results, especially in vitiligo. In the near future, a better understanding of molecular processes involved in cutaneous pigmentation, the development of melanocyte cultures and transplantation techniques, and probably a genetic approach will bring new efficient therapies for pigmentary disorders.

References

[1] Ortonne JP, Nordlund JJ. The pigmentary system: physiology and physiopathology. New York: Oxford University Press; 1998.

[2] Schaffer JV, Bolognia JL. The treatment of hypopigmentation in children. Clin Dermatol 2003;21: 296–310.

[3] Grimes PE. Psoralen photochemotherapy for vitiligo. Clin Dermatol 1997;15:921–6.

[4] Njoo MD, Spuls PI, Bos JD, et al. Nonsurgical repigmentation therapies in vitiligo: meta-analysis of the literature. Arch Dermatol 1998;134:1532–40.

[5] Koster W, Wiskemann A. Phototherapy with UV-B in vitiligo. Z Hautkr 1990;65:1022–9.

[6] Mofty ME, Zaher H, Esmat S, et al. PUVA and PUVB in vitiligo: are they equally effective? Photodermatol Photoimmunol Photomed 2001;17:159–63.

[7] Ortonne JP. Vitiligo and other disorders of hypopig-

mentation. In: Bolognia JL, et al, editors. Dermatology, vol. I, chapter 66. New York: Mosby; 2003. p. 947–73.

[8] Nordlund JJ, Ortonne JP. Vitiligo vulgaris. In: Nordlund JJ, et al, editors. The pigmentary system. chapter 37. New York: Oxford University Press; 1998. p. 513–50.

[9] Schallreuter KU, Wood JM, Lemke KR, et al. Treatment of vitiligo with a topical application of pseudocatalase and calcium in combination with short-term UVB exposure: a case study on 33 patients. Dermatology 1995;190:223–9.

[10] Lotti T, Menchini G, Andreassi L. UV-B radiation microphototherapy: an elective treatment for segmental vitiligo. J Eur Acad Dermatol Venereol 1999;13: 102–8.

[11] Menchini G, Tsoureli-Nikita E, Hercogova J. Narrow-band UV-B micro-phototherapy: a new treatment for vitiligo. J Eur Acad Dermatol Venereol 2003;17: 171–7.

[12] Leone G, Iacovelli P, Paro Vidolin A, et al. Monochromatic excimer light 308 nm in the treatment of vitiligo: a pilot study. J Eur Acad Dermatol Venereol 2003;17:531–7.

[13] Spencer JM, Nossa R, Ajmeri J. Treatment of vitiligo with the 308-nm excimer laser: a pilot study. J Am Acad Dermatol 2002;46:727–31.

[14] Baltas E, Csoma Z, Ignacz F, et al. Treatment of vitiligo with the 308-nm xenon chloride excimer laser. Arch Dermatol 2002;138:1619–20.

[15] Taneja A, Trehan M, Taylor CR. 308-nm excimer laser for the treatment of localized vitiligo. Int J Dermatol 2003;42:658–62.

[16] Esposito M, Soda R, Costanzo A, et al. Treatment of vitiligo with the 308 nm excimer laser. Clin Exp Dermatol 2004;29:133–7.

[17] Ostovari N, Passeron T, Zakaria W, et al. Treatment of vitiligo by 308-nm excimer laser: an evaluation of variables affecting treatment response. Lasers Surg Med 2004;35:152–6.

[18] Alexiades-Armenakas MR, Bernstein LJ, Friedman PM, et al. The safety and efficacy of the 308-nm excimer laser for pigment correction of hypopigmented scars and striae alba. Arch Dermatol 2004;140:955–60.

[19] Smith DA, Tofte SJ, Hanifin JM. Repigmentation of vitiligo with topical tacrolimus. Dermatology 2002;205: 301–3.

[20] Grimes PE, Soriano T, Dytoc MT. Topical tacrolimus for repigmentation of vitiligo. J Am Acad Dermatol 2002;47:789–91.

[21] Lepe V, Moncada B, Castanedo-Cazares JP, et al. A double-blind randomized trial of 0.1% tacrolimus vs 0.05% clobetasol for the treatment of childhood vitiligo. Arch Dermatol 2003;139:581–5.

[22] Westerhof W, Nieuweboer-Krobotova L, Mulder PG, et al. Left-right comparison study of the combination of fluticasone propionate and UV-A vs. either fluticasone propionate or UV-A alone for the long-term treatment of vitiligo. Arch Dermatol 1999;135:1061–6.

[23] Hartmann A, Henning Hamm CL, Bröcker EB, et al. Narrow-band UVB 311 nm vs. broad-band UVB

therapy in combination with topical calcipotriol vs. placebo in vitiligo. Int J Dermatol 2004 [Online publication]. Available at: http://blackwell-synergy.com.

[24] Castanedo-Cazares JP, Lepe V, Moncada B. Repigmentation of chronic vitiligo lesions by following tacrolimus plus ultraviolet-B-narrow-band. Photodermatol Photoimmunol Photomed 2003;19:35–6.

[25] Passeron T, Ostovari N, Zakaria W, et al. Topical tacrolimus and 308 nm excimer laser: a synergistic combination for the treatment of vitiligo. Arch Dermatol 2004;140:1291–3.

[26] Kawelek AZ, Spencer JM, Phelps RG. Combined excimer laser and topical tacrolimus for the treatment of vitiligo: a pilot study. Dermatol Surg 2004;30: 130–5.

[27] Tanghetti EA, Gillis PR. Clinical evaluation of B clear and protopic treatment for vitiligo. Lasers Surg Med 2003;32:37.

[28] Hartmann A, Brocker EB, Becker JC. Hypopigmentary skin disorders: current treatment options and future directions. Drugs 2004;64:89–107.

[29] Njoo MD, Westerhof W, Bos JD, et al. A systematic review of autologous transplantation methods in vitiligo. Arch Dermatol 1998;134:1543–9.

[30] Yaar M, Gilchrest BA. Vitiligo: the evolution of cultured epidermal autografts and other surgical treatment modalities. Arch Dermatol 2001;137:348–9.

[31] Falabella R. Surgical therapies for vitiligo. Clin Dermatol 1997;15:927–39.

[32] Guerra L, Capurro S, Melchi F, et al. Treatment of stable vitiligo by timed surgery and transplantation of cultured epidermal autografts. Arch Dermatol 2000; 136:1380–9.

[33] Westerhof W, Boersma B. The minigrafting test for vitiligo: detection of stable lesions for melanocyte transplantation. J Am Acad Dermatol 1995;33: 1061–2.

[34] Falabella R, Arrunategui A, Barona MI, et al. The minigrafting test for vitiligo: detection of stable lesions for melanocyte transplantation. J Am Acad Dermatol 1995;32:228–32.

[35] Na GY, Seo SK, Choi SK. Single hair grafting for the treatment of vitiligo. J Am Acad Dermatol 1998;38: 580–4.

[36] McGovern TW, Bolognia J, Leffell DJ. Flip-top pigment transplantation: a novel transplantation procedure for the treatment of depigmentation. Arch Dermatol 1999;135:1305–7.

[37] Gauthier Y, Surleve-Bazeille JE. Autologous grafting with noncultured melanocytes: a simplified method for treatment of depigmented lesions. J Am Acad Dermatol 1992;26:191–4.

[38] Olsson MJ, Juhlin L. Melanocyte transplantation in vitiligo. Lancet 1992;340:981.

[39] Olsson MJ, Juhlin L. Clinical findings and therapeutic methods in vitiligo: patient's own melanocytes produce new pigmentation. Lakartidningen 1995;92: 1341–4.

[40] Falabella R, Escobar C, Borrero I. Treatment of

refractory and stable vitiligo by transplantation of in vitro cultured epidermal autografts bearing melanocytes. J Am Acad Dermatol 1992;26:230–6.

[41] Kaufmann R, Greiner D, Kippenberger S, et al. Grafting of in vitro cultured melanocytes onto laser-ablated lesions in vitiligo. Acta Derm Venereol 1998; 78:136–8.

[42] Zachariae H, Zachariae C, Deleuran B, et al. Auto-transplantation in vitiligo: treatment with epidermal grafts and cultured melanocytes. Acta Derm Venereol 1993;73:46–8.

[43] Olsson MJ, Moellmann G, Lerner AB, et al. Vitiligo: repigmentation with cultured melanocytes after cryo-storage. Acta Derm Venereol 1994;74:226–8.

[44] Halder RM, Pham HN, Breadon JY, et al. Micro-pigmentation for the treatment of vitiligo. J Dermatol Surg Oncol 1989;15:1092–8.

[45] Mosher DB, Parrish JA, Fitzpatrick TB. Monobenzyl-ether of hydroquinone: a retrospective study of treatment of 18 vitiligo patients and a review of the literature. Br J Dermatol 1977;97:669–79.

[46] Silvan M. The psychological aspects of vitiligo. Cutis 2004;73:163–7.

[47] Njoo MD, Vodegel RM, Westerhof W. Depigmentation therapy in vitiligo universalis with topical 4-methoxy-phenol and the Q-switched ruby laser. J Am Acad Dermatol 2000;42:760–9.

[48] Stratigos AJ, Katsambas AD. Optimal management of recalcitrant disorders of hyperpigmentation in dark-skinned patients. Am J Clin Dermatol 2004;5:161–8.

[49] Jimbow K, Obata H, Pathak MA, et al. Mechanism of depigmentation by hydroquinone. J Invest Dermatol 1974;62:436–49.

[50] Spencer MC. Hydroquinone bleaching. Arch Dermatol 1961;84:131–4.

[51] Katsambas AD, Stratigos AJ. Depigmenting and bleaching agents: coping with hyperpigmentation. Clin Dermatol 2001;19:483–8.

[52] Briganti S, Camera E, Picardo M. Chemical and instrumental approaches to treat hyperpigmentation. Pigment Cell Res 2003;16:101–10.

[53] Researching Committee of Rucinol. The study on the efficacy of Rucinol (4-N-butylresorcinol) in chloasma. Nishinihon J Dermatol 1999;61–6.

[54] Akasaka T, Ohurazaka H, Nishioheda G, et al. Topically applied 0.3% 4-N-butylresorcinol decrease pigmentation after laser therapy. Environ Dermatol 2002; 9:11–5.

[55] Bleehen SS. The treatment of hypermelanosis with 4-isopropylcatechol. Br J Dermatol 1976;94:687–94.

[56] Jimbow K. N-acetyl-4-S-cysteaminylphenol as a new type of depigmenting agent for the melanoderma of patients with melasma. Arch Dermatol 1991;127: 1528–34.

[57] Verallo-Rowell VM, Verallo V, Graupe K, et al. Double-blind comparison of azelaic acid and hydro-quinone in the treatment of melasma. Acta Derm Venereol Suppl (Stockh) 1989;143:58–61.

[58] Nakagawa M, Kawai K. Contact allergy to kojic acid in skin care products. Contact Dermatitis 1995; 32:9–13.

[59] Kameyama K, Sakai C, Kondoh S, et al. Inhibitory effect of magnesium L-ascorbyl-2-phosphate (VC-PMG) on melanogenesis in vitro and in vivo. J Am Acad Dermatol 1996;34:29–33.

[60] Huh CH, Seo KI, Park JY, et al. A randomized, double-blind, placebo-controlled trial of vitamin C iontophoresis in melasma. Dermatology 2003;206: 316–20.

[61] Espinal-Perez LE, Moncada B, Castanedo-Cazares JP. A double-blind randomized trial of 5% ascorbic acid vs. 4% hydroquinone in melasma. Int J Dermatol 2004; 43:604–7.

[62] Griffiths CE, Finkel LJ, Ditre CM, et al. Topical tretinoin (retinoic acid) improves melasma: a vehicle-controlled, clinical trial. Br J Dermatol 1993;129: 415–21.

[63] Kimbrough-Green CK, Griffiths CE, Finkel LJ, et al. Topical retinoic acid (tretinon) for melasma in black patients: a vehicle-controlled clinical trial. Arch Dermatol 1994;130:727–33.

[64] Rafal ES, Griffiths CE, Ditre CM, et al. Topical tretinoin (retinoic acid) treatment for liver spots associated with photodamage. N Engl J Med 1992;326: 368–74.

[65] Bulengo-Ransby SM, Griffiths CE, Kimbrough-Green CK, et al. Topical tretinoin (retinoic acid) therapy for hyperpigmented lesions caused by inflammation of the skin in black patients. N Engl J Med 1993;328: 1438–43.

[66] Romero C, Aberdam E, Larnier C, et al. Retinoic acid as modulator of UVB-induced melanocyte differentiation: involvement of the melanogenic enzymes expression. J Cell Sci 1994;107(Pt 4):1095–103.

[67] Sefton J, Kligman AM, Kopper SC, et al. Photo-damage pilot study: a double-blind, vehicle-controlled study to assess the efficacy and safety of tazarotene 0.1% gel. J Am Acad Dermatol 2000;43:656–63.

[68] Kang S, Goldfarb MT, Weiss JS, et al. Assessment of adapalene gel for the treatment of actinic keratoses and lentigines: a randomized trial. J Am Acad Dermatol 2003;49:83–90.

[69] Amer M, Metwalli M. Topical liquiritin improves melasma. Int J Dermatol 2000;39:299–301.

[70] Yokota T, Nishio H, Kubota Y, et al. The inhibitory effect of glabridin from licorice extracts on melanogenesis and inflammation. Pigment Cell Res 1998;11: 355–61.

[71] Saliou C, Kitazawa M, McLaughlin L, et al. Antioxidants modulate acute solar ultraviolet radiation-induced NF-kappa-B activation in a human keratinocyte cell line. Free Radic Biol Med 1999;26: 174–83.

[72] Ando H, Ryu A, Hashimoto A, et al. Linoleic acid and alpha-linolenic acid lightens ultraviolet-induced hyper-pigmentation of the skin. Arch Dermatol Res 1998; 290:375–81.

[73] Ando H, Watabe H, Valencia JC, et al. Fatty acids

regulate pigmentation via proteasomal degradation of tyrosinase: a new aspect of ubiquitin-proteasome function. J Biol Chem 2004;279:15427–33.

[74] Taylor SC, Torok H, Jones T, et al. Efficacy and safety of a new triple-combination agent for the treatment of facial melasma. Cutis 2003;72:67–72.

[75] Ortonne JP, Camacho F, Wainwright N, et al. Safety and efficacy of combined use of 4-hydroxyanisole (mequinol) 2% /tretinoin 0.01% solution and sunscreen in solar lentigines. Cutis 2004;74(4):261–4.

[76] Fleischer Jr AB, Schwartzel EH, Colby SI, et al. The combination of 2% 4-hydroxyanisole (Mequinol) and 0.01% tretinoin is effective in improving the appearance of solar lentigines and related hyperpigmented lesions in two double-blind multicenter clinical studies. J Am Acad Dermatol 2000; 42:459–67.

[77] Graupe K, Verallo-Rowell VM, Verallo V, et al. Combined use of 20% azelaic acid cream and 0.05% tretinoin cream in the topical treatment of melasma. J Dermatol Treat 1996;7:235–7.

[78] Kakita LS, Lowe NJ. Azelaic acid and glycolic acid combination therapy for facial hyperpigmentation in darker-skinned patients: a clinical comparison with hydroquinone. Clin Ther 1998;20:960–70.

[79] Lim JT. Treatment of melasma using kojic acid in a gel containing hydroquinone and glycolic acid. Dermatol Surg 1999;25:282–4.

[80] Njoo MD, Menke HE, Pavel S, et al. N-acetyl-cysteine as a bleaching agent in the treatment of melasma: a letter to the editor. J Eur Acad Dermatol Venereol 1997;9:86–7.

[81] Mahe A, Ly F, Aymard G, et al. Skin diseases associated with the cosmetic use of bleaching products in women from Dakar, Senegal. Br J Dermatol 2003; 148:493–500.

[82] Perez-Bernal A, Munoz-Perez MA, Camacho F. Management of facial hyperpigmentation. Am J Clin Dermatol 2000;1:261–8.

[83] Goldberg DJ, Meine JG. Treatment of facial telangiectases with the diode-pumped frequency-doubled Q-switched Nd:YAG laser. Dermatol Surg 1998;24: 828–32.

[84] Lim JT, Tham SN. Glycolic acid peels in the treatment of melasma among Asian women. Dermatol Surg 1997; 23:177–9.

[85] Grimes PE. The safety and efficacy of salicylic acid chemical peels in darker racial-ethnic groups. Dermatol Surg 1999;25:18–22.

[86] Kunachak S, Leelaudomlipi P, Wongwaisayawan S. Dermabrasion: a curative treatment for melasma. Aesthetic Plast Surg 2001;25:114–7.

[87] Pandya AG, Guevara IL. Disorders of hyperpigmentation. Dermatol Clin 2000;18:91–8.

[88] Todd MM, Rallis TM, Gerwels JW, et al. A comparison of 3 lasers and liquid nitrogen in the treatment of solar lentigines: a randomized, controlled, comparative trial. Arch Dermatol 2000;136:841–6.

[89] Bjerning P, Christiansen K. Intense pulsed light source for treatment of small melanocytic nevi and solar lentigines. J Cut Laser Ther 2000;2:177–81.

[90] Stratigos AJ, Dover JS, Arndt KA. Laser treatment of pigmented lesions—2000: how far have we gone? Arch Dermatol 2000;136:915–21.

[91] Li YT, Yang KC. Comparison of the frequency-doubled Q-switched Nd:YAG laser and 35% trichloroacetic acid for the treatment of face lentigines. Dermatol Surg 1999;25:202–4.

[92] Taylor CR, Anderson RR. Ineffective treatment of refractory melasma and postinflammatory hyperpigmentation by Q-switched ruby laser. J Dermatol Surg Oncol 1994;20:592–7.

[93] Nouri K, Bowes L, Chartier T, et al. Combination treatment of melasma with pulsed CO_2 laser followed by Q-switched alexandrite laser: a pilot study. Dermatol Surg 1999;25:494–7.

[94] Manaloto RM, Alster T. Erbium:YAG laser resurfacing for refractory melasma. Dermatol Surg 1999; 25:121–3.

[95] Holme SA, Beattie PE, Fleming CJ. Cosmetic camouflage advice improves quality of life. Br J Dermatol 2002;147:946–9.

[96] Levy SB. Tanning preparations. Dermatol Clin 2000; 18:591–6.

[97] Suga Y, Ikejima A, Matsuba S, et al. Medical pearl: DHA application for camouflaging segmental vitiligo and piebald lesions. J Am Acad Dermatol 2002;47: 436–8.

[98] Ongenae K, Van Geel N, De Schepper S, et al. Management of vitiligo patients and attitude of dermatologists towards vitiligo. Eur J Dermatol 2004; 14:177–81.

[99] Yang CH, Shen SC, Lee JC, et al. Seeing the gene therapy: application of gene gun technique to transfect and decolour pigmented rat skin with human agouti signalling protein cDNA. Gene Ther 2004;11: 1033–9.

ELSEVIER
SAUNDERS

DERMATOLOGIC
CLINICS

Dermatol Clin 23 (2005) 227 – 243

Management of Hair Loss

Elizabeth K. Ross, MD*, Jerry Shapiro, MD, FRCPC

*Division of Dermatology, University of British Columbia, and Vancouver Coastal Health Research Institute,
835 West 10th Avenue, Vancouver, BC V5Z 4E8, Canada*

Patients with scalp hair loss seek medical attention for various reasons. Some patients are anguished by their condition, and treatment is the prime motivation for the visit. Others worry that their hair loss is a sign of something medically dire and want appeasement. Still others arrive at the clinic appointment with seemingly unrelated scalp complaints (eg, intractable pruritus in those individuals with active lichen planopilaris) only to learn of their hair loss incidentally. In this broad patient context, an individualized management plan is required. Key components to its successful realization are patient education on the nature and course of the disease, prognosis, and treatment options, tempered by compassionate counseling. This article discusses therapeutic options and management strategies for male and female pattern hair loss (MPHL and FPHL; androgenetic alopecia), telogen effluvium (TE), and alopecia areata (AA).

Male pattern hair loss

Therapy approved by the US Food and Drug Administration

Topical minoxidil (Rogaine) and oral finasteride (Propecia) are the only treatments for MPHL that have been approved by the US Food and Drug Administration (FDA) [1]. Their use is indicated in men older than 18 years with mild to moderate

---

Dr. Shapiro is a consultant for Pfizer, Inc., and Merck & Co, Inc.
* Corresponding author.
E-mail address: ekr37@yahoo.com (E.K. Ross).

MPHL. Well-controlled studies substantiate these agents' efficacy [2–7]. Slowed hair loss, stabilization, or increased scalp coverage can be appreciated with either agent by 3 to 6 months of treatment, and are clearly evident by 1 year. Dense regrowth is uncommon. Early intervention, when thinning is first noticed and hairs are incompletely miniaturized, optimizes outcome. Neither agent can regrow hair in areas of total hair loss (bald areas). In responders, treatment must be continued indefinitely to maintain benefit. The extent of benefit wanes slightly with long-term use [2,6]. Stopping treatment results in a return to pretreatment status by 6 months with minoxidil [2] and by 12 months with finasteride [4].

Minoxidil

Two randomized, double-blind, placebo-controlled studies have evaluated efficacy of 5% versus 2% minoxidil topical solution [2,3]. In men aged 18 to 49 years with mild to moderate vertex hair loss, the 5% formulation is significantly superior [2]. Based on global photographic review, after 48 weeks of twice-daily treatment with 5% minoxidil, a mean of 57% of 139 patients had regrowth, compared with 41% of 142 patients and 23% of 71 patients in the 2% minoxidil and placebo-treated groups, respectively. The quality of regrowth was rated as mild to moderate in most individuals, with greater improvement seen in those using the 5% concentration. Hair counts and patient rating of scalp coverage and treatment benefit were also significantly better with the higher strength formulation. Peak hair counts occurred at 16 weeks with both concentrations. In a smaller study on 36 men aged 18 to 40 years who had mild to moderate frontoparietal hair loss, a trend toward greater improvement was seen with the 5% dose based on hair weights, but this result was not statistically significant [3]. After 96 weeks of treatment with 5% minoxidil, target-area hair weights increased by 35%, compared with an increase of 25% with 2% minoxidil. Untreated and placebo-controlled groups lost 6% in hair weight per year.

Instructions on how to use minoxidil and possible side effects will help to ensure its correct use. The patient should be told that minoxidil is a scalp, not a hair, solution [8]. Up to 1 mL of solution should be applied to dry affected scalp using a calibrated dropper (not a spray), twice daily. Patients who still have substantial hair should apply the solution along the length of five evenly spaced parts made in the treatment area, spreading it gently outward. Care should be taken to avoid deposition of the drug on hair as this can impart a greasy, flaky appearance, which can result in reduced compliance, particularly in women. Hair grooming products (eg, gels, mousse) can be used subsequently. The drug should be left on the scalp for at least 4 hours to maximize absorption. Patients should be forewarned that increased shedding is expected within a few weeks of starting treatment [8] and may last for a few months; during this time, they will not go "bald." Application site reactions occur in up to 6% of patients [8] and are largely caused by contact dermatitis or aggravation of underlying inflammatory disorders, such as seborrheic dermatitis or psoriasis [9]. Propylene glycol, rather than minoxidil, is usually the culprit. The use of a tar shampoo, topical corticosteroid scalp solution, or 2% minoxidil, which contains less propylene glycol, may control the problem [9]. Alternatively, a less reactive solvent for compounding minoxidil may

be tried (eg, butylene glycol); however, the efficacy of this method has not been formally tested [9]. Patch test kits are available from Pfizer (Morris Plains, New Jersey). Minimal systemic absorption of minoxidil can occur with topical use, but serum levels are well below those that produce hemodynamic effects [8]. A large-scale 1-year observational study on patients who used 2% or 5% topical minoxidil showed no increased risk of cardiovascular events compared with controls [10].

Finasteride

Large-scale randomized, double-blind, placebo-controlled studies showed that finasteride (1 mg/d) can effectively halt or reverse the progression of mild to moderate MPHL in men aged 18 to 60 years [4–7]. In men aged 18 to 41 years with mild to moderate vertex hair loss, global photographic review showed regrowth in 66% (30% slightly improved, 36% moderately or greatly improved) of the finasteride-treated group compared with 7% of placebo-treated controls, after 2 years of treatment [4]. In the ensuing 3 years of treatment, the level of improvement declined slightly but remained well above baseline in 90% of men [6]. Older men (aged 41–60 y) with mild to moderate hair loss predominantly affecting the vertex were less likely to respond (regrowth in 39% of men after 2 years of finasteride use; regrowth in 4% of those using placebo) [7]. In men aged 18 to 41 years with mild to moderate frontal hair loss treated with finasteride for 1 year, 37% had mild to moderate regrowth (placebo, 7%) (Fig. 1) [5].

The most common side effects are decreased libido, decreased semen volume, and erectile dysfunc-

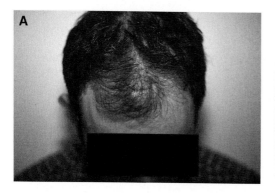
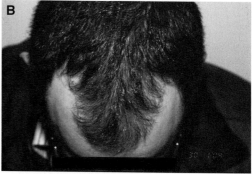

Fig. 1. An excellent response to treatment with oral finasteride in a 31-year-old man with pattern hair loss. Compared with his pretreatment status (*A*), significant regrowth is seen in the midfrontal scalp after 18 months of therapy (*B*). (*From* Ross E, Shapiro J. A practical approach to non-scarring alopecia: male pattern hair loss. Contemp Dermatol 2004;2(1):1–8; with permission.)

tion, with each occurring in fewer than 2% of men younger than 41 years [4–6] and slightly more often in older men [7]. These sexual side effects often abate with continued treatment and resolve completely within days to weeks if treatment is stopped [4,6]. Breast cancer has been reported in a few patients with higher dose (5 mg/d) finasteride (Proscar) [11,12], but the epidemiologic significance and causal relationship is unknown. A significantly lower prevalence of prostate cancer (25%), but a higher histologic grade (6.4% [drug] versus 5.1% [placebo], with a Gleason score of 7–10) also has been reported with daily use of 5-mg finasteride in a recent large-scale 7-year placebo-controlled study on men aged 55 or older with clinically normal prostates [13]. The clinical behavior of these cancers is unknown. The relevance to men with MPHL treated with one fifth of the dose has not been assessed; guidelines for determination of baseline and screening serum prostate-specific antigen (PSA) in these men have not been developed, and testing should be done according to the physician's discretion. For evaluative purposes, the value of the PSA obtained on routine screening should be doubled in men older than 41 years [15].

Finasteride is taken once daily, with or without food [11,14]. Because it is metabolized in the liver, caution is advised when treating patients with liver disease. There are no known drug interactions.

Combined use of finasteride and topical minoxidil

Small-scale, variably controlled studies conducted on a primate model for androgenetic alopecia and on young men with mild to moderate MPHL suggest that combination therapy may be more effective than monotherapy, but further investigation is needed [15,16].

Therapy not approved by the US Food and Drug Administration

The list of non–FDA-approved therapeutic agents is extensive, with many claims of efficacy unsubstantiated by formal clinical trials [17,18]. A detailed review is outside the scope of this article. A few interventions with suggestive benefit bear mentioning, however. Small-scale studies on 2% ketoconazole shampoo (used 2 to 4 times weekly) [16,19] show some efficacy when used alone [19] or with finasteride in young men with mild to moderate pattern hair loss [16]. Reports of a synergistic effect with combined use of topical tretinoin and minoxidil are also intriguing but require verification by larger controlled studies [20]. Concerns about increased irritation, possible systemic absorption of drug, and difficulties related to the use of both agents together [21] are somewhat prohibitive.

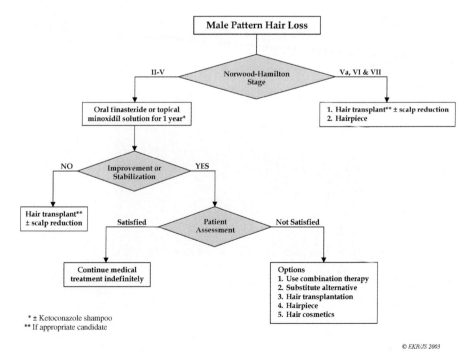

Fig. 2. An algorithmic approach for management of MPHL. © EKR/JS 2003.

230 ROSS & SHAPIRO

Management

In general, pretreatment work-up in men with MPHL is not necessary. A biopsy is rarely indicated. In men who are vegetarians, a serum ferritin level may be evaluated (see details on management in the "Telogen effluvium" section) [1,22]. Men with the global variant of MPHL may warrant evaluation of thyroid-stimulating hormone (TSH) levels [1].

A suggested algorithm for therapeutic management of MPHL is shown in Fig. 2. In those individuals with mild to moderate MPHL (Norwood-Hamilton type II–V), monotherapy with finasteride or 5% minoxidil is recommended for 1 year, with initial follow-up visits at 6 and 12 months, and annually thereafter in treatment responders. A pretreatment photograph should be taken to help track outcome. In those individuals with no perceptible improvement or stabilization after 1 year of treatment, the other, untried agent may be substituted. Overlapping regimens for the first 3 months is recommended [1]. Hair gained with first agent may still be shed but at a less rapid rate [23]. Patients who benefit from monotherapy may further improve with combined use of finasteride and minoxidil [16]. A 6- to 12-month trial of twice-weekly ketaconazole shampoo may also be added and discontinued thereafter in nonresponders. Hair transplantation is another important option. Hair transplantation can enhance cosmesis in those individuals who have responded to medical therapy but remain dissatisfied with their appearance, and in those who eschew medical therapy outright (Fig. 3) [21,24]. The ideal candidate has dense occipital scalp hair (typical donor bank). Cosmetic powders and topical preparations that match hair color (eg, Toppik, Nanogen, Le Couvré), lightening of hair color, creative styling, extensions, and partial hairpieces can also be used to camouflage visible scalp.

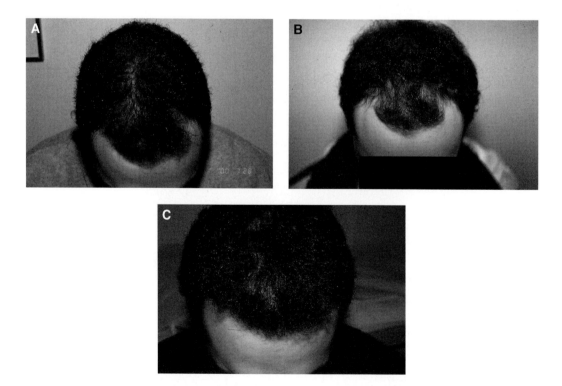

Fig. 3. Example of enhanced improvement derived from combined use of oral finasteride (1 mg/d) and hair transplantation in the management of MPHL. At age 19, this man was first treated with oral finasteride. Compared with his baseline photograph (*A*), there is no progression of hair loss in the centroparietal scalp after 2 years of treatment. Unlike the patient shown in Fig. 1, however, hair loss in the midfrontal scalp continued to worsen (*B*). Because the patient remained dissatisfied with his appearance and was an excellent candidate, he elected to undergo hair transplantation, continuing finasteride to preserve benefit in the centroparietal scalp. A total of 1270 follicular unit grafts were transplanted to the frontal scalp with the result as shown (*C*). (*From* Ross E, Shapiro J. A practical approach to non-scarring alopecia: male pattern hair loss. Contemp Dermatol 2004;2(1): 1–8; with permission.)

For men with advanced MPHL (Norwood-Hamilton type Va, VI, and VII) who have a good donor site, hair transplantation with or without scalp reduction can significantly improve cosmesis [21]. For patients who are not interested in a surgical remedy or who are poor candidates, a hairpiece is the best option.

The off-label use of topical minoxidil may be justified in adolescents with pattern hair loss whose psychosocial well-being is affected by their condition [25]. Retrospective, uncontrolled studies suggest that the treatment is effective in this age group [25]. The effect of finasteride on MPHL in males younger than 18 years is unknown.

Female pattern hair loss

Therapy approved by the US Food and Drug Administration

For the treatment of FPHL, 2% topical minoxidil is the only FDA-approved medication [26]. Its use is indicated in women older than 18 years with mild to moderate hair loss (Ludwig stage I or II). In a well-designed 32-week study, investigator global assessment determined that twice-daily 2% minoxidil stimulated mild to moderate regrowth in 63% of 157 women compared with 39% of 151 women treated with vehicle (Fig. 4) [26]. Results may be less impressive in those individuals with underlying hyperandrogenism [27]. In addition to contact dermatitis, hypertrichosis typically affecting the peripheral face develops in up to 7% of treated women [28]. This condition may diminish with continued treatment over the course of a year, and resolves completely within a few months once treatment is stopped

[21,28]. Pre-existing facial hair, higher dosing, and age older than 50 years are predisposing factors [28]. Care should be taken to avoid manual or fomite (eg, pillows) spread of minoxidil to sites other than the scalp, although the effect is largely believed to result from local absorption. Minoxidil should not be used in pregnant or nursing women, although no adverse pregnancy outcomes were reported in a large-scale 1-year observational study [10].

Therapy not approved by the US Food and Drug Administration

Non–FDA-approved therapeutic agents include 5% topical minoxidil solution and antiandrogen therapy with androgen receptor antagonists (cyproterone actetate, spironolactone, flutamide) or finasteride. The therapeutic value of oral contraceptive agents (OCAs) in FPHL is unknown. Those OCAs with moderate to high androgenic potency may, in fact, aggravate or unmask occult FPHL, as can starting and stopping use, through induction of TE [1,29]. The new generation of OCA with antiandrogenic progestogens (drosperinone [30], chlormadinone acetate [31], dienogest [31]) may have a place in the therapeutic armamentarium of FPHL but require further study. Early reports of remarkable response rates with chlormadinone acetate are intriguing [31]. Only drosperinone, in a dose equivalent to 25 mg of spironolactone and combined with ethinyl estradiol (Yasmin), is available in the United States [30].

5% Minoxidil

In a 48-week, well-designed study on the comparative efficacy of 5% versus 2% topical minoxidil in the treatment of mild to moderate FPHL, no sig-

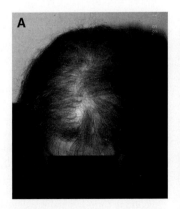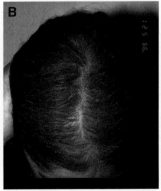

Fig. 4. Beneficial effect of topical minoxidil in a 46-year-old woman with Ludwig stage II pattern hair loss. Compared with baseline (*A*), there is remarkable regrowth after only 4 months of twice-daily treatment with 5% topical minoxidil, marked by enhanced scalp coverage and a diminished midline part width (*B*).

nificant difference in scalp coverage could be appreciated by investigator global assessment; however, patient satisfaction was significantly enhanced with use of the higher concentration [32]. Its use should be considered in those minimally responsive to the 2% formulation.

Antiandrogen therapy

Most of the antiandrogen therapies have not been rigorously studied in FPHL [1]. In general, better results are seen in women with hyperandrogenism [1,27,33]. The role of menopausal status and scalp site in therapeutic response is unknown. Nine months or more may be required before a benefit is appreciated [34]. Side effects are generally greater with cyproterone acetate (CPA) and spironolactone. Because feminization of the male fetus is a concern, concomitant use of an OCA is mandatory in women of childbearing age [1]. A pretreatment screening serum pregnancy test is also recommended.

Cyproterone acetate

CPA is not available in the United States. It is usually combined with ethinyl estradiol for added antiandrogenic effect and contraception [1,31,34]. Higher dosages of CPA may be more effective [1,27,31]. So-called "reverse sequential regimens" include 100 mg/day of CPA on days 5 to 15 of the menstrual cycle and 50 μg of ethinyl estradiol on days 5 to 25 [1]. Alternatively, 50 mg/day of CPA on days 1 to 10 of the cycle and 35 μg of ethinyl estradiol on days 1 to 21 may be given [31]. Serum vitamin B12 levels may fall with treatment and require supplementation [34]. Baseline and biannual monitoring is suggested.

Spironolactone

This agent may reduce shedding in those individuals without hyperandrogenism and may promote some hair growth in those with hyperandrogenism [1,21,34]. Dosages greater than 150 mg/day are usually required [34]. Periodic monitoring of serum potassium, especially early in treatment, and blood pressure and weight is recommended [35]. The use of this agent is contraindicated in women with renal insufficiency or hyperkalemia, and in those with a personal or family history of breast cancer because suprahuman doses (25–250 times) in rats induced malignant mammary tumors [35].

Flutamide

There are incidental reports of improvement of FPHL in women with hirsutism treated with fluta-mide [18]. Dosages vary from 250 to 500 mg/day, or 250 mg twice daily [18,33,34]. A recent comparative study in hyperandrogenic premenopausal women with FPHL treated with flutamide (250 mg/d), CPA, or finasteride showed that flutamide alone was efficacious, producing a small but definite reduction (21%) in Ludwig score [33]. Elevated liver transaminases occur in up to 32% of patients [34]. Hepatotoxicity that can lead to death has been reported in less than 1% of patients at dosages greater than 750 mg/day [34].

Finasteride

In a large-scale placebo-controlled study that did not stratify patients according to androgen status, 1 mg of finasteride taken daily for 1 year was shown to be of no benefit to postmenopausal women with FPHL [36]. In an isolated case report, however, higher dose finasteride (5 mg/d) was shown to induce significant regrowth in a postmenopausal, nonhyperandrogenic woman with FPHL, who was treated for 1 year [37]. Results of treatment with finasteride in women with androgen excess, based on two small, uncontrolled studies using different dosing regimens, are conflicting [33,38]. Further studies are needed. Finasteride is contraindicated in women of child-bearing potential [11,14].

Management

Before the initiation of treatment, other forms of hair loss that can coexist with or mimic FPHL should be assessed. A scalp biopsy should be done if the diagnosis is uncertain. Suspect causes of TE, which can worsen or unmask FPHL, should be corrected, when possible [1,29]. Serum ferritin levels should be measured in premenopausal women and vegetarians and optimized with iron supplementation if necessary (see "Telogen effluvium" section) [1,22]. Over-the-counter androgen supplements should be discontinued [1]. Androgenic progestogen content in OCA and hormone replacement therapy (HRT) should be minimized.

Once this pretreatment work-up is complete, patients should be stratified according to androgen status and then severity of hair loss (Fig. 5). In women without hyperandrogenism, the approach is straightforward. For women with clinical hyperandrogenism, serum androgen testing should be done according to individual presentation [39]. In cases of suspected polycystic ovary syndrome (PCOS), diagnosed in a significant proportion of these affected women, a serum free testosterone level should be

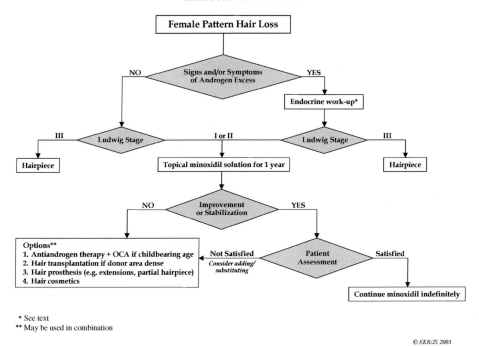

Fig. 5. An algorithmic approach for management of FPHL. © EKR/JS 2003.

obtained [40]. A more complete screening panel for hyperandrogenism consists of a serum total and free testosterone, dehydroepiandrosterone sulfate, prolactin, luteinizing hormone, follicle-stimulating hormone, and 17-hydroxyprogesterone levels, and is best done in the morning after fasting, during the first 7 days of the menstrual cycle [39]. Concomitant referral to an endocrinologist is recommended for two reasons: (1) seronegative patients may have enzyme deficiencies that require additional testing or results may be falsely negative; (2) treatment should be based on cause rather than piecemeal correction of dermatologic manifestations [39]. With appropriate management of the underlying endocrine disorder, the cutaneous manifestations of hyperandrogenism may be reversed [18,39]. Indeed, in patients with PCOS, regulation of menses and control of hyperinsulinemia can reduce or prevent acne and hirsutism [39] and may theoretically halt if not reverse FPHL. Lifestyle alterations, such as balanced weight loss and exercise, may be sufficient to induce this change [39]. Minoxidil can be instituted while the endocrine work-up is underway, in patients with Ludwig stage I or II FPHL [21]. Because the benefit may not be as great as is seen in nonhyperandrogenic controls [27], added or alternative use of antiandrogen therapy may be warranted before a full year of treatment is completed. In all patients, baseline photographs (typically

of the midline part) should be taken to track treatment response.

In patients who fail medical therapy or who desire further improvement and are appropriate candidates, hair transplantation should be discussed. Patient expectations should match projected results. In general, the best candidate has Ludwig stage II FPHL or anterior hairline recession. A patient with Ludwig I FPHL is unlikely to be satisfied with the surgical outcome because post-transplant hair density is often insufficient to impart the appearance of added fullness. Although studies are lacking in women, combination medical and surgical treatment may enhance outcome [24]. Tinted cosmetics, hair lightening, creative styling, and hair prostheses can also help to camouflage the defect.

Telogen effluvium

In established cases of TE, a detailed history and examination underlies successful management. Resolving disease, marked by normal levels of shedding, a negative pull test, and signs of synchronized regrowth on examination (hairs of equal length throughout the scalp), requires no intervention. In patients with ongoing TE, triggers that predate the onset of hair loss by approximately 1 to 3 months should be solicited [29,41]. Medication is a common culprit. In women, starting and stopping sex hormone therapy (eg, OCAs, HRT) is often causal. Other triggers include the following: parturition, major illness, surgery, rapid weight loss or poor nutrition, thyroid dysfunction, high fever, hemorrhage, acute psychosocial stressors (eg, death of a loved one, bankruptcy, divorce), and contact dermatitis from hair dyes [29,41,42]. In patients with chronic TE (duration, >6 mo), the precipitant is often not identified [43].

Patients who experience TE after an acute event (eg, parturition, surgery) will resolve spontaneously. In the remaining patients, steps should be taken to eliminate all possible triggers. Blood tests should be done to determine ferritin levels in menstruating women, vegetarians, and in those with a history of anemia; if levels are below 40 ug/L, iron supplementation should arguably be instituted [22,29]. Repeat testing is done every 4 to 6 months until stores are adequately repleted [41]. If indicated, TSH, and rapid plasma reagin (RPR) to rule out syphilis, should be obtained and abnormalities corrected [29,41]. In addition to these laboratory tests, exogenous causes of TE should be removed. Unnecessary supplements, vitamins (eg, vitamin A), and herbals should be discontinued. Over-the-counter and prescription medications that have a high chance of causing TE should be substituted with benign alternatives, when possible. Hormone therapies should be stabilized [29,41]. Nutrition should be optimized, particularly in those with inherited deficiencies, those on parenteral alimentation, and in vegetarians [29]. Diets for weight loss should be balanced, with daily caloric intake greater than 1200 kcal/day [29]. Recently, the current authors have seen a few cases of TE related to the Atkins diet, which occurred after a period of significant weight loss (>2 lb/wk). Once these factors have been addressed, observational monitoring and reassurance are usually all that is required. Regrowth is expected within 3 to 6 months after the trigger has been removed—at most, 1 year [41]. Exceptions include those individuals with certain chronic debilitating conditions (eg, organ transplant recipients; Elizabeth K. Ross, MD, Jerry Shapiro, MD, FRCPC, personal observation, 2004) in whom the cause is often multifactorial and practically irreversible, and those with chronic TE who can experience bouts of increased shedding for years [43]. In patients with underlying pattern hair loss, growth may not return to baseline levels [41]. For patients with persistent TE for more than 6 months, empiric use topical minoxidil twice daily may speed regrowth [41]. Patients should be forewarned about transient worsening from minoxidil-induced TE.

Alopecia areata

There are no FDA-approved treatments for AA. Corticosteroids, topical immunotherapy, anthralin, topical minoxidil, and psoralen plus ultraviolet A (PUVA) comprise the more frequently cited modalities. None is curative nor reliably effective. The recommendation for the use of any one therapeutic agent is hampered by the lack of long-term, randomized, double-blind, placebo-controlled studies of sufficient power and duration. This situation is further compounded by the failure of many studies to control for rates of spontaneous remission or to stratify patients according to type of disease, among other prognostic factors. Because most patients resolve within 1 year without any intervention [44], half-head/half-lesion studies are essential to establishing treatment effect. A precise definition of "response," often omitted, aids in interpretation of results. And yet, despite this complexity, there are several treatments that do seem to work in some patients with AA. A recent evidence-based evaluation of the therapeutic literature by the British Association of Dermatologists provides guidance [45]. Although the current authors are largely in agreement with the recommendations contained therein, there are some points of departure based largely on assimilation of new data published after this report and the authors' anecdotal experience.

Corticosteroids

Topical corticosteroids

Controlled studies on treatment of AA with standard topical corticosteroid lotions, creams, and ointments have shown some benefit, but this benefit occurs infrequently and the extent of hair regrowth is usually suboptimal [46,47]. Different formulations or adding occlusion produces better results, presumably through enhanced skin penetration and delivery of drug to the hair bulb [46,48–50]. In a multicenter, randomized, investigator-blinded study on 61 patients with limited, patchy AA (<26% hair loss), 0.12% betamethasone valerate foam was found to be significantly superior to 0.05% betamethasone dipropionate lotion when used twice daily for 12 weeks [46]. At 8 weeks post treatment, 61% of patients treated with the foam had more than 75% regrowth, compared with 27% of those treated with the lotion. Matched potencies and unilateral treatment would have strengthened this finding. Occlusion of non-foam topical corticosteroids also improves outcome [49,50]. In the double-blind, half-head, placebo-controlled arm of a two-part study, 54% (7 of 13) of patients treated with 0.2% fluocinolone cream (1–2 g twice daily, with occlusion at night) showed unilateral regrowth after 3 to 6 months, compared with 0% with vehicle [49]. Although the quality of regrowth was not characterized in this study arm, when results were combined with those seen in the single-blind arm, complete or near-complete restoration of hair occurred in 65% of treatment responders. All children younger than 10 years and older patients with disease for less than 1 year responded favorably to treatment. Unexpectedly, patchy AA and alopecia totalis (AT) were equally treatment responsive. The benefit of this approach in severe disease was subsequently reinforced by Tosti et al [50], who showed that 8 of 28 patients with chronic, treatment-refractory AT or alopecia universalis (AU) had a cosmetically acceptable outcome after 6-month treatment with 0.05% clobetasol propionate ointment, nightly, under occlusion [50]. The effect was durable in 18% of patients.

Drawbacks to this approach include an up to 4-month delay before regrowth appears and a high rate of relapse (38%–63%) during treatment and after treatment has ceased [49,50]. In addition, painful folliculitis and acne develop in a significant number of patients [46,48–50]. This result is less likely with use of the foam. Temporary cessation of treatment usually alleviates the problem. Rarely, telangiectasias and mild atrophy develop. There is no evidence of systemic absorption by biochemical and clinical parameters in patients older than 17 years who are treated with occlusion of an ultrapotent corticosteroid on the entire scalp for 6 months [50]. The risk in children has not been adequately investigated.

Intralesional corticosteroids

There are some variably controlled studies and anecdotal reports that validate the efficacy of intralesional corticosteroids in the treatment of AA, as marked by tufts of newly grown hair at drug injection sites exclusively [51–54]. In North America, this is mainstay therapy for limited scalp AA. Triamcinolone acetonide (Kenalog) is primarily used, at concentrations of 5 to 10 mg/mL, diluted in isotonic saline [52–54]. Abell and Munro [53] showed that biweekly injections of 5 mg/mL of triamcinolone acetonide for 12 weeks (maximum dose/session, 30 mg) induced regrowth at injected sites in 71% (47 of 66) of patients with subtotal AA and in 28% (15 of 18) of patients with AT, compared with 7% (1 of 15) of those injected with isotonic saline alone. In an uncontrolled study, Kubeyinje [54] reported similar results in 40 patients with subtotal AA, noting

that patients with fewer than five patches measuring less than 3 cm in diameter were particularly treatment responsive. At the University of British Columbia (UBC) Hair Treatment Centre, intralesional Kenalog (ILK) is routinely used to treat limited scalp AA, with good regrowth often seen after three to four visits. Every 4 to 6 weeks, 0.1 mL aliquots of triamcinolone acetonide (5 mg/mL; maximum volume, 3 mL) are injected at 1-cm intervals into the deep dermis in areas of alopecia and clinically active hair-bearing sites using a 0.5-in 30-gauge needle. Repeat treatments are administered to sites adjacent to newly grown hair. Treatment-induced regrowth persists for weeks to months [51–54]. ILK for beard and eyebrow AA is also effective (2.5 mg/mL; maximum, 0.5 mL to each eyebrow and 1 mL to beard), as noted by others as well [53]. Pretreatment with a short-acting topical anesthetic can help to minimize the pain with injection, or the physician can use a needle-free device [53]. Adverse effects include transient atrophy or, if the same site is injected repeatedly, permanent atrophy in addition to hypo/depigmentation and telangiectasias. In addition, there is an isolated report of anaphylaxis from ILK used to treat scalp AA [55] and a report of ipsilateral amaurosis in three patients with frontotemporal AA who were injected with less soluble corticosteroid suspensions (eg, hydrocortisone) using the fanning technique [56].

Systemic corticosteroids

There is empiric evidence that systemic steroids (oral, IV, or intramuscular) are effective in some patients with AA, but formal, controlled studies are lacking [57–61]. Protracted daily or alternate-day therapy has been supplanted by short-taper or pulse delivery of corticosteroids to minimize harmful side effects. In a two-arm uncontrolled study, Olsen et al [58] reported that 12% (5 of 43) to 28% (9 of 32) of patients with 1% to 99% scalp AA regrew 50% or more of their hair after a 6-week prednisone taper (starting at 40 mg) [58]. Common side effects included weight gain and mood changes. In an open study on treatment of patchy AA (30%–50% involvement), a single pulse of methylprednisolone (250 mg IV twice daily for 3 consecutive days) resulted in 50% or more regrowth in 65% (13 of 20) of patients after 1 month, with continued improvement thereafter [59]. Conflicting outcomes have been reported in ophiasis, AT, and AU, and in those with chronic disease [58–61]. Treatment withdrawal often results in loss of hair gained, within weeks. Although the current authors do not use systemic corticosteroids to treat AA, there are advocates for a short-course therapy in cases of rapidly advancing AA, as a stopgap measure in anticipation of spontaneous remission [58,59,61].

Topical immunotherapy with diphenylcyclopropenone and squaric acid dibutylester

Primary reports in the literature on treatment of AA with allergic contact immunotherapy outnumber those of any other therapeutic agent. For extensive AA, this approach is standard in Europe and Canada and has been used safely and effectively for over two decades. Two agents are used: diphenycyclopropenone (DPCP) and squaric acid dibutylester (SADBE). Both are unlicensed for therapeutic use. Neither agent is mutagenic by Ames testing [62,63]; however, one precursor of DPCP is mutagenic, as is potentially a photochemically activated intermediate [62]. Accordingly, commercial supplies of DPCP should ideally be screened for contaminants, and the purified product then stored in amber bottles to prevent degradation by light [62]. A local ethics committee should be asked for consent to use this treatment.

This therapy's efficacy has been largely demonstrated by half-head studies. Reported response rates have varied widely but seem to be similar for both agents, averaging 50% to 60% [64]. In the largest case series to date (N = 148), treatment of scalp AA with DPCP resulted in cosmetically acceptable regrowth in 100% of patients with 25% to 49% hair loss, 88% of patients with 50% to 74% hair loss, 60% of patients with 75% to 99% hair loss, and 17% of patients with AT or AU [65]. Regrowth was apparent in most patients after 3 to 12 months of treatment. Relapse occurred frequently (62%) during and after treatment (median time, 31 mo). A durable response was seen in 29% of patients (Fig. 6).

Other studies have confirmed that limited disease responds best to treatment [65–69]. When scalp involvement is less than 40%, however, equally good outcomes are seen with 1% topical minoxidil or placebo, attesting to the high rates of spontaneous remission seen in this type of disease [70]. The use of DPCP or SADBE should thus be reserved for more severe disease. In addition to severity, childhood on-

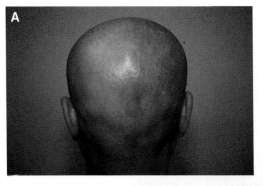
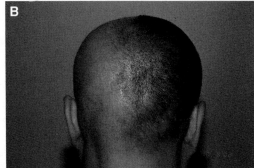
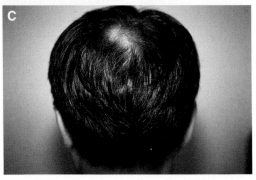

Fig. 6. Excellent result with diphencyprone in a 55-year-old man with near-total AA for 8 months. (*A*) After 10 weeks of treatment on the right side of the scalp, a mild eczematous reaction and some regrowth can be appreciated. (*B*) After 20 weeks of treatment on the right side and 4 weeks of treatment on the contralateral side. (*C*) Results after 13 months of treatment. After 7 months of continued, intermittent therapy, a few new patches of AA developed, and weekly treatments were reinstituted.

set, chronicity, nail changes, and atopic eczema have been shown to be significant negative prognostic indicators in some, but not all, studies [65–69,71,72].

Erythema, pruritus, and fine scaling are intrinsic to treatment. Induction of a mild eczematous reaction is sufficient to elicit benefit [68,73]. The most common adverse effects include regional lymphadenopathy, blistering, and pruritus that disrupts sleep [72,74]. Other adverse effects include pigmentary changes (postinflammatory hyperpigmentation or hypopigmentation, a combination of the two called "dyschromia in confetti," and vitiligo), which may prohibit use in darker skinned individuals, who are particularly prone [65]; facial and scalp edema; autoeczematization; contact urticaria; yellow discoloration of gray hair; dermatographism; eruptive lentigines; and consort dermatitis [64,65,72,74,75]. Flulike symptoms, fever, erythema multiformelike reactions, and one case of anaphylaxis have been reported with DPCP [72].

There is no evidence of systemic absorption of DPCP or teratogenicity in animal models or in cases of accidental pregnancy [62,74]. Nonetheless, women should use contraception during treatment and immediately discontinue the use of DPCP in the event of pregnancy [64,74]. No long-term side effects have been reported with either DPCP or SADBE [64,72].

Before commencing treatment, risks and benefits of treatment are reviewed in detail with the patient, and an informed consent is signed. At the UBC Hair Treatment Centre, patients older than 10 years with 50% or more hair loss are eligible for treatment with DPCP. Treatment is administered in the clinic. The patient is first sensitized with a 2% dose applied to a small area of the scalp. Two weeks later, weekly half-head treatments are started, beginning with a dilute solution of DPCP. The DPCP is left on the scalp for 48 hours and then washed off. Care is taken to avoid sun exposure during this period of time. On return, the concentration of DPCP is adjusted incrementally, based on the intensity of the reaction provoked by the previous week's treatment (range, 0.0001%–2%). The goal is to maintain low-grade erythema and pruritus. Once established, weekly applications of the eliciting dose are continued until unilateral regrowth is apparent. Treatment is then extended to the other side (see Fig. 5). The early onset of terminal hair regrowth and lower eliciting dose are predictors of a good response [65]. The development of tolerance precludes further treatment; switching to SADBE can be productive [72]. The reader is referred to other sources for greater detail on methodology [67,68,71, 72,74].

Anthralin

There are a few variably controlled studies on treatment of AA with anthralin [76–78]. In a partly controlled study, Schmoeckel et al [76] reported cosmetically acceptable regrowth after an unspecified treatment duration in 75% (18 of 24) of patients with patchy AA and in 25% (2 of 8) of patients with AT treated with anthralin once daily in concentrations sufficient to produce erythema and pruritus (range, 0.2%–0.8%). New hair was visible by 8 weeks. The photographs shown of two patients with extensive AA who underwent half-head treatment show a definite unilateral effect. The induction of an overt dermatitis seems to be essential to therapeutic response [77]. Because of the documented results in the former study, and anecdotal success with anthralin in a small proportion of patients (Jerry Shapiro, MD, FRCPC, personal observation), this agent is used as second-line therapy at the UBC Hair Treatment Centre. Patients are instructed to apply 0.5%–1% anthralin cream to bare areas for 20 to 30 minutes daily over 2 weeks, gradually increasing daily exposure time by 10 to 15 minutes at 2-week intervals, up to 1 hour total, until low-grade erythema and pruritus develop. Once achieved, daily treatment at this exposure time is continued for 3 months and stopped thereafter in nonresponders. In responders, the entire involved scalp is then treated until cosmetically acceptable regrowth is seen, which may take 6 months or longer. Attempts to gradually taper treatment frequency are made thereafter. Hands should be washed well after each application, avoiding eye contact with the drug. The treated area should be protected from the sun. Irritation and staining of treated skin are expected. Adverse effects include staining of unaffected skin, fabrics, and fair hair, which prohibits use in some individuals [45,74]. Folliculitis, regional lymphadenopathy, severe itching, and blistering can also develop [74,76].

Psoralen plus ultraviolet A

There are no controlled studies on the use of PUVA to treat AA. Success rates vary widely, with excellent (60%–100%) regrowth reported in up to 53% of patients treated for 2 to 3 months, including those with severe forms of the condition [79–82]. Protocols involve oral or topical formulations of psoralen used in combination with either localized scalp or total body UVA irradiation, with no clear difference in response based on approach. The cessation of therapy commonly results in relapse, which may be less likely when treatments are slowly tapered rather than abruptly stopped [82]. Adverse events include burn, nausea with use of oral psoralen, and pruritus

[80,81]. The need for long-term maintenance therapy raises concern about future skin cancers. Because of this concern and the fact that rates of spontaneous remission approximate rates of treatment success in these uncontrolled studies, the authors rarely use this therapeutic modality.

Minoxidil

There are several small, adequately controlled studies on the use of topical minoxidil to treat AA, largely conducted over 15 years ago [83–90]. Results vary widely. Different formulations of minoxidil were used, with no comparative studies on bioavailability. In a randomized, double-blind, placebo-controlled crossover study by Fenton and Wilkinson [83], twice-daily application of topical 1% minoxidil ointment or lotion, compounded from crushed tablets, was shown to be significantly superior to vehicle. After 3 months of treatment, regrowth was present in 73% (11 of 15) of drug-treated patients compared with 7% (1 of 15) of controls, and eventuated in a cosmetically acceptable result in 81% of patients by 6 months. AT

and AU were less responsive. In a half-head study using the same treatment protocol with 1% minoxidil ointment, Maitland et al [90] were unable to verify this high treatment response rate, observing cosmetically acceptable regrowth in only 1 of 15 patients with patchy AA that was clearly attributable to treatment [90]. Results with higher doses of minoxidil, used primarily in solution form, also have been mixed [85–89]. Most controlled studies on 3% minoxidil have shown no significant benefit in AT or AU [85–87], but efficacy in patients with subtotal AA, the cohort that responded best to 1% minoxidil in the study by Fenton and Wilkinson [83], has been limitedly explored. A small-scale study found that 5% minoxidil, when used twice daily for 3 months, was significantly superior to placebo [88], but when cosmetically acceptable coverage was the endpoint measured, no distinct advantage was observed [89]. Side effects are as mentioned in the section on MPHL. Absorption data for children are unknown. The current authors use 5% minoxidil solution to treat patients with patchy AA or ophiasis at doses pre-

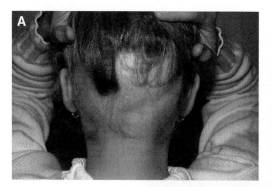
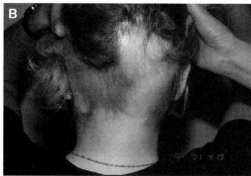
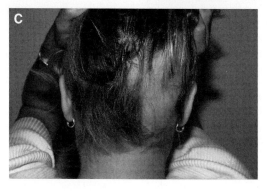

Fig. 7. Synergistic effect of dual treatment with short-contact anthralin and 5% topical minoxidil therapy. This 34-year-old woman with long-standing ophiasis, who had been unresponsive to monotherapy, showed marked regrowth when both agents were used together. (*A*) Baseline. (*B*) After 11 weeks of treatment with 5% topical minoxidil on alternate nights and 1% anthralin cream for 1 hour every third day, applied only to the left occipital scalp. (*C*) Results after 6 months of unilateral treatment.

scribed for pattern hair loss, usually in combination with another compatible topical agent (see *Combination therapy* section below).

Combination therapy

There are a few reports of enhanced benefit derived from combination therapy. In an incompletely detailed study, treatment with 0.05% betamethasone dipropionate and 5% topical minoxidil was found to be superior to the use of either agent alone or placebo [91]. In a well-designed half-head study on a small group of patients with severe AA, adjunctive use of twice-daily 5% topical minoxidil solution with DPCP for 24 weeks did not improve outcome [92]. Injections of ILK to persistent patches of AA in DPCP responders, however, did significantly improve cosmesis [65]. The combined use of anthralin and minoxidil also has been reported to produce an additive effect. In an uncontrolled study on 45 patients with severe refractory AA who had a poor response to monotherapy, twice-daily use of 5% minoxidil with overlying 0.5% anthralin cream at night resulted in cosmetically acceptable regrowth in 11% of patients by 6 months [93]. Serum and urine levels of minoxidil were increased, but systemic

symptoms were absent. The current authors have used this approach in a patient with ophiasis with good effect (Fig. 7).

Management

At the patient's first visit, the nature of the condition, prognosis, and risk–benefit ratio of appropriate treatments should be explained in detail. Questions and concerns should be addressed with compassion and honesty. Sufficient time should be allotted to discuss the impact of alopecia on the patient's psychologic well-being. Information on the National Alopecia Areata Foundation (www.alope ciaareata.org) and local support groups should be offered. Although the threshold for the use of cosmetic aids varies among patients, scalp prostheses and other camouflage techniques should be sensitively broached with patients who have hair loss of more than 50% or rapidly advancing disease, taking care to assure the patient that their use does not imply that the patient's hair loss is permanent.

Because of the capricious nature of the disease and the failure of any one therapy to fundamentally

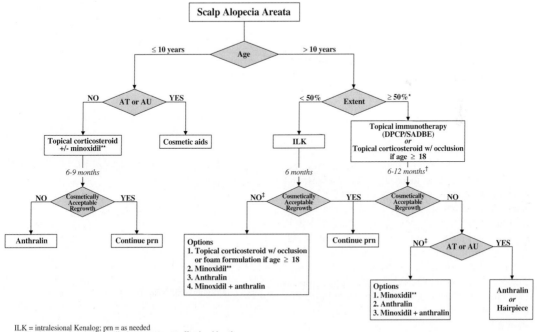

ILK = intralesional Kenalog; prn = as needed
* Consider use of a hairpiece until adequate treatment effect is achieved.
** The authors use 5% topical minoxidil solution exclusively.
† Acceptable response may occur earlier with topical corticosteroid regimen.
‡ In partial responders, compatible agents may be used in combination (see text).

© EKR/JS 2004

Fig. 8. An algorithmic approach for management of AA.

alter its course, no treatment is an important option to offer all patients. This option is particularly relevant to young children for whom the choice of easily tolerated therapies with proven safety is limited. For those who do want treatment, the half-head or half-lesion approach is recommended, to rule out spontaneous remission. With the exception of DPCP and SADBE [64,65], results can be assessed by 3 to 4 months. In responders, treatment is extended to the remaining involved scalp, and once cosmetically acceptable regrowth is achieved (typically, 6–12 mo), attempts to discontinue treatment by slow taper should be made. Partial responders may be offered an alternative agent or may use a second, compatible agent in combination with the first. Nonresponders require use of a different modality.

An algorithmic approach to treatment of AA is shown in Fig. 8. Patients should be stratified according to age and then by extent of disease. In school-age children aged 10 years and younger who have partial scalp hair loss, twice-daily use of a medium-potency topical corticosteroid alone or in combination with twice-daily 5% minoxidil solution is recommended. Short-contact anthralin is a second-line therapeutic agent; potential systemic absorption makes its combined use with minoxidil in this young cohort somewhat prohibitive. AT or AU is probably best managed with the use of cosmetic aids. In patients older than 10 years with involvement of less than 50%, ILK is often effective. Alternative modalities include the nightly use of a potent topical corticosteroid with occlusion (which may prove impractical in those with substantial remaining hair) or foam formulation twice daily, in patients older than 18 years, and 5% minoxidil solution twice daily or short-contact anthralin, which can be used in patients aged 11 to 18 years as well. Acceptable combination regimens are topical corticosteroids with 5% minoxidil, and short-contact anthralin with 5% minoxidil, taking care to monitor for irritation and signs of absorption, particularly in younger patients and patients with more extensive disease. For patients with hair loss of 50% or more, the choice of DPCP, SADBE or clobetasol propionate nightly with occlusion depends on patient age and availability for clinic visits. In responders, ILK is used to treat persistent patches of alopecia. Second-line therapy is topical minoxidil or short-contact anthralin. If combination therapy is used, the surface area exposed should be limited for reasons discussed previously. For motivated patients with refractory AT or AU, a 3- to 4-month trial of short-contact anthralin may be tried. However, the use of a hairpiece may be the best option.

Summary

Because the individual experience of hair loss varies, a customized management plan is required for each patient. The patient should be actively engaged in the development of this plan. For the motivated patient who wants treatment, the selection of modality depends on age, extent of alopecia, comorbid factors, expected outcomes, and patient preference. In patients with mild to moderate pattern hair loss, effective medical and surgical approaches are available; these can be used alone or in combination to further enhance improvement. In patients with advanced pattern hair loss, hair transplantation and hair prostheses should be discussed. The elimination of an identifiable trigger usually underlies the effective management of TE, although this is not always possible. Patients with AA are particularly challenging to manage because of the unpredictable nature of the disease and the lack of a therapeutic cure. A flexible approach is essential, based on changing needs of the patient and evolution of the disease. The initial use of half-head/lesion treatment will control for spontaneous remission. Regardless of the cause of hair loss, the option to forgo treatment is important to discuss with all patients, as is the use of cosmetic means for correction. An open-minded and steadfast approach to management, guided by each patient's needs and expectations, will ensure its success.

Acknowledgments

The authors thank Anne Lee-Fraizer for her helpful and expert assistance with the figure graphics and bibliography.

References

[1] Olsen EA, Messenger AG, Shapiro J, et al. Recommended guidelines for the evaluation and treatment of male and female pattern hair loss. J Am Acad Dermatol 2005;52:301–11.
[2] Olsen EA, Dunlap FE, Funicella T, et al. A randomized clinical trial of 5% topical minoxidil versus 2% topical minoxidil and placebo in the treatment of androgenetic alopecia in men. J Am Acad Dermatol 2002;47:377–85.
[3] Price VH, Menefee E, Strauss PC. Changes in hair weight and hair count in men with androgenetic alopecia, after application of 5% and 2% topical minoxidil, placebo, or no treatment. J Am Acad Dermatol 1999;41:717–21.

[4] Kaufman KD, Olsen EA, Whiting D, et al. Finasteride in the treatment of men with androgenetic alopecia. J Am Acad Dermatol 1998;39:578–89.

[5] Leyden J, Dunlap F, Miller B, et al. Finasteride in the treatment of men with frontal male pattern hair loss. J Am Acad Dermatol 1999;40:930–7.

[6] Finasteride Male Pattern Hair Loss Group. Long-term (5-year) multinational experience with finasteride 1 mg in the treatment of men with androgenetic alopecia. Eur J Dermatol 2002;12:38–49.

[7] Whiting DA, Olsen EA, Savin R, et al. Efficacy and tolerability of finasteride 1 mg in men aged 41 to 60 years with male pattern hair loss. Eur J Dermatol 2003;13:150–60.

[8] Olsen EA, Shapiro J. Managing the patient with androgenetic alopecia: current concepts in diagnosis and treatment (slides and lecture notes). Presented at the Rogaine Speakers Bureau, Pharmacia Corporation, 2001.

[9] Friedman ES, Friedman PM, Cohen DE, Washenik K. Allergic contact dermatitis to topical minoxidil solution: etiology and treatment. J Am Acad Dermatol 2002;46:309–12.

[10] Shapiro J. Safety of topical minoxidil solution: a one-year, prospective, observational study. J Cutan Med Surg 2003;7:322–9.

[11] Monograph on Proscar. Merck & Co., Inc: Whitehouse Station (NJ); April 2004.

[12] Green L, Wysowski DK, Fourcroy JL. Gynecomastia and breast cancer during finasteride therapy. N Engl J Med 1996;335(11):823.

[13] Thompson IM, Goodman PJ, Tangen CM, et al. The influence of finasteride on the development of prostate cancer. N Engl J Med 2003;349(3):213–22.

[14] Monograph on Propecia. Merck & Co., Inc: Whitehouse Station (NJ); October 2003.

[15] Diani AR, Mulholland MJ, Shull KL, et al. Hair growth effects of oral administration of finasteride, a steroid 5α-reductase inhibitor, alone and in combination with topical minoxidil in the balding stumptail macaque. J Clin Endocrinol Metab 1992;74(2):345–50.

[16] Khandpur S, Suman M, Reddy BS. Comparative efficacy of various treatment regimens for androgenetic alopecia in men. J Dermatol 2002;29:489–98.

[17] Meidan VM, Touitou E. Treatments for androgenetic alopecia and alopecia areata: current options and future prospects. Drugs 2001;61(1):53–69.

[18] Olsen EA. Pattern hair loss in men and women. In: Olsen EA, editor. Disorders of hair growth: diagnosis and treatment. 2nd edition. New York: McGraw-Hill; 2003. p. 321–63.

[19] Piérard-Franchimont C, De Doncker P, Cauwenbergh G, Piérard GE. Ketoconazole shampoo: effect of long-term use in androgenic alopecia. Dermatology 1998; 196:474–7.

[20] Bazzano GS, Terezakis N, Galen W. Topical tretinoin for hair growth promotion. J Am Acad Dermatol 1986; 15:880–93.

[21] Shapiro J. Androgenetic alopecia: pathogenesis, clinical features and practical medical treatment. Hair loss: principles of diagnosis and management of alopecia. London: Martin Dunitz; 2002. p. 83–121.

[22] Kantor J, Kessler LJ, Brooks DG, Cotsarelis G. Decreased serum ferritin is associated with alopecia in women. J Invest Dermatol 2003;121:985–8.

[23] Tosti A, Iorizzo M, Vincenzi C. Finasteride treatment may not prevent telogen effluvium after minoxidil withdrawal. Arch Dermatol 2003;139:1221–2.

[24] Avram MR, Cole JP, Gandelman M, et al. The potential role of minoxidil in the hair transplantation setting. Dermatol Surg 2002;28:894–900.

[25] Price VH. Androgenetic alopecia in adolescents. Cutis 2003;71:115–21.

[26] DeVillez RL, Jacobs JP, Szpunar CA, Warner ML. Androgenetic alopecia in the female. Arch Dermatol 1994;130:303–7.

[27] Vexiau P, Chaspoux C, Boudou P, et al. Effects of minoxidil 2% vs. cyproterone acetate treatment on female androgenetic alopecia: a controlled, 12-month randomized trial. Br J Dermatol 2002;146:992–9.

[28] Dawber RPR, Rundegren J. Hypertrichosis in females applying minoxidil topical solution and in normal controls. J Eur Acad Dermatol Venereol 2003;17:271–5.

[29] Fiedler VC, Gray AC. Diffuse alopecia: telogen hair loss. In: Olsen EA, editor. Disorders of hair growth: diagnosis and treatment. 2nd edition. New York: McGraw-Hill; 2003. p. 303–21.

[30] Schwetz BA. New oral contraceptive. JAMA 2001; 286:527.

[31] Raudrant D, Rabe T. Progestogens with antiandrogenic properties. Drugs 2003;63(5):463–92.

[32] Lucky AW, Piacquadio DJ, Ditre CM, et al. A randomized, placebo-controlled trial of 5% and 2% topical minoxidil solutions in the treatment of female pattern hair loss. J Am Acad Dermatol 2004;50:541–53.

[33] Carmina E, Lobo RA. Treatment of hyperandrogenic alopecia in women. Fertil Steril 2003;79:91–5.

[34] Diamanti-Kandarakis E. Current aspects of antiandrogen therapy in women. Curr Pharm Des 1999;5: 707–23.

[35] Sawaya ME. Antiandrogens and androgen inhibitors. In: Wolverton SE, editor. Comprehensive dermatologic drug therapy. Philadelphia: WB Saunders; 2001. p. 385–402.

[36] Price VH, Roberts JL, Hordinsky M, et al. Lack of efficacy of finasteride in postmenopausal women with androgenetic alopecia. J Am Acad Dermatol 2000;43: 768–76.

[37] Thai KE, Sinclair RD. Finasteride for female androgenetic alopecia. Br J Dermatol 2002;147:812–3.

[38] Shum KW, Cullen DR, Messenger AG. Hair loss in women with hyperandrogenism: four cases responding to finasteride. J Am Acad Dermatol 2002;47:733–9.

[39] Goodman NF, Bledsoe MB, Cobin RH, et al. American Association of Clinical Endocrinologists medical guidelines for the clinical practice for the diagnosis and treatment of hyperandrogenic disorders. Endocr Pract 2001;7(2):120–34.

[40] Lobo RA. What are the key features of importance in polycystic ovary syndrome? Fertil Steril 2003;80(2): 259–61.

[41] Shapiro J. Telogen effluvium: acute and chronic. In: Hair loss: principles of diagnosis and management of alopecia. London: Martin Dunitz; 2002. p. 121–35.

[42] Tosti A, Piraccini BM, van Neste DJJ. Telogen effluvium after allergic contact dermatitis of the scalp. Arch Dermatol 2001;137:187–90.

[43] Whiting DA. Chronic telogen effluvium: increased scalp hair shedding in middle-aged women. J Am Acad Dermatol 1996;35:899–906.

[44] Gip L, Lodin A, Molin L. Alopecia areata. A follow-up investigation of outpatient material. Acta Dermatol Venereol 1969;49:180–8.

[45] MacDonald Hull SP, Wood ML, Hutchinson PE, Sladden M, Messenger AG. Guidelines for the management of alopecia areata. Br J Dermatol 2003;149: 692–9.

[46] Mancuso G, Balducci A, Casadio C, et al. Efficacy of betamethasone valerate foam formulation in comparison with betamethasone dipropionate lotion in the treatment of mild-to-moderate alopecia areata: a multicenter, prospective, randomized, controlled, investigator-blinded trial. Int J Dermatol 2003;42:572–5.

[47] Charuwichitratana S, Wattanakrai P, Tanrattanakorn S. Randomized double-blind placebo-controlled trial in the treatment of alopecia areata with 0.25% desoximetasone cream. Arch Dermatol 2000;136:1276–7.

[48] Leyden JL, Kligman AM. Treatment of alopecia areata with steroid solution. Arch Dermatol 1972;106:924.

[49] Pascher F, Kurtin S, Andrade R. Assay of 0.2 percent fluocinolone acetonide cream for alopecia areata and totalis. Dermatologica 1970;141:193–202.

[50] Tosti A, Piraccini BM, Pazzaglia M, Vincenzi C. Clobetasol propionate 0.05% under occlusion in the treatment of alopecia totalis/universalis. J Am Acad Dermatol 2003;49:96–8.

[51] Orentreich N, Sturm HM, Weidman AI, Pelzig A. Local injection of steroids and hair regrowth in alopecias. Arch Dermatol 1960;82:894–902.

[52] Porter D, Burton JL. A comparison of intra-lesional triamcinolone hexacetonide and triamcinolone acetonide in alopecia areata. Br J Dermatol 1971;85:272–3.

[53] Abell E, Munro DD. Intralesional treatment of alopecia areata with triamcinolone acetonide by jet injector. Br J Dermatol 1973;88:55–9.

[54] Kubeyinje EP. Intralesional triamcinolone acetonide in alopecia areata amongst 62 Saudi Arabs. East Afr Med J 1994;71:674–5.

[55] Downs AM, Lear JT, Kennedy CT. Anaphylaxis to intradermal triamcinolone acetonide. Arch Dermatol 1998;134:1163–4.

[56] Selmanowitz VJ, Orentreich N. Cutaneous corticosteroid injection and amaurosis. Analysis for cause and prevention. Arch Dermatol 1974;110:729–34.

[57] Michalowski R, Kuczynska L. Long-term intramuscular triamcinolone acetonide therapy in alopecia areata

[58] Olsen EA, Carson SC, Turney EA. Systemic steroids with or without 2% topical minoxidil in the treatment of alopecia areata. Arch Dermatol 1992;128:1467–73.

[59] Friedli A, Labarthe MP, Engelhardt E, Feldmann R, Salomon D, Saurat JH. Pulse methylprednisolone therapy for severe alopecia areata: an open prospective study of 45 patients. J Am Acad Dermatol 1998;39: 597–602.

[60] Burton JL, Shuster S. Large doses of glucocorticoid in the treatment of alopecia areata. Acta Dermatol Venereol 1975;55:493–6.

[61] Friedli A, Salomon D, Saurat JH. High-dose pulse corticosteroid therapy: is it indicated for severe alopecia areata? Dermatology 2001;202:191–2.

[62] Wilkerson MG, Connor TH, Henkin J, Wilkin JK, Matney TS. Assessment of diphenylcyclopropenone for photochemically induced mutagenicity in the Ames assay. J Am Acad Dermatol 1987;17:606–11.

[63] Happle R, Kalveram KJ, Buchner U, Happle KE, Goggelmann W, Summer KH. Contact allergy as a therapeutic tool for alopecia areata: application of squaric acid dibutylester. Dermatologica 1980;161:289–97.

[64] Rokhsar CK, Shupack JL, Vafai JJ, Washenik K. Efficacy of topical sensitizers in the treatment of alopecia areata. J Am Acad Dermatol 1998;39:751–61.

[65] Wiseman MC, Shapiro J, MacDonald N, Lui H. Predictive model for immunotherapy of alopecia areata with diphencyprone. Arch Dermatol 2001;137: 1063–8.

[66] van der Steen PH, van Baar HM, Happle R, Boezeman JB, Perret CM. Prognostic factors in the treatment of alopecia areata with diphenylcyclopropenone. J Am Acad Dermatol 1991;24:227–30.

[67] Micali G, Cicero RL, Nasca MR, Sapuppo A. Treatment of alopecia areata with squaric acid dibutylester. Int J Dermatol 1996;35:52–6.

[68] Orecchia G, Malagoli P, Santagostino L. Treatment of severe alopecia areata with squaric acid dibutylester in pediatric patients. Pediatr Dermatol 1994;11:65–8.

[69] Schuttelaar ML, Hamstra JJ, Plinck EP, et al. Alopecia areata in children: treatment with diphencyprone. Br J Dermatol 1996;135:581–5.

[70] Tosti A, De Padova MP, Minghetti G, Veronesi S. Therapies versus placebo in the treatment of patchy alopecia areata. J Am Acad Dermatol 1986;15:209–10.

[71] Tosti A, Guidetti MS, Bardazzi F, Misciali C. Long-term results of topical immunotherapy in children with alopecia totalis or alopecia universalis. J Am Acad Dermatol 1996;35:199–201.

[72] Higgins E, du Vivier A. Topical immunotherapy: unapproved uses, dosages, or indications. Clin Dermatol 2002;20:515–21.

[73] Orecchia G, Perfetti L. Alopecia areata and topical sensitizers: allergic response is necessary but irritation is not. Br J Dermatol 1991;124:509.

[74] Shapiro J. Alopecia areata: pathogenesis, clinical

features, diagnosis and practical management. In: Hair loss: principles of diagnosis and management of alopecia. London: Martin Dunitz; 2002. p. 19–83.

[75] Tosti A, Piraccini BM, Misciali C, Vincenzi C. Lentiginous eruption due to topical immunotherapy. Arch Dermatol 2003;139:544–5.

[76] Schmoeckel C, Weissmann I, Plewig G, Braun-Falco O. Treatment of alopecia areata by anthralin-induced dermatitis. Arch Dermatol 1979;115:1254–5.

[77] Nelson DA, Spielvogel R. Anthralin therapy for alopecia areata. Int J Dermatol 1985;24:606–7.

[78] Fiedler-Weiss VC, Buys CM. Evaluation of anthralin in the treatment of alopecia areata. Arch Dermatol 1987;123:1491–3.

[79] Lassus A, Eskelinen A, Johansson E. Treatment of alopecia areata with three different PUVA modalities. Photodermatology 1984;1:141–4.

[80] Healy E, Rogers S. PUVA treatment for alopecia areata—does it work? A retrospective review of 102 cases. Br J Dermatol 1993;129:42–4.

[81] Taylor CR, Hawk JL. PUVA treatment of alopecia areata partialis, totalis and universalis: audit of 10 years' experience at St John's Institute of Dermatology. Br J Dermatol 1995;133:914–8.

[82] Whitmont KJ, Cooper AJ. PUVA treatment of alopecia areata totalis and universalis: a retrospective study. Australas J Dermatol 2003;44:106–9.

[83] Fenton DA, Wilkinson JD. Topical minoxidil in the treatment of alopecia areata. BMJ 1983;287:1015–7.

[84] Vestey JP, Savin JA. A trial of 1% minoxidil used topically for severe alopecia areata. Acta Dermatol Venereol 1986;66:179–80.

[85] Price VH. Double-blind, placebo-controlled evaluation of topical minoxidil in extensive alopecia areata. J Am Acad Dermatol 1987;16:730–6.

[86] Fransway AF, Muller SA. 3 percent topical minoxidil compared with placebo for the treatment of chronic severe alopecia areata. Cutis 1988;41:431–5.

[87] Ranchoff RE, Bergfeld WF, Steck WD, Subichin SJ. Extensive alopecia areata. Results of treatment with 3% topical minoxidil. Cleve Clin J Med 1989;56:149–54.

[88] Fiedler-Weiss VC, West DP, Buys CM, Rumsfield JA. Topical minoxidil dose-response effect in alopecia areata. Arch Dermatol 1986;122:180–2.

[89] Price VH. Topical minoxidil in extensive alopecia areata, including 3-year follow-up. Dermatologica 1987;175(Suppl 2):36–41.

[90] Maitland JM, Aldridge RD, Main RA, White MI, Ormerod AD. Topical minoxidil in the treatment of alopecia areata. BMJ 1984;288:794.

[91] Fiedler VC. Alopecia areata: current therapy. J Invest Dermatol 1991;96:69S–70S.

[92] Shapiro J, Tan J, Ho V, Tron V. Treatment of severe alopecia areata with topical diphenylcyclopropenone and 5% minoxidil: a clinical and immunopathologic evaluation. J Invest Dermatol 1995;104:36S.

[93] Fiedler VC, Wendrow A, Szpunar GJ, Metzler C, DeVillez RL. Treatment-resistant alopecia areata. Response to combination therapy with minoxidil plus anthralin. Arch Dermatol 1990;126:756–9.

ELSEVIER
SAUNDERS

Dermatol Clin 23 (2005) 245 – 258

DERMATOLOGIC
CLINICS

Topical Immunotherapy: What's New

Daniel N. Sauder, MD*, Mona Z. Mofid, MD

*Department of Dermatology, Johns Hopkins University School of Medicine, 601 North Caroline Street, Room 6068,
Baltimore, MD 21205-0900, USA*

In the past several years, there have been major therapeutic advances in dermatology, especially in topical immune response modifiers (IRMs). The skin represents a potent immune organ and plays an important role in the innate and adaptive immune responses, and modulation of these responses can be crucial to influencing numerous dermatoses. IRMs target the immune system (eg, inflammatory cells, cytokines, receptors) to combat a disease process. There is a wide range of these modifiers, including microbial products, natural and synthetic agents, and immune system–derived proteins [1], which target the pathophysiology and biochemical pathways in the disease process. These agents include both proinflammatory and immunosuppressive molecules and have been used to treat many dermatologic conditions. As with many dermatologic therapies, their use has spanned indications approved by the US Food and Drug Administration (FDA) and off-label indications, which have ranged from inflammatory diseases to neoplasms.

The proinflammatory agents include the Toll-like receptor (TLR) agonists (eg, imiquimod and resiquimod) and interferon (eg, interferon α [IFN-α]) and act to boost innate and acquired immune response in part by shifting the balance of the T-helper 1/T-helper 2 (Th1/Th2) paradigm. Immunosuppressive agents target the body's inflammatory or immune response and include the following: topical and intralesional corticosteroids (which dermatologists have been using for decades); the newer anti–tumor necrosis factor (anti-TNF) agents being used for psoriasis

(eg, infliximab and etanercept); and anti-CD4$^+$ T-cell agents, including calcineurin inhibitors and mycophenolate. By targeting the immune system, immunomodulators potentially have prolonged therapeutic effects because they engage the immune memory, which can then recognize and respond to the disease long-term. Topical therapies offer several advantages over systemic therapies, both practically and therapeutically. The ease of application is advantageous, and pharmacologically topical therapies confer a localized effect with a much lower risk of adverse systemic effects [2,3]. This article discusses several of the newer topical agents that leverage the body's immune system to treat dermatologic conditions and that have many promising and novel therapeutic applications (Box 1).

What are Toll-like receptors and how do they work?

The immune system can be subdivided into the innate immune system and the adaptive or acquired immune system. The innate immune system relies on phagocytic cells to recognize pathogens (either by complement fixation or by binding to specific receptor recognition molecules); this action then activates pathways, including natural killer cells (NKs). The adaptive or acquired arm of the immune response relies on the recognition of foreign antigen presentation by major histocompatibility complex (MHC) classes I and II (MHC I, MHC II) and by antigen-presenting cells (APCs), such as the epidermal Langerhans' cells (LCs).

Although somewhat primitive compared with the adaptive immune response, the innate response is

---

* Corresponding author.
E-mail address: dsauder@jhmi.edu (D.N. Sauder).

derm.theclinics.com

Box 1. Topical immune response modifiers in dermatology

Toll-like receptor agonists
  Imiquimod 5% cream (Aldara)
  Resiquimod

Immunosuppressive agents
  Topical corticosteroids
  Calcineur inhibitors: macrolactams
    Tacrolimus 0.03%,
      ointment (Protopic) 0.1%
    Pimecrolimus 1% cream (Elidel)

---

able to react rapidly and nonspecifically. The innate immune system uses a series of receptors termed *pattern-recognition receptors* to detect the presence of pathogens, tissue injury, and malignancy, and to allow the host to orchestrate a rapid response. That recognition in mammals, directed by macrophages and dendritic cells, allows diverse signaling pathways to be activated and is a crucial component of the innate defense. The action of the innate immune system is mediated in part by activation through TLRs. Toll receptors were initially identified in the fruit fly, *Drosophila melanogaster*, and were noted to play a key role in its antifungal defenses [4]. The mammalian homologs of Toll receptors, TLRs, are expressed on APCs (eg, macrophages and dendritic cells). TLRs are a family of type I transmembrane receptors that are pattern-recognition receptors and that are activated by conserved structures on microbes and certain host molecules. At least 10 TLR genes have been identified in mice and humans [5]. Their extracellular amino-terminus has a leucine-rich repeat, whereas the carboxy-terminal cytoplasmic tail harbors a conserved region known as the Toll/interleukin 1 (IL-1) receptor domain, which exhibits remarkable similarity to the cytoplasmic region of the IL-1 superfamily of receptors and triggers a common intracellular signal transduction cascade [6]. The engagement of the TLRs with their ligands elicits a pathogen-specific cellular immune response that ultimately provokes various proinflammatory and antimicrobial responses, such as the induction of cytokines and chemokines, in addition to the recruitment of neutrophils to the site of defense [7]. This stimulation depends on the protein MyD88, which, when activated, recruits protein kinases and transcription factors and activates nuclear factor κB (NF-κB), which then stimulates the production of key cytokines, such as IFN-α, TNF-α, IL-1, IL-6, and

IL-12 [8]. This process allows for critical intervention in the influence of the adaptive Th1-type and Th2 immune responses by up-regulating the Th1 immune response and down-regulating the Th2 immune response.

Th cells are CD4+ cells that recognize antigenic peptides in association with their MHC class II molecules. There are several Th cells that have been described and that have been categorized primarily on the basis of their cytokine secretion patterns. The differentiation of their cytokine secretion pattern is used to separate Th1 from Th2 cells. Th1 cytokines preferentially induce cell-mediated or innate immunity and, although they secrete several cytokines, they are typified by IL-2, IFN-γ and TNF-β. Psoriasis is a typical Th1-mediated disease. Th2 cytokines preferentially induce humoral immunity and are typified by secreting cytokines IL-4, IL-5, IL-6, IL-9, IL-10, and IL-13. This process favors antibody production; Th2 responses are often associated mainly with allergic diseases, such as the acute phase of atopic dermatitis (AD). It is important to recognize that numerous dermatoses are T-cell mediated and may favor, but are not exclusive to, a Th1- or Th2-mediated pathway.

TLRs have been detected in human neutrophils and macrophages and dendritic, dermal endothelial, mucosal epithelial, B, and T cells [9]. They alert the immune system to the presence of a pathogen. In addition, TLRs function as sentinels in the mammalian immune response affecting both innate and cell-mediated immunity; therefore, influencing the TLRs in certain dermatologic conditions can offer opportunities for the development of new remedies.

Toll-like receptor agonists

Imiquimod 5% cream (Aldara) was approved by the FDA for the treatment of external genital and perianal warts in adults in 1997; in 2004, this drug received FDA approval for the treatment of actinic keratoses (AKs) of the face and scalp followed by approval for the treatment of superficial basal cell carcinoma on the body, neck, arms, or legs. It is the first member of the imidazoquinolinamine family of TLR agonists and acts primarily at TLR-7 (Fig. 1) [8]. Imiquimod's exact mechanism of action in viral, neoplastic, and immunoregulatory diseases has not yet been fully elucidated; however, it has been shown to stimulate the innate immune response by increasing NKC activity, in addition to the production of cytokines and nitric oxide from dendritic cells of monocyte/macrophyte origin in addition to the

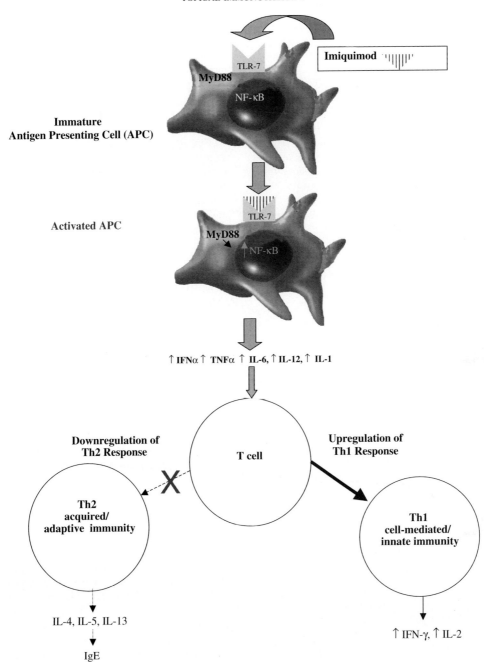

Fig. 1. Imiquimod's mechanism of action at the TLR, a simplified approach.

induction, proliferation, and differentiation of B lymphocytes [9]. Specifically, imiquimod's activation of TLR-7 stimulates the NF-κB cascade, which in turn stimulates secretion of proinflammatory cytokines (eg, IFN-α, TNF-α, IL-6) [10–12]. The stimulation of IFN-α by dendritic cells and mono-cytes promotes CD4+ Th1 cytokines, inducing the production of cytokines, including IFN-γ and IL-2, and down-regulating the Th2 response. IFN-α and IFN-γ also act to inhibit production of IL-4 and IL-5 by Th2 cells [10,13]. IFN-γ and IL-2 furthermore activate CD8+ cells to become cytotoxic T cells, allowing them to kill virus-infected and tumor cells (Box 2) [10,13].

LCs play an important role in the immune response and are the relevant APCs in the epidermis because they recognize, engulf, and process antigens; migrate to regional lymph nodes; and induce activation of specific lymphocytes. Studies have shown that imiquimod enhances the maturation of LCs into potent APCs and enhances their mobility for migration to draining lymph nodes where they are able to present antigen to T lymphocytes and induce true

---

Box 2. Mechanism of actions of imiquimod

- Increasing NKC activity
- Maturation of LCs to APCs
- Increased migration of dendritic cells to lymph nodes
- Induction of proliferation and differentiation of B lymphocytes
- Activation of macrophages to secrete cytokines by means of TLR-7-MyD88–dependent signaling cascade
    Major cytokines stimulated by activation of the TLR-7
    IFN-α
    TNF-α
    IL-6
    Additional cytokines involved
    IL-1, IL-5, IL-8, IL-10, and IL-12
    IL-1 receptor antagonist
    Granulocyte colony–stimulating factor
    Granulocyte-macrophage colony–stimulating factor
    Macrophage inflammatory protein 1α and 1β
    Macrophage chemotactic protein 1
- Up-regulating Th1 pathway and down-regulating Th2 pathway; increasing IFN-γ and IL-2 production
- Stimulation of cytotoxic T cells [15,86]
- Induction of immunologic memory, potentially preventing disease recurrence [87]
- Induction of cell surface expression FasR on tumor cells, leading to apoptosis [88]
- Alteration of expression of caspase 3 and DNA fragment factor in keloids [39]

T-cell–mediated immunity [10,14,15]. Therefore, several possible explanations exist for topical imiquimod's effectiveness in treating many dermatologic diseases.

Imiquimod in the treatment of viral disease

Human papillomavirus (HPV) is a nonenveloped, double-stranded DNA virus that infects the basal keratinocytes in the epidermis of skin or mucosa. More than 100 genotypes of HPV have been identified [16], and viral infections with HPV have been responsible for various cutaneous diseases, including precancerous and malignant conditions, which often prove challenging and cumbersome for clinicians to treat [17] and difficult, time-consuming, and often painful for the patient undergoing treatment. HPV infects keratinocytes but does not induce LCs to present viral antigens; in addition, it often lies relatively dormant, making it especially evasive and difficult for the host to elicit an effective immune response. It is hypothesized that patients infected with HPV may lack a memory T-cell population able to target HPV, that they lack HPV-specific T cells that are able to migrate to the site of infection or to secrete the necessary cytokines to mount an effective antiviral response [1,9,18]. Because an immune response is often required to mount an effective antiviral response against HPV, many of the current therapies are not effective.

Imiquimod received its initial indication for the treatment of condylomata acuminata in 1997 and has been used in varying dosing regimens with impressive results. Since then, imiquimod 5% cream has been used outside of its indication with varying degrees of success to treat numerous other viral and HPV-induced conditions, as both monotherapy and as adjunctive therapy. It has been used in combination with other topical agents and traditional destructive techniques and has been used in conditions ranging from plantar warts to epidermodysplasia verruciformis. Imiquimod also has been used successfully to treat molluscum contagiosum, where one study showed complete remission in 53% of patients, including adults and children (Box 3) [19].

Furthermore, there have been many encouraging studies reported using imiquimod 5% cream to treat nongenital cutaneous warts in HIV-infected and other immunosuppressed patients [20]. Research in organ transplant recipients has been done in which the incidence of viral warts, depending on the level of the patient's immunosuppression, ranges from 24% to 53% [20]. Because these patients are immunosup-

Box 3. Conditions reported to be responsive to topical imiquimod as monotherapy or in combination with other therapies

Viral-induced
HPV-associated
Plantar warts [89 – 91]
Common warts [92,93]
Flat warts [94,95]
Butcher's warts [96]
Condylomata acuminata/anogenital warts [97 – 100]

HPV-induced associated with malignancy
Intraepithelial neoplasia [101 – 103]
Bowenoid papulosis [86,104,105]
Erythroplasia of Queyrat [86]
Epidermodysplasia verruciformis [106]
Verrucous carcinoma/Buschke-Lowenstein tumor [107]

Other viral
Genital herpes [108 – 110]
Molluscum contagiosum (poxvirus) [41,111]

Neoplastic
AK [112 – 114]
Actinic cheilitis [115]
Squamous cell carcinoma (SCC)
SCC in situ [116 – 118]
Bowen's disease [116,118]
Keratoacanthoma-type [119,120]
Invasive [117,121]
Basal cell carcinoma (BCC)
Superficial [122,123]
Nodular [124]
Multiple BCCs in patients with xeroderma pigmentosum [32,125]
Multiple BCCs in patients with basal cell nevus syndrome [33]
Melanoma
Lentigo maligna [38,126,127]
Melanoma skin metastases [128,129]
Extramammary Paget's disease [130 – 132]
Cutaneous T-cell lymphoma [133]

Immune-mediated
Localized morphea [134]
Chronic discoid lupus erythematosus [135]

Other
Keloids [39,136]
Granuloma annulare [137,138]
Infantile hemangioma [139]
Porokeratosis of Mibelli [140,141]
Leishmaniasis [142]

pressed, viral warts are of different prognostic importance, because not only are the patients more susceptible to opportunistic pathogens but spontaneous regression is low. Some transplant patients may be poor candidates for traditional destructive or systemic therapies because their treatments are often complicated by impaired wound healing and increased susceptiblity to skin infections. Recent studies have suggested that most transplant recipients will develop HPV-induced warts with an increased likelihood of malignant progression to SCC [20] and that these patients have an increased frequency of SCC, up to 150-fold more than that of the general population [20]. It has been hypothesized that the transformation of viral warts to malignant lesions is in part caused by ultraviolet radiation (UV-) – induced immunosuppression (which causes mutations in cellular DNA and impairs the cellular immune system) in concert with the HPV infection [21] and that 40% of transplant patients will develop premalignant or malignant skin tumors within 5 years of receiving their new organ [21]. By enabling a localized immune response that targets HPV in these patients, there have been decreases in the malignant transformation contributed to by HPV, which significantly alters the progression of AKs to SCC, thereby increasing the survival and decreasing the morbidity in these patients [21].

Imiquimod as an antineoplastic agent

There are several topical agents on the market for the treatment of AKs, including 5-fluorouracil (Efudex, Carac), diclofenac (Solaraze), photodynamic therapy (Levulan), chemical peels, and topical retinoids. Traditional treatment modalities, including cryosurgery, curettage, and chemical destruction, also remain at the forefront; however, it is advantageous not only to treat apparent lesions but to destroy subclinical lesions as well.

AKs are squamoproliferative lesions of keratinocytes in the epidermis, and UV radiation is believed to be the impetus for this neoplastic transformation. AKs account for approximately 14% of visits to dermatologists in the United States, and it is believed that 0.25% to 1% of these lesions will convert to SCC each year [22,23]. AKs are the most important risk factor for those individuals predisposed to the development of SCC, with their presence most likely being an early stage in a biologic continuum [24]. Studies have shown that on sun-damaged skin, up to 60% of SCCs begin as AKs. This finding is histologically supported by evidence that AKs were contiguous with the SCC in 97% of these cases [25,26]. Imiquimod not only has immunomodulatory effects but has shown antineoplastic activity in vitro in human keratinocyte and SCC cell lines [11,27] by inducing skin tumor cell–specific apoptosis [28]. The activation of the immune response may enhance tumor recognition and may allow localized targeting of tumor cells by means of the promotion of cell infiltration (eg, T cells, NKCs) at the tumor site, leading to tumor clearance or shrinkage and the up-regulation of the Th1 system. These findings can also help explain imiquimod's antineoplastic effects [10,11].

BCC is the most common malignancy among white individuals worldwide, and UV radiation plays several key roles in the development of BCC. UV radiation has been shown to produce DNA damage and immunosuppression by altering antigen-presenting ability and the generation of immunosuppressive cytokines (IL-10, TNF-α) [28]. Because topical imiquimod exhibits antitumor activity, it is rational to consider this agent as a nonsurgical treatment option for BCCs [29]. Several studies have shown efficacy in the treatment of BCCs, both superficial and nodular (in varying dosing regimens and durations), with topical imiquimod [30,31]. Successful outcomes in patients predisposed to numerous BCCs, as with xeroderma pigmentosum [32] and basal cell nevus syndrome, also have been reported [33,34].

How does imiquimod work in basal cell carcinoma?

The release of IFN-α and other immune cytokines results in the activation of the innate immune system. Activated macrophages and dendritic cells can release oxygen-reactive intermediates, leading to apoptosis of tumor cells, which suggests that T-cell activation is not the major factor in imiquimod's efficacy [35]. There have been some studies that lend additional insight into the drug's antineoplastic activity, however. Fas receptors (FasR, CD-95) are members of the TNF receptor family and are a group of receptors involved in apoptosis [36]. Tumor cells are able to avoid apoptotic signaling by reducing their expression of FasR, which contributes to their longevity; moreover, these tumor cells are able to strongly express FasL, which likely induces apoptosis in infiltrating antitumor T lymphocytes [36]. The binding of FasR to its ligand (FasL) activates a cascade, which includes caspase activation and ultimately leads to cell death; the FasR–FasL interaction has been shown to play a role in cancer development [37]. Studies have revealed that BCC cells typically do not express FasR but show that IFN-α (induced by imiquimod) is able to induce the expression of FasR

on BCCs. Furthermore, the interaction between the Fasr and FasL is hypothesized to lead to apoptosis [36]. This imiquimod-induced FasR-mediated apoptosis is likely a key component in the drug's effectiveness in the treatment of BCC.

In addition to studies showing the efficacy of topical imiquimod in AKs, SCCs, and BCCs, Naylor et al [38] have published data on its use in the treatment of lentigo maligna, where they demonstrated that 93% of patients (26 of 28) treated with imiquimod 5% cream daily for 3 months achieved a complete response. Lentigo maligna has often proved challenging to treat because of the extent of the lesion, patient age, and high recurrence rates, and therefore a nonsurgical intervention, such as topical imiquimod, may have a significant impact on the disease, either as monotherapy or adjuvant therapy. In addition, if topical imiquimod is able to induce immunologic memory against melanoma cells, this process could contribute to a reduction in the recurrence rate.

Imiquimod and future use

Imiquimod is an IMR that is able to enhance the immune function by stimulating both the innate and adaptive arms of the immune system and has antiviral, antiproliferative, antiangiogenic, and immune-enhancing properties. It has been found to be effective in the treatment of numerous conditions. In keloids, which exhibit aberrant expression of apoptotic genes, imiquimod has been shown to alter the gene expression of markers as previously shown in its efficacy in BCC [39]. Jacob et al [39] have identified genes associated with apoptosis, including caspase 3 and DNA fragment factor-45, or *DFFA*, whose expression is altered by imiquimod in keloids and which may suggest a mechanism of action for imquimod's antiproliferative effect on these lesions.

Many studies have shown topical imiquimod to be well tolerated. The most common side effects include erythema, pruritus, burning, and pain [40,41]. The lack of systemic side effects correspond with the low rate of systemic absorption, which was observed to be less than 1% in the urine after one application of cream [11]. The only contraindication is in the case of hypersensitivity, which is rare [40].

Resiquimod (R-848), a second-generation imidazoquinolinamine, is currently under investigation for the treatment of various conditions, including herpes simplex virus [42], but it is likely that other IRMs will be developed for more specific dermatologic applications.

Imiquimod's place in the therapeutic armamentarium, as monotherapy and in combination with other topical, destructive, and systemic therapies, is promising and continued developments in understanding the mechanism and future applications are evolving rapidly. Clinicans should be cautioned, however, that many reported successes using topical imiquimod have been secondary to combination therapy, and the possibility of a host response unrelated to the use of the medication always remains a possibility. Studies using imiquimod as a treatment for various benign, premalignant, and malignant diseases are promising.

Immunosuppressive treatments

Physicians have used steroids as immunosuppressive therapy since 1949 when synthetic cortisone was first used to treat rheumatoid arthritis; the development of topical hydrocortisone rapidly followed in the early 1950s [43]. For decades, topical corticosteroids have been the mainstay of treatment for various dermatologic conditions, including AD, psoriasis, and alopecia; however, their use often has been limited by their potential for side effects, which include cutaneous atrophy, telangiectasias, and perioral dermatitis. The newer topical agents have provided increased options to bypass these and other potential side effects of topical steroids.

Cyclosporine was the first anti–T-cell immunosuppressive agent to be used clinically in transplantation medicine and was introduced in the early 1980s [44]. Cyclosporine, a lipophilic polypeptide, binds to the immunophilin cyclophilin. It is a calcineurin inhibitor that is structurally and functionally different from the macrolactam family of compounds. The cyclosporine-cyclophilin complex calcineurin, which is a calcium-dependent phosphatase, is necessary for the activation of the nuclear factor of activated T cells (NF-AT) transcription factor [44]. When activated, NF-AT binds to the IL-2 gene promotor (in addition to others), which initiates transcription and thus IL-2 production. This process suppresses T-cell activation and proliferation, reducing the T-cell–mediated response. Cyclosporine is poorly absorbed through the skin, however, and is not effective as a topical agent. [45] There are at present two effective topical calcineurin inhibitors.

Calcineurin inhibitors

The macrolactam immunomodulators, isolated from various species of *Streptomyces*, are antifungal derivatives and encompass a group of topical immunosuppressive drugs that target activated T-cell responses to protein antigens. Their mechanism of action is similar to that of cyclosporine in that they block calcineurin; however, they interact with the macrophilin immunophilins and not cyclophilin. The topical calcineurin inhibitors currently used in the treatment of dermatologic diseases include tacrolimus and pimecrolimus; in addition, they have gained favor in the treatment of AD because they do not have steroidal side effects [46]. Furthermore, because of their lipophilic characteristics, systemic absorption is limited, which allows nonsystemic, localized treatment (Table 1).

Tacrolimus

Tacrolimus (FK506) in its oral form was used in transplant patients for many years to prevent organ transplant rejection. Its topical form (Protopic) was approved by the FDA in 2001 for the treatment of AD, which is estimated to affect 20% of the worldwide population [47]. Tacrolimus binds to the FK-binding protein or macrophilin 12. The resulting complex blocks calcineurin activation of NF-AT and transcription of NF-AT–dependent genes, including IL-2 [48,49], IL-4, and IL-5, and in some cells, IL-8 [47]. In a preclinical animal model of induced allergic-contact dermatitis, tacrolimus reduced levels of IL-1α and IL-1β, granulocyte-macrophage colony–stimulating factor (GM-CSF), TNF-α, macrophage inflammatory protein 2, and IFN-γ RNA [50]. In addition, in an ex vivo study in human peripheral blood mononuclear cells, tacrolimus inhibited both Th1 (eg, IL-2, IFN-γ) and Th2 cytokines (eg, IL-4, IL-5) and IL-3 and GM-CSF. Its inhibition of cytokine production was equal or superior to mid-potency topical steroids. Furthermore, studies have indicated that the percutaneous absorption of tacrolimus decreases with continued treatment, leading to a favorable long-term safety and tolerability profile [46].

Tacrolimus is currently available in the US market in ointment form in concentrations of 0.03% and 0.1%. It is indicated for short-term and intermittent long-term therapy in the treatment of children and adults with moderate to severe AD. Preliminary data from several studies have demonstrated that tacrolimus ointment is more effective than pimecrolimus cream in the treatment of AD in both adults and children [51]. Although it seems to be more potent than the other topical calcineurin inhibitors, however, application site reactions are more common (Fig. 2).

Table 1
Topical calcineurin inhibitors

Inhibitors	Tacrolimus	Pimecrolimus
Trade name	Protopic	Elidel
Vehicle	Ointment	Cream
Quantity dispensed	30 g, 60 g, 100 g	30 g, 60 g, 100 g
FDA approved	Feb 2001	March 2002
FDA indication	Moderate to severe AD	Mild to moderate AD
Age indication	0.03%, ages 2–15 y	Indicated for patients ≥ 2 y
	0.1%, ages >15 y	

These reactions include pruritus and erythema, usually during the first few days of treatment; they are generally transient and only occasionally result in the discontinuation of treatment [52]. Some patients have found that refrigerating the medication, keeping it cool, helps to decrease these side effects.

Tacrolimus has been used outside of its indication for many other dermatologic conditions, including seborrheic dermatitis [53,54], contact dermatitis [55], rosacea [56], bullous pemphigoid [57,58], Hailey-Hailey disease [59], granuloma faciale [60], vulvar/anogenital lichen sclerosus [61,62], and oral lichen planus. In addition, using tacrolimus ointment in combination with other agents, such as midpotency topical corticosteroids, can often yield more effective results than treatment with either agent alone [63].

Pimecrolimus

Pimecrolimus (ASM981, Elidel) was approved by the FDA in 2002. Pimecrolimus, also a calcineurin inhibitor in the macrolactam family, is an ascomycin deriviative. It is structurally similar to tacrolimus and also binds to macrophilin 12; however, it has a threefold lower binding affinity [64]. It has been shown to prevent the release of proinflammatoy cytokines in mast cells [65] and also acts to prevent calcineurin dephosphorylation of NF-AT. Pimecrolimus has shown comparable efficacy to betamethasone-17-valerate in the treatment of allergic-contact dermatitis. Furthermore, because it is not a steroid, it does not lead to atrophogenic or other commonly associated adverse effects of topical corticosteroids (including the concern over hypothalamic–pituitary–adrenal axis suppression in children treated with moderate- and high-potency topical corticosteroids) [66,67]. Billich et al [68] found that pimecrolimus had a lower degree of percutaneous absorption as

compared with tacrolimus and much lower than corticosteroids, which is likely explained by its higher lipophilicity and higher molecular weight.

Pimecrolimus 1% cream is indicated for short-term and intermittent long-term therapy in the treatment of mild to moderate AD in patients older than 2 years and has been well tolerated in studies of children as young as 1 year [69,70]. Although this agent has similar local application-site reactions as tacrolimus, it seems to be better tolerated, which may affect patient compliance [71]. As with tacrolimus, pimecrolimus has been used off-label in numerous other inflammatory dermatologic conditions [72–74].

Because these agents are topical immunosuppressants, caution must be used in prescribing these medications off-label in the presence of infectious organisms, such as molluscum, herpes simplex virus, and varicella. Reported cases associated with its use have included tinea incognito [75] and eczema molluscatum [76].

Other topical immunosuppressant agents are currently under investigation. Mycophenolate mofetil, a semisynthetic morpholinoethyl ester of mycophenolic acid, is rapidly hydrolyzed to mycophenolic acid following digestion [77]. It confers immunosuppressive, antibacterial, antiviral, and antifungal activity, and noncompetitively inhibits eukaryotic inosine monophosphate dehydrogenase (IMP-DH) conversion of iosine-5-phosphate and xanthine-5-phosphate to guanosine-5- phosphate, which is a necessary precursor for RNA and DNA synthesis [77]. IMP-DH is a key enzyme in the de novo purine biosynthesis pathway. Therefore, by targeting cell types undergoing de novo purine synthesis, such as T and B lymphocytes, mycophenolate mofetil inhibits antibody production, antigen presentation, cytotoxic T-cell activation, fibroblast proliferation, and leukocyte influx [78,79]. The oral form is efficacious in the treatment of several dermatologic conditions, includ-

Fig. 2. Mechanism of action of calcineurin inhibitors in T cells. FKBP, FK binding protein; NF-ATc, NF-AT cytoplasmic; NF-ATn, NF-AT nuclear; P, phosphorylated.

Antigen Presenting Cell- T cell interaction leads to increased Ca^{2+} in T cell which binds calmodulin

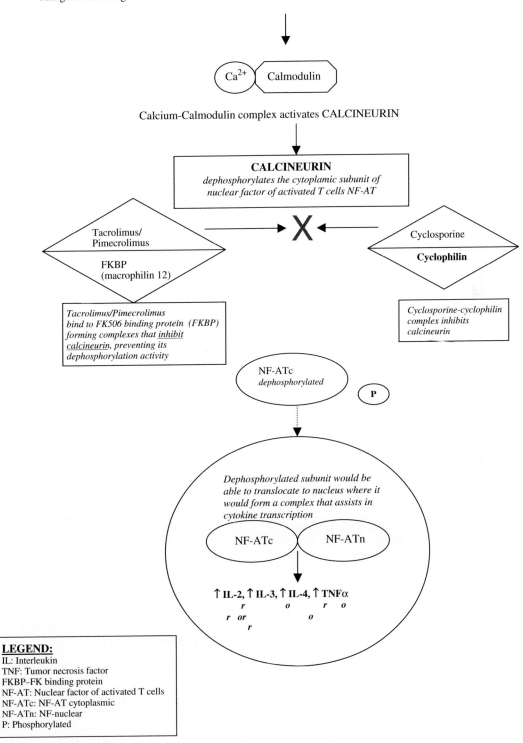

Calcium-Calmodulin complex activates CALCINEURIN

CALCINEURIN
dephosphorylates the cytoplamic subunit of nuclear factor of activated T cells NF-AT

Tacrolimus/Pimecrolimus

FKBP (macrophilin 12)

Cyclosporine

Cyclophilin

Tacrolimus/Pimecrolimus bind to FK506 binding protein (FKBP) forming complexes that <u>inhibit calcineurin</u>, preventing its dephosphorylation activity

Cyclosporine-cyclophilin complex inhibits calcineurin

NF-ATc
dephosphorylated

P

Dephosphorylated subunit would be able to translocate to nucleus where it would form a complex that assists in cytokine transcription

NF-ATc   NF-ATn

↑ IL-2, ↑ IL-3, ↑ IL-4, ↑ TNFα

LEGEND:
IL: Interleukin
TNF: Tumor necrosis factor
FKBP–FK binding protein
NF-AT: Nuclear factor of activated T cells
NF-ATc: NF-AT cytoplasmic
NF-ATn: NF-nuclear
P: Phosphorylated

ing immunobullous diseases [3,80], psoriasis [81,82], AD [3], eczema [83], and pyoderma gangrenosum [84]. The risk profile includes the development of malignancy, neutropenia, and infection [77]. Topical mycophenolate has been reported to be effective in treating psoriasis [85] and is currently under investigation for other dermatoses.

Summary

Further understanding of the pathogenesis of dermatologic conditions at a molecular level has led to targeted therapies. The topical IMRs have contributed significantly to the treatment of cutaneous diseases. New topical remedies, particularly the TLR agonists and calcineurin inhibitors, have added to the clinical armamentarium and further advanced clinicians' ability to treat a wide variety of benign, premalignant, and malignant conditions. Furthermore, these agents have in turn contributed further knowledge to an understanding of the disease process. The next decade will witness even greater advances in targeted immunotherapies for dermatologic disease.

References

[1] Hengge UR, Benninghoff B, Ruzicka T, Goos M. Topical immunomodulators—progress towards treating inflammation, infection, and cancer. Lancet Infect Dis 2001;1(3):189–98.

[2] Smith KJ, Germain M, Skelton H. Squamous cell carcinoma in situ (Bowen's disease) in renal transplant patients treated with 5% imiquimod and 5% 5-fluorouracil therapy. Dermatol Surg 2001;27(6): 561–4.

[3] Grundmann-Kollmann M, Korting HC, Behrens S, Kaskel P, Leiter U, Krahn G, et al. Mycophenolate mofetil: a new therapeutic option in the treatment of blistering autoimmune diseases. J Am Acad Dermatol 1999;40:957–60.

[4] Lemaitre B, Nicolas E, Michaut L, Reichhart JM, Hoffmann JA. The dorsoventral regulatory gene cassette spatzle/Toll/cactus controls the potent antifungal response in Drosophila adults. Cell 1996;20; 86(6):973–83.

[5] Chuang T, Ulevitch RJ. Identification of hTLR10: a novel human Toll-like receptor preferentially expressed in immune cells. Biochim Biophys Acta 2001;1518(1–2):157–61.

[6] Takeda K, Akira S. Microbial recognition by Toll-like receptors. J Dermatol Sci 2004;34(2):73–82.

[7] Armant MA, Fenton MJ. Toll-like receptors: a family of pattern-recognition receptors in mammals. Genome Biol 2002;3(8):reviews 3011.1–reviews 3011.6.

[8] Gaspari AA, Sauder DN. Immunotherapy of basal cell carcinoma: evolving approaches. Dermatol Surg 2003;29:1027–34.

[9] Sauder DN. Imiquimod: modes of action. Br J Dermatol 2003;149(Suppl 66):5–8.

[10] Hemmi H, Kaisho T, Takeuchi O, Sato S, Sanjo H, Hoshino K, et al. Small anti-viral compounds activate immune cells via the TLR7 MyD88-dependent signaling pathway. Nat Immunol 2002;3(2):196–200.

[11] Sauder DN. Immunomodulatory and pharmacologic properties of imiquimod. J Am Acad Dermatol 2000; 43:S6–11.

[12] Miller RL, Tomai MA, Harrison CJ, Bernstein DI. Immunomodulation as a treatment strategy for genital herpes: review of the evidence. Int Immunopharmacol 2002;2(4):443–51.

[13] Burns Jr RP, Ferbel B, Tomai M, Miller R, Gaspari AA. The imidazoquinolines, imiquimod and R-848, induce functional, but not phenotypic, maturation of human epidermal Langerhans' cells. Clin Immunol 2000;94(1):13–23.

[14] Suzuki H, Wang B, Shivji GM, Toto P, Amerio P, Tomai MA, et al. Imiquimod, a topical immune response modifier, induces migration of Langerhans cells. J Invest Dermatol 2000;114(1):135–41.

[15] Petrow W, Gerdsen R, Uerlich M, Richter O, Bieber T. Successful topical immunotherapy of bowenoid papulosis with imiquimod. Br J Dermatol 2001; 145(6):1022–3.

[16] Kirnbauer R, Lenz P, Okun M. Human papillomavirus. In: Bolognia JL, Jorizzo JL, Rapini RP, editors. Dermatology. Philadelphia: Mosby; 2003. p. 1217.

[17] Koutsky LA, Galloway DA, Holmes KK. Epidemiology of genital human papillomavirus infection. Epidemiol Rev 1988;10:122–63.

[18] Hengge UR, Cusini M. Topical immunomodulators for the treatment of external genital warts, cutaneous warts and molluscum contagiosum. Br J Dermatol 2003;149(Suppl 66):15–9.

[19] Hengge UR, Esser S, Schultewolter T, Behrendt C, Meyer T, Stockfleth E, et al. Self-administered topical 5% imiquimod for the treatment of common warts and molluscum contagiosum. Br J Dermatol 2000; 143(5):1026–31.

[20] Leffell DJ. The scientific basis of skin cancer. J Am Acad Dermatol 2000;42:18–22.

[21] Stockfleth E, Ulrich C, Meyer T, Christophers E. Epithelial malignancies in organ transplant patients: clinical presentation and new methods of treatment. Recent Results Cancer Res 2002;160:251–8.

[22] Gupta AK, Cooper EA, Feldman SR, Fleischer Jr AB. A survey of office visits for actinic keratosis as reported by NAMCS, 1990–1999. National Ambulatory Medical Care Survey. Cutis 2002;70S:8–13.

[23] Jeffes EW, Tang EH. Actinic keratosis. Current treatment options. Am J Clin Dermatol 2000;1:167–79.

[24] Salasche SJ. Epidemiology of actinic keratoses and squamous cell carcinoma. J Am Acad Dermatol 2000; 42:4–7.

[25] Hurwitz RM, Monger LE. Solar keratosis: an evolving squamous cell carcinoma. Benign or malignant? Dermatol Surg 1995;21(2):184.

[26] Marks R, Renne G, Selwood TS. Malignant transformation of solar keratosis to squamous cell carcinoma. Lancet 1998;1:795–7.

[27] Beg AA. Endogenous ligands of Toll-like receptors: implications for regulating inflammatory and immune responses. Trends Immunol 2002;23(11):509–12.

[28] Grossman D, Leffell DJ. The molecular basis of nonmelanoma skin cancer: new understanding. Arch Dermatol 1997;133(10):1263–70.

[29] Greenway HT, Cornell RC, Tanner DJ, Peets E, Bordin GM, Nagi C. Treatment of basal cell carcinoma with intralesional interferon. J Am Acad Dermatol 1986;15(3):437–43.

[30] Geisse JK, Rich P, Pandya A, Gross K, Andres K, Ginkel A, et al. Imiquimod 5% cream for the treatment of superficial basal cell carcinoma: a double-blind, randomized, vehicle-controlled study. J Am Acad Dermatol 2002;47(3):390–8.

[31] Sterry W, Ruzicka T, Herrera E, Takwale A, Bichel J, Andres K, et al. Imiquimod 5% cream for the treatment of superficial and nodular basal cell carcinoma: randomized studies comparing low-frequency dosing with and without occlusion. Br J Dermatol 2002;147(6):1227–36.

[32] Weisberg NK, Varghese M. Therapeutic response of a brother and sister with xeroderma pigmentosum to imiquimod 5% cream. Dermatol Surg 2002;28(6): 518–23.

[33] Kagy MK, Amonette R. The use of imiquimod 5% cream for the treatment of superficial basal cell carcinomas in a basal cell nevus syndrome patient. Dermatol Surg 2000;26:577–8.

[34] Beutner KR, Geisse JK, Helman D, Fox TL, Ginkel A, Owens ML. Therapeutic response of basal cell carcinoma to the immune response modifier imiquimod 5% cream. J Am Acad Dermatol 1999;41(6): 1002–7.

[35] Dummer R, Urosevic M, Kempf W, Hoek K, Hafner J, Burg G. Imiquimod in basal cell carcinoma: how does it work? Br J Dermatol 2003;149(Suppl 66):57–8.

[36] Berman B, Sullivan T, De Araujo T, Nadjii M. Expression of Fas-receptor on basal cell carcinomas after treatment with imiquimod 5% cream or vehicle. Br J Dermatol 2003;149(Suppl 66):59–61.

[37] Krammer PH. CD95's deadly mission in the immune system. Nature 2000;407:789–95.

[38] Naylor MF, Crowson N, Kuwahara R, Teague K, Garcia C, Mackinnis C, et al. Treatment of lentigo maligna with topical imiquimod. Br J Dermatol 2003; 149(Suppl 66):66–70.

[39] Jacob SE, Berman B, Nassiri M, Vincek V. Topical application of imiquimod 5% cream to keloids alters expression genes associated with apoptosis. Br J Dermatol 2003;149(Suppl 66):62–5.

[40] Rudy SJ. Imiquimod (Aldara): modifying the immune response. Dermatol Nurs 2002;14(4):268–70.

[41] Bayerl C, Feller G, Goerdt S. Experience in treating molluscum contagiosum in children with imiquimod 5% cream. Br J Dermatol 2003;149(Suppl 66):25–9.

[42] Jones T. Resiquimod 3M. Curr Opin Investig Drugs 2003;4(2):214–8.

[43] Sulzberger MB, Witten VH, Smith CC. Hydrocortisone (compound F) free alcohol ointment. JAMA 1953;152(15):1456.

[44] Bornhovd E, Burgdorf WH, Wollenberg A. Macrolactam immunomodulators for topical treatment of inflammatory skin diseases. J Am Acad Dermatol 2001;45(5):736–43.

[45] Lauerma AI, Surber C, Maibach HI. Absorption of topical tacrolimus (FK506) in vitro through human skin: comparison with cyclosporin A. Skin Pharmacol 1997;10(5–6):230–4.

[46] Bos JD. Non-steroidal topical immunomodulators provide skin-selective, self-limiting treatment in atopic dermatitis. Eur J Dermatol 2003;13(5):455–61.

[47] Truong S, et al. Utilization of topical steroids and topical immmunomodulators in the United States. J Am Acad Dermatol 2004;50(3):88.

[48] Schreiber SL, Crabtree GR. The mechanism of action of cyclosporin A and FK506. Immunol Today 1992; 13(4):136–42.

[49] Wesselborg S, Fruman DA, Sagoo JK, Bierer BE, Burakoff SJ. Identification of a physical interaction between calcineurin and nuclear factor of activated T cells (NFATp). J Biol Chem 1996;271(3):1274–7.

[50] Homey B, Assmann T, Vohr HW, Ulrich P, Lauerma AI, Ruzicka T, et al. Topical FK506 suppresses cytokine and costimulatory molecule expression in epidermal and local draining lymph node cells during primary skin immune responses. J Immunol 1998; 160(11):5331–40.

[51] Clinical comparison pushes AD treatment toward potency chart. Dermatol Times. February 7, 2004. Available at: http://www.dermatologytimes.com.

[52] Paller A, Eichenfield LF, Leung DY, Stewart D, Appell M. A 12-week study of tacrolimus ointment for the treatment of atopic dermatitis in pediatric patients. J Am Acad Dermatol 2001;44(Suppl 1): S47–57.

[53] Meshkinpour A, Sun J, Weinstein G. An open pilot study using tacrolimus ointment in the treatment of seborrheic dermatitis. J Am Acad Dermatol 2003; 49(1):145–7.

[54] Braza TJ, DiCarlo JB, Soon SL, McCall CO. Tacrolimus 0.1% ointment for seborrhoeic dermatitis: an open-label pilot study. Br J Dermatol 2003;148(6): 1242–4.

[55] Saripalli YV, Gadzia JE, Belsito DV. Tacrolimus ointment 0.1% in the treatment of nickel-induced allergic contact dermatitis. J Am Acad Dermatol 2003;49(3):477–82.

[56] Bamford JT, Elliott BA, Haller IV. Tacrolimus effect on rosacea. J Am Acad Dermatol 2004;50(1): 107–8.

[57] Chu J, Bradley M, Marinkovich MP. Topical tacrolimus is a useful adjunctive therapy for bullous pemphigoid. Arch Dermatol 2003;139(6):813–5.

[58] Ko MJ, Chu CY. Topical tacrolimus therapy for localized bullous pemphigoid. Br J Dermatol 2003; 149(5):1079–81.

[59] Umar SA, Bhattacharjee P, Brodell RT. Treatment of Hailey-Hailey disease with tacrolimus ointment and clobetasol propionate foam. J Drugs Dermatol 2004; 3(2):200–3.

[60] Ludwig E, Allam JP, Bieber T, Novak N. New treatment modalities for granuloma faciale. Br J Dermatol 2003;149(3):634–7.

[61] Assmann T, Becker-Wegerich P, Grewe M, Megahed M, Ruzicka T. Tacrolimus ointment for the treatment of vulvar lichen sclerosus. J Am Acad Dermatol 2003;48(6):935–7.

[62] Bohm M, Frieling U, Luger TA, Bonsmann G. Successful treatment of anogenital lichen sclerosus with topical tacrolimus. Arch Dermatol 2003;139(7): 922–4.

[63] Guttman C. Atopic dermatitis duo. Dermatol Times. February 1, 2004. Available at: http://dermatologytimes.com.

[64] Reitamo S, Remitz A, Kyllonen H, Saarikko J. Topical noncorticosteroid immunomodulation in the treatment of atopic dermatitis. Am J Clin Dermatol 2002;3(6):381–8.

[65] Zuberbier T, Chong SU, Grunow K, Guhl S, Welker P, Grassberger M, et al. The ascomycin macrolactam pimecrolimus (Elidel, SDZ ASM 981) is a potent inhibitor of mediator release from human dermal mast cells and peripheral blood basophils. J Allergy Clin Immunol 2001;108(2):275–80.

[66] Rutledge BJ. Combo useful for pediatric dermatitis. Dermatol Times. May 1, 2004;35. Available at: http://dermatologytimes.com.

[67] Gupta AK, Chow M. Pimecrolimus: a review. J Eur Acad Dermatol Venereol 2003;17(5):493–503.

[68] Billich A, Aschauer H, Aszodi A, Stuetz A. Percutaneous absorption of drugs used in atopic eczema: pimecrolimus permeates less through skin than corticosteroids and tacrolimus. Int J Pharmacol 2004;269(1):29–35.

[69] Eichenfield LF, Lucky AW, Boguniewicz M, Langley RG, Cherill R, Marshall K, et al. Safety and efficacy of pimecrolimus (ASM 981) cream 1% in the treatment of mild and moderate atopic dermatitis in children and adolescents. J Am Acad Dermatol 2002; 46(4):495–504.

[70] Kapp A, Papp K, Bingham A, Folster-Holst R, Ortonne JP, Potter PC, et al. Flare Reduction in Eczema with Elidel (infants) multicenter investigator study group. Long-term management of atopic dermatitis in infants with topical pimecrolimus, a consteroid anti-inflammatory drug. J Allergy Clin Immunol 2002;110(2):277–84.

[71] Rutledge BJ. Pimecrolimus cream shows better tolerability. Dermatol Times. May 1, 2004. Available at: http://www.dermatologytimes.com.

[72] Crutchfield III CE. Pimecrolimus: a new treatment for seborrheic dermatitis. Cutis 2002;70(4):207–8.

[73] Brownell I, Quan LT, Hsu S. Topical pimecrolimus in the treatment of seborrheic dermatitis. Dermatol Online J 2003;9(3):13. Available at: http://dermatology.edlib.org/93/case_reports/seborrhea/brownell.html.

[74] Mayoral FA, Gonzalez C, Shah NS, Arciniegas C. Repigmentation of vitiligo with pimecrolimus cream: a case report. Dermatology 2003;207(3):322–3.

[75] Siddaiah N, Erickson Q, Miller G, Elston DM. Tacrolimus-induced tinea incognito. Cutis 2004; 73(4):237–8.

[76] Wetzel S, Wollenberg A. Eczema molluscatum in tacrolimus treated atopic dermatitis. Eur J Dermatol 2004;14(1):73–4.

[77] Liu V, Mackool BT. Mycophenolate in dermatology. J Dermatol Treatment 2003;14(4):203–11.

[78] Allison AC, Eugui EM. Purine metabolism and immunosuppressive effects of mycophenolate mofetil (MMF). Clin Transplant 1996;10(1 Pt 2):77–84.

[79] Mehling A, Grabbe S, Voskort M, Schwarz T, Luger TA, Beissert S. Mycophenolate mofetil impairs the maturation and function of murine dendritic cells. J Immunol 2000;165(5):2374–81.

[80] Katz KH, Marks Jr JG, Helm KF. Pemphigus foliaceus successfully treated with mycophenolate mofetil as a steroid-sparing agent. J Am Acad Dermatol 2000;42(3):514–5.

[81] Nousari HC, Anhalt GJ, Morison WL. Mycophenolate in psoralen-UV-A desensitization therapy for chronic actinic dermatitis. Arch Dermatol 1999; 135(9):1128–9.

[82] Grundmann-Kollmann M, Mooser G, Schraeder P, Zollner T, Kaskel P, Ochsendorf F, et al. Treatment of chronic plaque-stage psoriasis and psoriatic arthritis with mycophenolate mofetil. J Am Acad Dermatol 2000;42(5 Pt 1):835–7.

[83] Neuber K, Schwartz I, Itschert G, Dieck AT. Treatment of atopic eczema with oral mycophenolate mofetil. Br J Dermatol 2000;143(2):385–91.

[84] Nousari HC, Lynch W, Anhalt GJ, Petri M. The effectiveness of mycophenolate mofetil in refractory pyoderma gangrenosum. Arch Dermatol 1998; 134(12):1509–11.

[85] WohlrabK J, Plaetzer JM, Neubert WC. Topical application of mycophenolate mofetil in plaque-type psoriasis. Br J Dermatol 2001;144:1263–4.

[86] Loo WJ, Holt PJ. Bowenoid papulosis successfully treated with imiquimod. J Eur Acad Dermatol Venereol 2003;17(3):363–5.

[87] Kaspari M, Gutzmer R, Kiehl P, Dumke P, Kapp A, Brodersen JP. Imiquimod 5% cream in the treatment of human papillomavirus-16-positive erythroplasia of Queyrat. Dermatology 2002;205(1):67–9.

[88] Meyer T, Nindl I, Schmook T, Ulrich C, Sterry W, Stockfleth E. Induction of apoptosis by Toll-like

receptor-7 agonist in tissue cultures. Br J Dermatol 2003;149(Suppl 66):9 – 14.

[89] Yesudian PD, Parslew RA. Treatment of recalcitrant plantar warts with imiquimod. J Dermatol Treatment 2002;13(1):31 – 3.

[90] Tucker SB, Ali A, Ransdell BL. Plantar wart treatment with combination imiquimod and salicylic acid pads. J Drugs Dermatol 2003;2(2):124 – 6.

[91] Sparling JD, Checketts SR, Chapman MS. Imiquimod for plantar and periungual warts. Cutis 2001;68(6): 397 – 9.

[92] Micali G, Dall'Oglio F, Nasca MR. An open label evaluation of the efficacy of imiquimod 5% cream in the treatment of recalcitrant subungual and periungual cutaneous warts. J Dermatol Treatment 2003;14(4): 233 – 6.

[93] Juschka U, Hartmann M. Topical treatment of common warts in an HIV-positive patient with imiquimod 5% cream. Clin Exp Dermatol 2003; 28(Suppl 1):48 – 50.

[94] Khan DB, Jappe U. Successful treatment of facial plane warts with imiquimod. Br J Dermatol 2002; 147(5):1018.

[95] Oster-Schmidt C. Imiquimod: a new possibility for treatment-resistant verrucae planae. Arch Dermatol 2001;137(5):666 – 7.

[96] Poochareon V, Berman B, Villa A. Successful treatment of butcher's warts with imiquimod 5% cream. Clin Exp Dermatol 2003;28(Suppl 1):42 – 4.

[97] Senatori R, Dionisi B, Lippa P, Inghirami P. Topical imiquimod cream in the treatment of external anogenital warts: personal experience [in Italian]. Minerva Ginecol 2003;55(6):541 – 6.

[98] Haidopoulos D, Diakomanolis E, Rodolakis A, Vlachos G, Elsheikh A, Michalas S. Safety and efficacy of locally applied imiquimod cream 5% for the treatment of condylomata acuminata of the vulva. Arch Gynecol Obstet 2003 [Epub ahead of print].

[99] Cox JT. Extensive condyloma acuminata treated with imiquimod 5% cream: a case report. Clin Exp Dermatol 2003;28(Suppl 1):51 – 4.

[100] Vilata JJ, Badia X. Effectiveness, satisfaction and compliance with imiquimod in the treatment of external anogenital warts. Int J STD AIDS 2003; 14(1):11 – 7.

[101] Campagne G, Roca M, Martinez A. Successful treatment of a high-grade intraepithelial neoplasia with imiquimod, with vulvar pemphigus as a side effect. Eur J Obstet Gynecol Reprod Biol 2003; 109(2):224 – 7.

[102] Travis LB, Weinberg JM, Krumholz BA. Successful treatment of vulvar intraepithelial neoplasia with topical imiquimod 5% cream in a lung transplanted patient. Acta Dermatol Venereol 2002;82(6):475 – 6.

[103] Diakomanolis E, Haidopoulos D, Stefanidis K. Treatment of high-grade vaginal intraepithelial neoplasia with imiquimod cream. N Engl J Med 2002; 347(5):374.

[104] Richter ON, Petrow W, Wardelmann E, Dorn C, Kupka M, Ulrich U. Bowenoid papulosis of the vulva—immunotherapeutical approach with topical imiquimod. Arch Gynecol Obstet 2003;268(4):333 – 6.

[105] Richter ON, Kubler K, Schmolling J, Kupka M, Reinsberg J, Ulrich U, et al. Oxytocin receptor gene expression of estrogen-stimulated human myometrium in extracorporeally perfused non-pregnant uteri. Mol Hum Reprod 2004;10(5):339 – 46.

[106] Arlette JP. Treatment of Bowen's disease and erythroplasia of Queyrat. Br J Dermatol 2003; 149(Suppl 66):43 – 9.

[107] Heinzerling LM, Kempf W, Kamarashev J, Hafner J, Nestle FO. Treatment of verrucous carcinoma with imiquimod and CO2 laser ablation. Dermatology 2003;207(1):119 – 22.

[108] Danielsen AG, Petersen CS, Iversen J. Chronic erosive herpes simplex virus infection of the penis in a human immunodeficiency virus-positive man, treated with imiquimod and famciclovir. Br J Dermatol 2002;147(5):1034 – 6.

[109] Slade HB, Schacker T, Conant M, Thoming C. Imiquimod and genital herpes. Arch Dermatol 2002; 138(4):534 – 5.

[110] Christensen B, Hengge UR. Recurrent urogenital herpes simplex—successful treatment with imiquimod? Sex Transm Infect 1999;75(2):132 – 3.

[111] Skinner Jr RB. Treatment of molluscum contagiosum with imiquimod 5% cream. J Am Acad Dermatol 2002;47:S221 – 4.

[112] Lebwohl M, Dinehart S, Whiting D, Lee PK, Tawfik N, Jorizzo J, et al. Imiquimod 5% cream for the treatment of actinic keratosis: results from two phase III, randomized, double-blind, parallel group, vehicle-controlled trials. J Am Acad Dermatol 2004; 50(5):714 – 21.

[113] Chen K, Yap LM, Marks R, Shumack S. Short-course therapy with imiquimod 5% cream for solar keratoses: a randomized controlled trial. Australas J Dermatol 2003;44(4):250 – 5.

[114] Tran H, Chen K, Shumack S. Summary of actinic keratosis studies with imiquimod 5% cream. Br J Dermatol 2003;149(Suppl 66):37 – 9.

[115] Smith KJ, Germain M, Yeager J, Skelton H. Topical 5% imiquimod for the therapy of actinic cheilitis. J Am Acad Dermatol 2002;47(4):497 – 501.

[116] Prinz BM, Hafner J, Dummer R, Burg G, Bruswanger U, Kempf W. Treatment of Bowen's disease with imiquimod 5% cream in transplant recipients. Transplantation 2004;77(5):790 – 1.

[117] Nouri K, O'Connell C, Rivas MP. Imiquimod for the treatment of Bowen's disease and invasive squamous cell carcinoma. J Drugs Dermatol 2003;2(6):669 – 73.

[118] Chen K, Shumack S. Treatment of Bowen's disease using a cycle regimen of imiquimod 5% cream. Clin Exp Dermatol 2003;28(Suppl 1):10 – 2.

[119] Peris K, Micantonio T, Fargnoli MC. Successful treatment of keratoacanthoma and actinic keratoses with imiquimod 5% cream. Eur J Dermatol 2003; 13(4):413 – 4.

[120] Bhatia N. Imiquimod as a possible treatment for keratoacanthoma. J Drugs Dermatol 2004;3(1): 71–4.

[121] Sidbury R, Neuschler N, Neuschler E, Sun P, Wang XQ, Miller R, et al. Topically applied imiquimod inhibits vascular tumor growth in vivo. J Invest Dermatol 2003;121(5):1205–9.

[122] Sullivan TP, Dearaujo T, Vincek V, Berman B. Evaluation of superficial basal cell carcinomas after treatment with imiquimod 5% cream or vehicle for apoptosis and lymphocyte phenotyping. Dermatol Surg 2003;29(12):1181–6.

[123] Geisse J, Caro I, Lindholm J, Golitz L, Stampone P, Owens M. Imiquimod 5% cream for the treatment of superficial basal cell carcinoma: results from two phase III, randomized, vehicle-controlled studies. J Am Acad Dermatol 2004;50(5):722–33.

[124] Huber A, Huber JD, Skinner Jr RB, Kuwahara RT, Haque R, Amonette RA. Topical imiquimod treatment for nodular basal cell carcinomas: an open-label series. Dermatol Surg 2004;30(3):429–30.

[125] Nagore E, Sevila A, Sanmartin O, Botella-Estrada R, Requena C, Serra-Guillen C, et al. Excellent response of basal cell carcinomas and pigmentary changes in xeroderma pigmentosum to imiquimod 5% cream. Br J Dermatol 2003;149(4):858–61.

[126] Powell AM, Russell-Jones R, Barlow RJ. Topical imiquimod immunotherapy in the management of lentigo maligna. Clin Exp Dermatol 2004;29(1): 15–21.

[127] Powell AM, Russell-Jones R. Amelanotic lentigo maligna managed with topical imiquimod as immunotherapy. J Am Acad Dermatol 2004;50(5):792–6.

[128] Loquai C, Nashan D, Metze D, Beiteke U, Ruping KW, Luger TA, et al. Imiquimod, pegylated interferon-alpha-2b and interleukin-2 in the treatment of cutaneous melanoma metastases [in German]. Hautarzt 2004;55(2):176–81.

[129] Hesling C, D'Incan M, Mansard S, Franck F, Corbin-Duval A, Chevenet C, et al. In vivo and in situ modulation of the expression of genes involved in metastasis and angiogenesis in a patient treated with topical imiquimod for melanoma skin metastases. Br J Dermatol 2004;150(4):761–7.

[130] Qian Z, Zeitoun NC, Shieh S, Helm T, Oseroff AR. Successful treatment of extramammary Paget's disease with imiquimod. J Drugs Dermatol 2003;2(1): 73–6.

[131] Zampogna JC, Flowers FP, Roth WI, Hassenein AM. Treatment of primary limited cutaneous extramammary Paget's disease with topical imiquimod monotherapy: two case reports. J Am Acad Dermatol 2002;47(Suppl 4):S229–35.

[132] Wang LC, Blanchard A, Judge DE, Lorincz AA, Medenica MM, Busbey S. Successful treatment of recurrent extramammary Paget's disease of the vulva with topical imiquimod 5% cream. J Am Acad Dermatol 2003;49(4):769–72.

[133] Do JH, McLaughlin SS, Gaspari AA. Topical imiquimod therapy for cutaneous T-cell lymphoma. Skin Med 2003;2(5):316–8.

[134] Man J, Dytoc MT. Use of imiquimod cream 5% in the treatment of localized morphea. J Cutan Med Surg 2004 [Epub ahead of print]. Available at: http://www. springerlink.com. Accessed May, 2004.

[135] Gerdsen R, Wenzel J, Uerlich M, Bieber T, Petrow W. Successful treatment of chronic discoid lupus erythematosus of the scalp with imiquimod. Dermatology 2002;205(4):416–8.

[136] Berman B, Villa A. Imiquimod 5% cream for keloid management. Dermatol Surg 2003;29(10):1050–1.

[137] Kuwahara RT, Skinner Jr RB. Granuloma annulare resolved with topical application of imiquimod. Pediatr Dermatol 2002;19(4):368–71.

[138] Kuwahara RT, Naylor MF, Skinner RB. Treatment of granuloma annulare with topical 5% imiquimod cream. Pediatr Dermatol 2003;20(1):90.

[139] Martinez MI, Sanchez-Carpintero I, North PE, Mihm Jr MC. Infantile hemangioma: clinical resolution with 5% imiquimod cream. Arch Dermatol 2002;138(7): 881–4.

[140] Harrison S, Sinclair R. Porokeratosis of Mibelli: successful treatment with topical 5% imiquimod cream. Australas J Dermatol 2003;44(4):281–3.

[141] Agarwal S, Berth-Jones J. Porokeratosis of Mibelli: successful treatment with 5% imiquimod cream. Br J Dermatol 2002;146(2):338–9.

[142] Arevalo I, Ward B, Miller R, Meng TC, Najar E, Alvarez E, et al. Successful treatment of drug-resistant cutaneous leishmaniasis in humans by use of imiquimod, an immunomodulator. Clin Infect Dis 2001;33(11):1847–51.

ELSEVIER
SAUNDERS

DERMATOLOGIC
CLINICS

Dermatol Clin 23 (2005) 259–300

The Use of Systemic Immune Moderators in Dermatology: An Update

Dana Kazlow Stern, MD[a], Jackie M. Tripp, MD[b],
Vincent C. Ho, MD[b], Mark Lebwohl, MD[c],*

[a]*Department of Dermatology, Mount Sinai Medical Center, Mount Sinai School of Medicine, 1 Gustave L. Levy Place,
Box 1048, New York, NY 10029-6574, USA*
[b]*Division of Dermatology, Department of Medicine, Vancouver Hospital and Health Sciences Center and
University of British Columbia, 835 West 10th Avenue, Vancouver, BC V5Z 4E8, Canada*
[c]*Department of Dermatology, The Mount Sinai School of Medicine, Mount Sinai Medical Center, Clinical Trials Center,
5 East 98th Street, 5th floor, New York, NY 10029-6574, USA*

When inflammatory dermatoses are severe or recalcitrant to topical therapies, dermatologists are occasionally required to prescribe immunomodulatory drugs. The first-line systemic anti-inflammatory therapy is the oral administration of corticosteroids, but frequently other immunomodulatory drugs are needed to control disease activity, while at the same time limiting or even eliminating the need for corticosteroids. These immunomodulatory therapies can be divided into two broad categories: the more traditional and well-known nonsteroidal immune-modifying drugs, also commonly referred to as the systemic therapies, and the newer immunobiologic agents.

The most common nonsteroidal immune-modifying drugs include the following agents: azathioprine, cyclophosphamide, cyclosporine, methotrexate, and mycophenolate mofetil (MMF). These agents are predominantly cytotoxic, but data seem to suggest that methotrexate has significant anti-inflammatory activity as well. The other category encompasses the plethora of newer immunobiologic agents that are being developed, the most well known of which include alefacept, efalizumab, etanercept, and infliximab. The current authors and others have previously reviewed the pharmacology, mode of action, and adverse effects of some of these agents [1–6]. The current article reviews new data concerning the pharmacology, mechanism of action, adverse effects, and dermatologic applications of these two categories of therapeutic agent. Familiarity with the disease-specific clinical efficacy of each of these medications and their dosages and side-effect profiles allows for the proper and efficacious use of these drugs to treat dermatologic disease.

Azathioprine

Inititially used as an immunosuppressant for renal transplantation, azathioprine has been available for more than 40 years, and because of its relatively favorable therapeutic index, it is one of the more commonly used immunomodulatory drugs in dermatology. Structurally, it is a synthetic purine analog formed by attaching an imidazole ring to 6-mercaptopurine (6-MP). This analog is a prodrug and is quickly converted to 6-MP by a nonenzymatic

Dr. Stern has been an investigator for Biogen Idec, Inc., Genentech, Inc., Amgen, Inc., and Centocor Inc. Dr. Lebwohl has been an investigator, speaker, and consultant for Centocor, Inc., Biogen Idec, Inc., Genentech, Inc., and Amgen Inc., and he has been a speaker and investigator for Abbott, Inc.

* Corresponding author.
E-mail address: mark.lebwohl@mssm.edu (M. Lebwohl).

nucleophilic attack by sulfhydryl compounds present in erythrocytes and body tissues.

Pharmacology

A comparison of the main pharmacologic attributes of the immunosuppressants discussed in this article is presented in Table 1. Azathioprine is rapidly absorbed after oral administration. The drug has a plasma half-life of only 3 hours because of its conversion to 6-MP. Active metabolites have a long half-life, however, allowing once-daily dosing. The 6-MP is metabolized by means of three competing pathways: thiopurine methyltransferase (TPMT) catalyzes S-methylation to 6-methyl mercaptopurine, an inactive compound. Xanthine oxidase catalyzes oxidation to the inactive 6-thiouric acid. Hypoxanthine-guanine phosphoribosyl transferase (HGPRT) catalyzes the conversion of 6-MP to the active 6-thioguanine metabolites. Erythrocyte levels of 6-thioguanine nucleotides correlate with absolute neutrophil counts [7], and steady-state levels may take days to years to achieve. A genetic polymorphism controls TPMT activity. In a recent review of more than 3000 patients, approximately 80% of the patients had normal TPMT activity, 9% had enzymatic activity that was above normal, and 10% displayed low activity [8]. It was also found that 0.45% (1:220) of the study population had no detectable enzyme activity. This ratio is higher than the previously reported 1 in 300 occurrence of undetectable TPMT levels in the population reported in other smaller studies. In renal transplant patients, low TPMT activity has been found to correlate with a higher incidence of leukopenia caused by azathioprine, and those with higher levels were found to be less immunosuppressed [9]. Patients with intermediate TPMT activity may be more likely to develop late-onset neutropenia [10].

The determination of pretreatment red blood cell TPMT activity has been advocated to detect those patients at risk for early-onset neutropenia [11]. This test can be accomplished using either a radiochemical assay of enzyme activity or by high-pressure liquid chromotography. Recently, the isolation and characterization of mutant alleles causing TPMT deficiency have enabled identification of more than 80% of all TPMT mutant alleles in white persons and have allowed the diagnosis of TPMT deficiency and heterozygosity based on genotype [12]. If the drug is used without pretreatment measurement of TPMT activity, it is now recommended that patients be counseled about the associated risks and the inadequacy of blood count monitoring as a method of

preventing early toxicity [13]. TPMT measurement is becoming more widely available, and one recent cost-effectiveness study has shown that polymerase chain reaction testing to identify TPMT polymorphisms before treatment represents good economic value in certain health care settings [14].

Other factors affect TPMT activity. Sulfasalazine and its metabolite 5-aminosalicylic acid inhibit TPMT activity, whereas 6-MP itself and diuretics can induce its activity [15]. Further, very low lymphocyte activities of 5-nucleotidase have been documented in transplant recipients with normal TPMT activity who developed neutropenia when given azathioprine. All patients require tailoring of this medication, guided by leukocyte and platelet counts.

The 6-thioguanine metabolites prevent the interconversion of purine bases and inhibit de novo biosynthesis of purine bases in an S-phase–specific fashion. This antiproliferative effect may not be solely responsible for the immunosuppressive action of azathioprine, because effects on natural killer cell (NKC) function, T-cell signaling, T-cell cytolytic activity, prostaglandin production, and neutrophil activity have been noted [1]. No significant changes in interleukin (IL) levels have been noted.

Adverse effects

Hematologic

Myelosuppression, manifesting as leukopenia, thrombocytopenia, or pancytopenia, is the most significant adverse effect of azathioprine. As stated previously, early toxicity, which is of rapid onset and severe, may be predicted by a knowledge of TPMT activity. Continued monitoring is required, because late-onset myelosuppression occurs more slowly and may be delayed for years. Significant leukopenia was seen in 10% of patients (3 of 29) who had pemphigus vulgaris treated at a mean dosage of 2 mg/kg per day for 4 to 12 years [16], and, in a survey of azathioprine use by dermatologists in the United Kingdom, 45% of respondents had observed significant myelosuppression [17].

Gastrointestinal

Nausea and vomiting are the most frequent side effects, occurring 12.4 times and 5.1 times per 100 patient-years, respectively, in patients receiving standard dosages for rheumatoid arthritis (RA), an average of 104 mg per day [18]. A recent study has shown that azathioprine-related gastrointestinal side effects are independent of TPMT polymorphism [19]. Hepatotoxicity was noted in 8% of patients receiving

Table 1
Pharmacology of the common immunosuppressants used in dermatology

Features	Azathioprine	Cyclophosphamide	Methotrexate	Cyclosporine	MMF
Mechanism of action	Cell cycle–specific antimetabolite, inhibition of neutrophil trafficking, inhibition of cellular cytotoxicity	Non–cell cycle–specific antimetabolite, selective macrophage inhibition, selective B-cell suppression	Cell cycle–specific antimetabolite, inhibition of neutrophil chemotaxis, inhibition of IL-1, IL-6, and IL-8 release	Inhibition of signal transduction and IL-2 production in lymphocytes	Cell cycle–specific antimetabolite, inhibition of Tc and B-cell proliferation
Rate of onset of clinical immunosuppression	Slow (4–8 wk)	Moderately rapid (2–4 wk)	Moderately rapid (2–4 wk)	Rapid (1–2 wk)	Slow (4–8 wk)
Route of administration	Per os	Per os/IV	Per os/SC/intramuscular/IV	Per os	Per os
Route of elimination	Hepatic metabolism and renal excretion	Hepatic metabolism and renal excretion	Renal excretion by active tubular secretion	Hepatic metabolism	Hepatic metabolism and renal excretion
Dose modification in presence of: Renal insufficiency	Moderate decrease in dosage may be required	Moderate decrease in dosage may be required	Relatively contraindicated, significant dose reduction necessary	No change in dosage necessary	Moderate decrease in dosage may be required
Hepatic insufficiency	No change in dose necessary	Moderate decrease in dosage may be required	Moderate decrease in dosage may be required	Significant dose alteration needed	No change in dose necessary
Major potential drug interactions	Allopurinol, warfarin	Allopurinol	Probenecid, NSAIDs, cotrimazole	Multiple (see text)	Acyclovir, iron, antacids, cholestyramine
Major toxicity	Bone marrow depression, carcinogenesis	Bone marrow depression, hemorrhagic cystitis, carcinogenesis	Hepatotoxicity, bone marrow depression, carcinogenesis	Hypertension, nephrotoxicity, carcinogenesis	Bone marrow depression, carcinogenesis

azathioprine and prednisolone for bullous pemphigoid [20].

Opportunistic infections

An increased susceptibility to opportunistic infections has been reported in patients receiving both azathioprine and corticosteroids, even in the absence of leukopenia. Eruptions of herpes simplex, herpes zoster, and verrucae may be more common [1].

Oncogenic potential

Azathioprine has been associated with an increased incidence of malignancy in renal transplant patients. Malignancies have included lymphomas, Kaposi's sarcoma, renal carcinomas, carcinomas of the cervix and vulva, and skin cancers [21]. An analysis of the risk of skin cancer in renal transplant recipients, with a multivariate analysis of subgroups on either long-term cyclosporine or azathioprine with or without corticosteroids, showed no differences between the groups, suggesting that the increased risk is associated with the drug-induced immunosuppression and is independent of the agents used to achieve this [22]. An analysis of 1191 patients who have multiple sclerosis (MS) identified patients who have cancer, matched them to patients who do not have cancer, and compared them in terms of exposure to azathioprine therapy [23]. MS patients given azathioprine were found to have a relative increase in cancer risk of 1.3 when treated less than 5 years, of 2.0 when treated 5 to 10 years, and of 4.4 when treated more than 10 years. Wide confidence intervals undermined these results, but overall, the long-term risk for these patients was low. A more recent retrospective study of 626 patients taking azathioprine who were observed for a mean duration of 6.9 years showed no increased risk of cancer diagnosis [24].

Hypersensitivity reactions

Several reports call attention to azathioprine hypersensitivity syndrome [25–28]. This syndrome has been reviewed comprehensively by Saway et al [29]. The time of onset is from 3 hours to 42 days after onset of medication use, with a mean of 14 days. Hypersensitivity syndrome is rare, with some 30 case reports in the literature. Manifestations may include the following: hypotension; shock; a maculopapular, urticarial, or vasculitic eruption; fever; acute hepatotoxicity; pancreatitis; rhabdomyolysis; acute renal failure; and pneumonitis. Recently, a higher incidence of acute febrile toxic reaction has been reported in 4 of 43 patients (9.3%) with RA who were on long-term methotrexate and in whom azathioprine in usual

dosages was added, suggesting a possible adverse drug interaction [30].

Miscellaneous

Azathioprine, used in conjunction with isotretinoin, has been reported to induce curling of hair [31]. Azathioprine and isotretinoin also have been associated independently with the development of curly hair. In addition, azathioprine administered following corneal transplantation has been reported to cause bilateral macular hemorrhage secondary to aplastic anemia [32].

Clinical use in dermatology

A 1997 survey of current practice in the use of azathioprine by dermatologists in the United Kingdom revealed that the most common indications for its use were the immunobullous disorders (pemphigoid and pemphigus, where it was used in conjunction with corticosteroids), atopic dermatitis and chronic actinic dermatitis (both more often in the absence of corticosteroids), and dermatomyositis (again as a steroid-sparing agent) [17]. Other common uses included pyoderma gangrenosum, systemic lupus erythematosus, psoriasis, lichen planus, and cutaneous lupus erythematosus. There remain very few controlled trials to support the drug's use in dermatology. The data supporting the adjuvant use of azathioprine in pemphigus were reviewed; these data consisted of seven studies totalling 105 patients with no significant difference in outcome between patients treated with cyclophosphamide or azathioprine [33]. Likewise, the use of azathioprine in pemphigoid has been variably shown to have a steroid-sparing effect [1], and in a study in which dosages of both corticosteroid and azathioprine were fixed [20], to result in more adverse effects. Azathioprine may be effective as a steroid-sparing agent in moderately severe systemic lupus, but there is conflicting evidence as to its efficacy in severe disease [1]. The efficacy of azathioprine in dermatomyositis-polymyositis also has been questioned [34].

A retrospective review of 35 patients who had severe, longstanding atopic dermatitis treated with azathioprine showed that 3 of 35 patients had severe nausea, which resulted in treatment discontinuation. The median difference in disability index before and after treatment was highly significant in the 32 patients who tolerated the drug [35]. More recently, a double-blind, randomized, placebo-controlled trial of azathioprine was performed in 37 adult patients who had severe atopic dermatitis (AD), and it similarly showed significant improvement in symptom scores.

There were, however, gastrointestinal side effects in 14 patients [36]. A favorable short-term response to azathioprine in four patients with intractable prurigo nodularis also has been reported [37].

The efficacy of azathioprine in controlling the ocular and extraocular manifestations of Behçet's disease was shown in a double-blind controlled trial [38]. The follow-up of this study showed that the beneficial effect of treatment favorably affected the long-term prognosis of these patients [39].

Azathioprine has been shown to be an effective steroid-sparing agent for generalized lichen planus [40] and also has been used successfully as monotherapy in two patients [41].

Usage guidelines

Azathioprine is contraindicated in patients with known hypersensitivity to the drug. Dosage adjustment, as guided by serial blood counts, may be required in patients with hepatic or renal insufficiency. The drug should not be used during pregnancy unless the benefits outweigh the risks. Both the parent drug and its metabolites can cross the placenta and act as potential teratogens. The magnitude of the teratogenic risk has been evaluated as minimal to small [42,43]. In contrast to the other cytotoxic agents, there is no evidence that azathioprine produces gonadotoxicity or infertility.

Drug interactions

Because allopurinol inhibits the metabolism of azathioprine by xanthine oxidase, the two drugs should not be used concurrently if possible. During concurrent therapy, the dosage of azathioprine should be decreased by at least two thirds, although this dosage reduces, but does not abolish, the risk of myelotoxicity [44]. In this clinical situation, the monitoring of 6-thioguanine levels would seem warranted [45].

Angiotensin-converting enzyme (ACE) inhibitors have been shown to potentiate anemia in renal transplant patients concurrently on azathioprine [46]. This finding seems to be caused by the erythropoietin-lowering effect of the ACE inhibitors rather than from a pharmacokinetic interaction between the two drugs [47]. To the current authors' knowledge, a clinically significant interaction has not been documented in a nonrenal transplant setting, although the current American College of Rheumatology guidelines advise against this combination [48]. Both azathioprine and trimethoprim-sulfamethoxazole are antimetabolites that have a synergistic effect in inhibiting bone marrow proliferation [49]. Again, however, no significant interaction was noted in renal transplant patients treated with concomitant therapy over 4 months [50]. Because of inhibition of TPMT activity, sulfasalazine may potentiate azathioprine toxicity. Finally, warfarin resistance has been noted in patients treated with azathioprine [51,52].

Dosage and monitoring

Azathioprine is supplied for oral use as scored 50-mg tablets. The usual starting dose is 1 to 2 mg/kg per day in single or two divided dosages. One recent study of 48 children receiving azathioprine for atopic dermatitis initiated therapy at dose levels of 2.5 to 3.5 mg/kg in those with a normal TPMT level [53]. Therapeutic response for azathioprine occurs in 6 to 8 weeks. After 6 to 8 weeks, the dose may be increased by 0.5 mg/kg at 4-week intervals according to white blood cell counts and clinical response, and generally should not exceed 3 mg/kg per day. If there is no beneficial response in 12 to 16 weeks, treatment using azathioprine should be discontinued. There are no formal consensus guidelines for monitoring azathioprine when used for dermatologic indications. The current authors' recommendations have been adapted from published guidelines in the dermatologic literature [54] and are presented in Table 2.

Cyclophosphamide

Cyclophosphamide is another cytotoxic agent used on occasion by dermatologists as an immune modulator. Because of the risk of bladder toxicity, myelotoxicity, gonadotoxicity, and malignancy, its use is reserved for serious and potentially life-threatening disorders in which the benefit outweighs the risks.

Pharmacology

Cyclophosphamide belongs to the nitrogen mustard family of alkylating agents. It was initially synthesized as an orally active form of chlorethamine (nitrogen mustard). It is well absorbed after oral administration, with peak plasma levels within 3 hours. The plasma half-life is 5 to 6 hours, with 12% to 14% of the drug being plasma bound [55]. The drug is metabolized by hepatic cytochrome P450 microsomal enzymes and oxidized to form the active metabolites phosphoramide mustard and acrolein. No consistent association between renal or hepatic insufficiency and cyclophosphamide toxicity has been found, and the drug can be metabolized independently of hepatic metabolism.

Table 2
Monitoring guidelines for the use of immunosuppressants

Drug [Ref.]	Monitoring tests	Frequency	Guidelines for dosage modification
Azathioprine [54]	CBC with differential WBC and platelets	Weekly ×4, every 2 wk ×2, then monthly	Decrease dose if WBC < 4 × 10⁹/L, platelets < 10¹¹/L, discontinue if WBC < 2.5 × 10⁹/L
Cyclophosphamide [54]	CBC with differential WBC and platelets	Weekly ×8, then monthly	Decrease dose if WBC < 4 × 10⁹/L, platelets < 10¹¹/L, discontinue if WBC < 2.5 × 10⁹/L
	Renal function tests: BUN, creatinine	Monthly	
	urinalysis	weekly ×8, then every 2 wk, urine cytology when > 50 g total dose monthly	Discontinue if hematuria
	Liver function tests	Monthly	
Methotrexate [105]	CBC with differential WBC and platelets	Weekly ×2, every 2 wk ×2, then monthly	Discontinue for 2–3 wk if WBC < 3.5 × 10⁹/L, discontinue if WBC < 2.5 × 10⁹/L or platelets < 10¹¹/L, increased MCV necessitates folate administration
	Renal function tests: BUN, creatinine	Every 3–4 mo	
	Liver function tests	Every 1–2 mo, ensure it is at least 1 week after most recent dose	If persistently elevated, withhold for 1–2 wk and repeat; if elevation persists for 2–3 mo perform liver biopsy
	Liver biopsy	If no risk factors, at cumulative doses of 1.5 g, 3 g, and 4 g. If risk factors, then first at 2–4 mo of therapy, then at cumulative doses of 1–1.5 g, 3 g, 4 g. After a cumulative dose of 4 g, biopsy every 1–1.5 g.	
Cyclosporine [189]	CBC with differential WBC and platelets	Every month, then every 2–3 mo	
	Renal function tests: BUN and creatinine (×3)	Biweekly ×6, then monthly	Decrease dose if creatinine increase is > 30% over baseline; if persistent over 2 evaluations, discontinue
	Blood pressure	Biweekly ×6, then monthly	
	Urinalysis	Biweekly ×2, then monthly	
	Liver function tests	Biweekly ×2, then monthly	
	Potassium, uric acid, magnesium, cholesterol, triglycerides	Biweekly ×2, then monthly	
	Creatinine clearance	Not done routinely	
MMF [207]	CBC with differential WBC and platelets	Weekly ×4, every 2 wk ×4, then monthly	Decrease dose or discontinue if neutropenic

For all immunosuppressants, lymph node examination, complete physical examination, stool guaiac, skin cancer examination, and PAP smear every 6 mo are recommended.

Abbreviations: BUN, blood urea nitrogen; CBC, complete blood (cell) count; MCV, molluscum contagiosum virus; WBC, white blood cell (count).

Phosphoramide mustard is the metabolite that alkylates DNA and inhibits DNA replication. Unlike azathioprine metabolites, the action of phosphoramide mustard is not S-phase specific and it can affect noncycling cells. There is a differential cytotoxicity to various lymphoid cell populations, with selective suppression of B cells [56]. Hence, this drug has its greatest effect in suppressing humoral immunity. Cyclophosphamide has a more variable response on cell-mediated immunity, and low-dose cyclophosphamide has been shown to potentiate immune responses in experimental systems. Immunostimulation has been related to increased IL-12 gene expression [57]. Variable effects on macrophages also have been noted [58].

Adverse effects

Hematologic

Myelosuppression, consisting primarily of leukopenia, is the most common adverse reaction and can be dose-limiting. After intravenous (IV) administration, the nadir occurs at 8 to 12 days and recovery takes 18 to 25 days. A similar lag is noted with oral therapy. During the leukopenia, the patient is at increased risk of infection by pathogenic and opportunistic organisms. Thrombocytopenia and anemia occur less frequently.

Gastrointestinal

Anorexia, nausea, and vomiting occur commonly with IV administration. These symptoms are dose-related and have been associated with the phosphoramide mustard metabolite. Oral ondansetron and dexamethasone have been shown to control nausea resistant to standard antiemetics in patients treated with IV cyclophosphamide for lupus nephritis [59]; however, a recent double-blind study of 258 patients undergoing emetic chemotherapy showed that a regimen of oral granisetron and oral dexamethasone did not achieve significantly better results than a course of metoclopramide, and that the former regimen was thus not cost-effective [60].

Urologic

Urologic adverse effects are one of the major toxicities of this drug and can include dysuria, urgency, hematuria, bladder fibrosis, and necrosis [61]. Death from hemorrhagic cystitis has occurred. Hemorrhagic cystitis can develop at significantly lower dosages and with shorter durations of therapy in patients treated intravenously rather than orally. At the dose commonly used in dermatology, the average

risk is 5% to 10% [62]. A review of 145 patients with Wegener's granulomatosis treated with oral cyclophosphamide at a dosage of 2 mg/kg, however, identified nonglomerular hematuria in 50% of patients (73 of 145) [63]. Nonglomerular hematuria occurred earlier in smokers and was chronic and recurrent in 38% of patients, even after discontinuation of the drug. Acrolein is the metabolite believed to be responsible for urotoxicity. Dehydration is an undisputed risk factor. High fluid intake and concurrent administration of mesna (sodium 2-mercaptoethane sulfonate) reduce the risk of this complication during IV administration. Mesna binds to acrolein in the bladder, producing an inactive compound that is eliminated in the urine. The relative efficacy of these two maneuvers is still a matter of debate [64].

Oncogenic potential

Patients taking long-term oral cyclophosphamide have up to a 45-fold increase in the incidence of bladder cancer [65]. The estimated incidence of transitional cell carcinoma of the urinary tract, after first exposure to cyclophosphamide in patients who have Wegener's granulomatosis, was 5% at 10 years and 16% at 15 years [63]. Nonglomerular hematuria identified a subgroup at increased risk but was not invariably present. In patients who had RA and who were receiving oral cyclophosphamide, a 4-fold increase in solid tumors and a 16-fold increase in lymphoreticular malignancies have been observed [66,67]. In a case-control study in which patients were followed up for 2 decades after treatment, the relative risk of cancer for those treated with cyclophosphamide was 1.5 and bladder cancer was noted as late as 17 years after discontinuation of the drug [68]. There was a recent report of a bladder carcinoma arising as late as 20 years after oral therapy with cyclophosphamide [69].

Reproductive toxicity

Azoospermia and amenorrhea have been noted after both oral and IV pulse therapy. The incidence is as high as 50%, and risk factors include age, longer period of treatment, and degree of marrow suppression. Male patients may consider a sperm bank before treatment. A study of men given testosterone before and during an 8-month cycle of cyclophosphamide for nephrotic syndrome suggests that this method may help preserve fertility [70]. Suppressing ovarian function with oral contraceptives may protect the ovary, and some advocate the use of coadministering gonadotropins [71].

Opportunistic infections

Pathogenic and opportunistic infections can occur during treatment. They may occur in the absence of leukopenia. In a series of 100 patients with systemic lupus erythematosus, infections occurred with equal prevalence in those who received IV (39%) or oral (40%) medication. Risk factors for severe infections included a white blood cell count of less than 3000 and sequential IV and oral therapy [72].

Miscellaneous

Anagen effluvium, mucositis, and hyperpigmentation have been reported. When used in higher dosages, cardiomyopathy, pneumonitis, pulmonary fibrosis, hepatotoxicity, and syndrome of inappropriate antidiuretic hormone also have been reported [61].

Clinical use in dermatology

Cyclophosphamide continues to be used for potentially life-threatening dermatoses that are resistant to other forms of treatment. These may include systemic necrotizing vasculitis, severe forms of systemic lupus, severe blistering disorders, multicentric reticulohistiocytosis, relapsing polychondritis, and pyoderma gangrenosum [2]. Cyclophosphamide is believed to be a more effective steroid-sparing agent than azathioprine in the treatment of resistant pemphigus, although there is no incontrovertible evidence in the literature to support this view [33]. There are also reports describing successful cyclosphosphamide therapy in recalcitrant pemphigus foliaceous [73] and pemphigus vulgaris [74]. IV pulse cyclophosphamide is being used more frequently by dermatologists based on its effectiveness in lupus erythematosus nephritis [75]. With adequate hydration and use of mesna, the incidence of hemorrhagic cystitis is lower than with oral therapy, and it is hoped that the risk of cancer is lowered as well. Using a combination of dexamethasone pulse, cyclophosphamide pulse, and oral cyclophosphamide, clinical remissions have been claimed in 61 of 79 patients who have pemphigus [76]. The combined use of IV pulse and oral cyclophosphamide was recently reported in ocular pemphigoid [77] and in resistant bullous pemphigoid [78] to decrease total cyclophosphamide dose. A patient who had recalcitrant herpes gestationis also has responded to pulse IV cyclophosphamide after delivery of the infant [79]. A report of a patient with toxic epidermal necrolysis responding to IV cyclophosphamide [80] adds to the four cases in the literature [81]. The feasibility of outpatient monthly oral bolus cyclophosphamide therapy has been documented in patients with active lupus erythematosus [82]. Patients were instructed to maintain a fluid intake of 2 to 3 L per day and were given concurrent oral mesna. The safety and patient acceptance remain to be documented. The comparative efficacy and toxicities of pulse versus continuous oral administration in dermatologic conditions also remain to be determined. Reports of the successful use of oral cyclophosphamide in scleromyxedema [83] and in multicentric histiocytosis (in combination with methotrexate and corticosteroids) [84] add to the anecdotal literature of the use of this drug in rare, recalcitrant dermatoses.

Usage guidelines

Cyclophosphamide is contraindicated in patients who have demonstrated hypersensitivity, in pregnancy, and during breast feeding.

Drug interactions

Allopurinol increases the toxicity of cyclophosphamide through an unknown mechanism. There is a potential risk of increasing the incidence of lung toxicity in those taking amiodarone [85]. Drugs that alter the P450 system may affect cyclophosphamide pharmacokinetics.

Dosage and monitoring

Cyclophosphamide is supplied for oral use as 25- and 50-mg tablets. The recommended oral dosage is 1 to 3 mg/kg per day (50–200 mg/d). This drug should be taken in the morning followed by adequate hydration throughout the day (3 L of fluid/d). In monthly IV pulse therapy, 0.5 to 1.0 g/m^2 is infused over 1 hour followed by vigorous IV hydration, and optional mesna usually at 160% of the cyclophosphamide dose separated into four doses at 0, 3, 6, and 9 hours. Some clinicians follow this treatment with daily oral cyclophosphamide at a dose of 50 mg/day. Further pulses are adjusted to obtain a white blood cell count nadir of 2 to 3×10^9 /L after 10 to 14 days. Monitoring guidelines are outlined in Table 2. It is recommended that all patients have a urinalysis every 3 to 6 months, even after the drug is discontinued, and that microscopic hematuria be evaluated by cystoscopy. Urine cytology should be done every 6 to 12 months, and routine cystoscopy should be considered every 1 to 2 years for all patients who have a history of microscopic hematuria [63].

Methotrexate

Methotrexate is a synthetic analog of folic acid that has been used in dermatologic therapy since 1951. Like azathioprine and cyclophosphamide, it has cytotoxic properties. There is now increasing evidence for separate mechanisms of anti-inflammatory activity.

Pharmacology

Methotrexate is usually given orally for the treatment of cutaneous disease but can be administered subcutaneously with similar kinetics [86]. Occasionally, this agent is given intramuscularly in the presence of gastrointestinal intolerance. There is marked variability in the bioavailability of oral methotrexate [87]. Approximately 35% to 50% of the drug is bound to albumin. Maximum blood levels occur 1 to 2 hours after oral and intramuscular administration [88,89]. Polyglutamate derivatives are formed intracellularly and are the principal bioactive metabolites that are long lasting. Hepatic oxidation forms 7-hydroxy-methotrexate, a minor metabolite. The serum half-life is 6 to 7 hours for the methotrexate but much longer for the polyglutamate derivatives. The drug is excreted by the kidney, with 80% of a dose eliminated unchanged within 24 hours. Methotrexate is filtered by the glomeruli and then undergoes bidirectional transport within the renal tubule. Enterohepatic recirculation occurs to a minor degree.

Methotrexate binds intracellularly to dihydrofolate reductase, thereby preventing the reduction of folate cofactors (the conversion of dihydrofolate to tetrahydrofolate) and inhibiting the thymidylate synthesis. Methotrexate polyglutamates further inhibit thymidylate synthase and other folate-dependent enzymes, such as aminoimidazole-carboxamide ribonucleoside (AICAR) transformylase. Purine synthesis, required for DNA, RNA, and protein synthesis, is thereby inhibited. The methylation of homocysteine to methionine is inhibited, affecting the synthesis of polyamines such as spermidine and spermine [90]. Methotrexate may directly inhibit epidermal cell proliferation by these mechanisms, although lymphoid and macrophage cell lines have been shown to be much more susceptible to the growth inhibitory and cytotoxic effects of methotrexate than epidermal cell lines [91]. Recently, it has been shown that the mechanism of action of methotrexate is highly dependent on the production of reactive oxygen species [92]. In addition, the antimetabolite effect of methotrexate is primarily S-phase specific. The inhibition of AICAR transformylase is believed to lead to intracellular accumulation of AICAR, which leads to release of adenosine into the extracellular space [90,93]. This process results, by way of interaction with specific cell surface adenosine receptors, in potent inhibition of polymorphonuclear chemotaxis and adherence and the inhibition of secretion of tumor necrosis factor α (TNF-α), IL-6, and IL-8 by monocyte/macrophages. This process may thus be responsible for the drug's anti-inflammatory effects. A recent study, however, downplays the role of adenosine release in the mechanism of action of methotrexate [94]. Inhibitory effects on IL-1, IL-2r, and the 5-lipoxygenase pathway also have been shown [95].

Adverse effects

Hematologic

Cytopenia occurs in 10% to 20% of patients on long-term methotrexate for psoriasis manifesting as leukopenia, thrombocytopenia, or pancytopenia [96]. Potential risk factors include renal insufficiency, increased mean corpuscular volume, older age, and concomitant use of trimethoprim-sulfamethoxazole or nonsteroidal anti-inflammatory drugs (NSAIDs) [97]. The use of either folic acid (1–5 mg/d) or folinic acid (leucovorin, 2.5–5 mg, 24 h after the methotrexate) has been advocated to reduce hematotoxicity and is indicated in patients who develop macrocytosis [98]. In a survey of British dermatologists, 75% use folate supplementation in patients on methotrexate for psoriasis, one fourth of this group use it for all patients on therapy, and three fourths use it only in certain circumstances, namely in patients with macrocytosis [99]. The survey also revealed the wide variety of opinion that exists regarding the indications and dosing regimens for folate supplementation during methotrexate therapy and pointed to the need for further studies to establish better guidelines.

Gastrointestinal

Nausea and vomiting are the most frequent adverse effects and are dose-related. Diarrhea and stomatitis may also occur. Folic acid administration, dose splitting, and parenteral administration may control symptoms [100]. Hepatotoxicity is a major concern, with a 7% overall risk of severe fibrosis/cirrhosis in patients with psoriasis but an apparent lower incidence in patients with RA [101,102]. Risk factors include age, total dose, obesity, heavy alcohol intake, diabetes, and daily dosage [103]. Reports of severe fibrosis continue to be published and fibrosis may occur despite serial normal liver function tests

[104]. Pretreatment complete blood count, liver function tests, and hepatitis A, B, and C serology should be performed [105,106]. Baseline and serial liver biopsies are also sometimes performed, but in the absence of certain risk factors, such as history of liver disease or alcoholism and elevated liver function tests, the usefulness of a baseline biopsy is not recommended [105,107,108]. It has been suggested that serial biopsies may not be required in the absence of abnormal liver function tests if the initial biopsy sample is normal [109] or if the weekly dose of the drug is 15 mg or less [108]. One recent study, which emphasized the use of methotrexate in developing countries, claimed that for certain short-term methotrexate regimens in the treatment of psoriasis, the need for liver biopsies can be safely minimized [110]. Serial liver function tests continue to be recommended [105], however, and several authors promote the serial use of serum type III procollagen aminopeptide (PIIINP) as a test for fibrinogenesis [104, 111]. A recent 10-year retrospective study of 70 patients with psoriasis who were taking methotrexate showed that the presence of repeatedly normal levels of PIIINP on serial blood examinations correlated to a minimal risk of developing liver toxicity [112]; however, this screening technique has not yet found common usage or availability.

Oncogenic potential

Methotrexate has been shown to be a significant independent risk factor (relative risk, 2.1) for developing squamous cell carcinoma (SCC) in patients with severe psoriasis [113], and this risk seems to be increased in patients with psoriasis who have undergone treatment with psoralen plus ultraviolet A (PUVA) [114]. Two patients with mixed-cellularity Hodgkin's disease have been reported in association with methotrexate use for psoriasis [115]. There also have been reports of an Epstein-Barr virus–associated lymphoproliferative disorder in patients on low-dose methotrexate [116–118]. Contrary to cyclophosphamide and azathioprine, methotrexate generally was not associated with an overall increased risk of lymphoma in a large-scale retrospective study of 16,263 patients with RA [119]. In addition, smaller retrospective studies found no increased risk of lymphoproliferative disease in patients with psoriasis on methotrexate [116].

Reproductive toxicity

Methotrexate is a known abortifacient and teratogen. Teratologists have recommended a delay of at least 12 weeks between drug discontinuation and conception in women [120]. Conception should be avoided during therapy and 3 months afterward by couples in which the man is taking the drug [105].

Opportunistic infections

Opportunistic infections are reported in patients on low-dose methotrexate; in patients with RA on methotrexate, these infections seem to be more common than in those treated with azathioprine, cyclophosphamide, or cyclosporine [121]. Live vaccines should not be administered to patients on methotrexate.

Miscellaneous

Idiosyncratic pneumonitis is rare in patients with psoriasis who are taking methotrexate, but it can be life threatening. A chest radiograph is warranted if pulmonary symptoms develop. Anaphylactoid reactions have been reported after low-dose methotrexate and can occur during initial exposure [122]. Painful erosion of psoriatic plaques is a cutaneous sign of methotrexate toxicity and occurred in two patients who had an alteration in methotrexate dosage and concomitant use of NSAIDs [123]. One report, however, described cutaneous ulceration that was attributed to methotrexate therapy in a patient without psoriasis [124]. Low-dose methotrexate may contribute to the development of stress fractures of long bone. One study recently reported on three patients on low-dose methotrexate with a triad of osseous pain, radiologic osteoporosis, and distal tibial stress fractures [125]. Alopecia, hyperpigmentation, UV burn recall, and toxic epidermal necrolysis also have been reported [89]. Central nervous system (CNS) toxicities, including headaches, dizziness, fatigue, and mood alterations, may occur.

Clinical use in dermatology

The most widely accepted use for methotrexate in cutaneous disease is for the treatment of severe or refractory psoriasis. It is also used for pityriasis rubra pilaris, sarcoidosis, chronic urticaria, dermatomyositis, and lymphoproliferative diseases, such as pityriasis lichenoides et varioliformis acuta, lymphomatoid papulosis, and cutaneous T-cell lymphoma [89]. A recent review of clinical experience with low-dose methotrexate to treat 113 patients with severe psoriasis at a Dutch center revealed that prolonged improvement was achieved in 81% of patients [96]. The drug has been found to be of value in psoriatic polyarthritis as well [126]. In a case series of patients with adult pityriasis rubra pilaris, the combined use of retinoids and methotrexate has been advocated for patients whose disease is resistant to retinoids. Of

11 patients, 9 experienced significant clinical improvement at 16 weeks [127]. Others have warned against this combination over concern for the potential of increased hepatotoxicity, however [128]. A review of the use of methotrexate in 45 patients with lymphomatoid papulosis and Ki-1 lymphoma revealed satisfactory long-term control in 87% of patients with doses of 25 mg or less given at 1- to 4-week intervals for up to several years [129].

The use of methotrexate as corticosteroid-sparing agent in inflammatory dermatoses continues to receive attention. Kasteler and Callen [130] reported on the successful use of methotrexate (2.5–30 mg/wk) as a corticosteroid-sparing agent in 13 patients with dermatomyositis and therapy-resistant cutaneous features. Although older reports suggest methotrexate should be avoided in the treatment of pemphigus vulgaris [131], it has been used at a dose of 5 to 10 mg per week as an efficacious steroid-sparing agent in an elderly population with bullous pemphigoid [132]. There is a single case report claiming a steroid-sparing effect of methotrexate in the treatment of pyoderma gangrenosum [133]. There also has been some benefit shown in the treatment of widespread morphea [134]. Finally, a case report of multicentric reticulohistiocystosis responding to low weekly dosages of methotrexate in addition to prednisone adds to the two cases in the literature [135].

Usage guidelines

Patients with a history of significant liver or kidney disease should be excluded. The reader is referred to the published guidelines for use in patients with psoriasis [105] and, for comparison, to the guidelines for use in RA [101]. Pregnancy is an absolute contraindication, and active infection, excessive alcohol consumption, patient unreliability, anemia, leukopenia, and thrombocytopenia are all relative contraindications.

Drug interactions

Methotrexate toxicity has been precipitated by probenecid, trimethoprim-sulfamethoxazole, omeprazole, and penicillins, possibly by interference with tubular secretion, and possibly by interference with plasma protein binding of the methotrexate. Nephrotoxic drugs, such as NSAIDs, can reduce the renal clearance of methotrexate. Trimethoprim-sulfamethoxazole and possibly sulfasalazine may increase bone marrow toxicity. Concurrent use of nonabsorbed oral antibiotics, such as vancomycin, may decrease gastrointestinal absorption of methotrexate [87].

Dosage and monitoring

Methotrexate is commonly given either as a single weekly dose or in three divided doses over 36 hours. Usual dosages are from 5 to 10 mg/m^2 per week (7.5–30 mg/wk). The drug is available orally as a 2.5-mg pill or can be given as a liquid (intended for injection). Monitoring guidelines are shown in Table 2.

Cyclosporine

Cyclosporine is a lipophilic cyclic undecapeptide isolated from the fungus *Tolypocladium inflatum.* It has been used for the treatment of severe psoriasis since the early 1980s and has more recently found application in other inflammatory dermatoses. Unlike the three previous immunomodulatory drugs, this drug's main effect is on the intracellular signal transduction pathways of cells that are primarily of the lymphoid lineage.

Pharmacology

Cyclosporine is insoluble in water. In a traditional formulation, given orally as a soft gelatin capsule, the absorption is erratic, with a bioavailability of approximately 30%, with high interpatient and intrapatient variability [136]. Peak blood levels occur after 2 to 4 hours, with an average serum half-life of 18 hours. Tissue concentrations are highest in adipose tissue and 80% of the drug is bound to lipoproteins. There is poor CNS penetration. The drug is metabolized by the cytochrome P450 3A system with bile excretion and enterohepatic recirculation. Metabolites are inactive and only 6% of the drug is excreted in the urine in the form of metabolites.

The microemulsion formulation of cyclosporine is now the standard formulation in Canada and Europe. It is absorbed more rapidly, with a peak serum concentration at 1 hour earlier than the original formulation, and has an increase in bioavailability, resulting in higher maximum concentrations and lower intrapatient and interpatient variability [137]. This effect is associated with an increase in clinical efficacy [138] and in a comparable safety profile. A decreased tolerability with a 1:1 dose conversion has been noted with an increase in reported gastrointestinal adverse effects [137]. A 1:1 dose conversion is still recommended when converting patients from the original formulation to the microemulsion formulation, however [139]. Use of the new formulation seems to result in an improved outcome at a lower dosage [140].Cyclosporine acts primarily on

T cells. The drug forms a complex with cyclophilin intracellularly, which then binds to and inhibits calcineurin. This process prevents the activation of nuclear factors involved in the transcription of genes encoding several cytokines, including IL-2 and interferon γ (IFN-γ) [141,142]. This process then results in the inhibition of T-cell activation and of T-cell–mediated potentiation of the immune response.

Adverse effects

Nephrotoxicity and hypertension

Cyclosporine can cause structural and functional changes in the kidney. Functional changes are caused by dose-related vasoconstriction in the renal microcirculation. Structural changes include an obliterative microangiopathy with tubular atrophy and interstitial fibrosis [143]. A recently proposed mechanism of nephrotoxicity is that cyclosporine, through the inhibition of the adaptive response to hypertonicity, interferes with the urinary concentration mechanism [144]. Risk factors include a daily dose of more than 5 mg/kg, persistent elevations of creatinine to more than 30% of baseline, and older age [145]. Structural changes may also correlate with drug-induced hypertension [146] and can even occur with low-dose cyclosporine [147,148]. Hypertension is seen in 10% to 15% of patients. This condition is reversible with drug discontinuation and can be controlled with calcium channel blockers [149,150]. Studies in animal models have shown that such supplements as magnesium [151], glycine [152], and L-arginine [153] may reduce the risk of nephrotoxicity.

Oncogenic potential

Cyclosporine is not mutagenic, but immunosuppression results in an increased risk of skin cancers and possibly lymphomas. There have been reports of lymphomas occurring while patients were taking cyclosporine [154], although some authors believe that these cases of lymphoma were not directly related to the cyclosporine, and that cyclosporine use in psoriasis does not necessarily convey an increased risk of lymphoma [155]. The increased risk in skin cancers has been estimated from 2.6-fold in patients with RA to 7.5-fold in patients with psoriasis [139]. A recent prospective study of 1252 patients with severe psoriasis on cyclosporine therapy showed a sixfold increase in cutaneous malignancy attributable to cyclosporine [156]. This study also noted that the increased risk for cutaneous malignancy was apparent after 2 years of therapy. Previous PUVA therapy and previous immunosuppressive therapy may be predisposing factors in the development of skin cancer in patients with psoriasis [156,157].

Miscellaneous

Hyperlipidemia, hyperkalemia, hypomagnesemia, and hyperuricemia can occur but are usually mild. Neurologic side effects can include hand tremors, paresthesias, dysesthesias, and headache. Mucocutaneous side effects include gingival hyperplasia, hypertrichosis, pilomatrix dysplasia, facial dysmorphism, acne, eruptive angiomas, and folliculitis. Transient nausea, vomiting, diarrhea, abdominal discomfort, and severe fatigue also have been noted.

Clinical use in dermatology

Cyclosporine has become an accepted treatment for severe psoriasis and atopic dermatitis. The efficacy of its use as maintenance therapy in severe psoriasis has been shown [158], and the safety of cyclosporine in the treatment of psoriasis for up to 2 years has been documented [159]. It is effective for psoriatic arthritis as well, although symptomatic improvement can be slow [160]. Strategies to minimize risk and optimize treatment include intermittent short-course therapy, rotational therapy, and short-term use for crisis management [139,161]. Cyclosporine is safe and effective for the short-term treatment of severe atopic dermatitis [162]. In an open trial, 65 of 100 patients completed 48 weeks of therapy with significant improvement at an average dose of 3 mg/kg per day [163]. A more recent study has shown that cyclosporine microemulsion is effective for the short-term treatment of severe atopic dermatitis using a bodyweight-independent dosing scheme [164]. The study results also showed that a starting dose of 150 mg per day was preferable to a starting dose of 300 mg per day, mainly because the former was observed to be much less nephrotoxic. As with psoriasis, relapses are the rule, but a fraction of patients have prolonged remissions [165]. The efficacy of cyclosporine at 3 mg/kg per day in recalcitrant hand dermatitis was similar to topical betamethasone dipropionate in a randomized double-blind study [166].

The use of cyclosporine in other dermatoses is based mostly on case reports and case series of successful outcomes. These have been summarized in review articles on the subject [167–169]. Cyclosporine is considered by some to be first-line treatment for pyoderma gangrenosum [168]. It is also excellent treatment for extensive cutaneous lichen planus and may result in prolonged remission even at very low dosages (1–5 mg/kg/d) [170]. Oral and genital lichen planus may be somewhat less responsive [1]. Reports of the efficacy of cyclosporine in the bullous disorders are mixed. In one report, long-lasting remissions were obtained in six patients with pemphigus vulgaris refractory to corticosteroids and other immunosuppressive agents [171]; however, a study comparing prednisone alone with prednisone plus cyclosporine and prednisone plus cyclophosphamide for the treatment of oral pemphigus found no significant difference between the groups [172]. A more recent study showed that combination treatment with corticosteroids and cyclosporine (at 5 mg/kg) offers no advantage over treatment with corticosteroids alone in patients with pemphigus [173]; however, some maintain that there is value in using cyclosporine as maintenance therapy for pemphigus [174]. Several case reports document the efficacy of cyclosporine as a steroid-sparing agent in bullous and cicatricial pemphigoid, and in epidermolysis bullosa acquisita [1]. Acute and juvenile dermatomyositis respond to cyclosporine, and the drug should be considered in severe or refractory disease [175]. Dramatic improvement also has been seen in the mucocutaneous manifestations of Behçet's disease [168]. Cyclosporine in addition to low-dose prednisone yielded cosmetically acceptable results in only two of eight patients treated for alopecia areata in a recent report without induction of durable remissions [176], and therefore does not seem warranted for this indication. Recent reports have suggested impressive responses in the treatment of severe cytophagic histiocytic panniculitis [177], toxic epidermal necrolysis [178], hidradenitis suppurativa [179], and prurigo nodularis [180]. Further study is warranted in these diseases. Also, there are reports of the successful use of cyclosporine in the following conditions: actinic reticuloid, Hailey-Hailey disease [181], granuloma annulare [182,183], chronic actinic dermatitis [184], recurrent Reiter's syndrome [185], eosinophilic cellulites [186], and Sweet's syndrome [187].

Usage guidelines

Guidelines for the use of cyclosporine in psoriasis have been published [139,188,189] and can be adopted for the use of cyclosporine in other dermatoses. Absolute contraindications are severe concurrent infection, uncontrolled hypertension, or renal insufficiency. Relative contraindications include the following: current or past malignancy, immunodeficiency, high risk of noncompliance, use of concomitant nephrotoxic drugs, gout, liver disease, and pregnancy [189].

Drug interactions

Cyclosporine, in either oral formulation, interacts with many drugs [139]. Most of the clinically relevant drug interactions with cyclosporine relate to competitive inhibition or induction of the cytochrome P450 3A microsomal enzymes. Anticonvulsant agents (phenytoin, phenobarbital, carbamazepine), antibiotics (rifampin, trimethoprim-sulfamethoxazole, nafcillin), and phenylbutazone can decrease cyclosporine levels; other antibiotics (erythromycin, doxycycline), antifungal agents (ketoconazole, itraconazole, fluconazole), calcium channel blockers (verapamil, diltiazem, nicardipine), steroid hormones, and diuretics (furosemide, thiazides) can increase cyclosporine levels. Several drugs may also synergistically increase cyclosporine nephrotoxicity (diuretics, NSAIDs, aminoglycosides, trimethoprim-sulfamethoxazole, amphotericin B, and melphalan).

Dosage and monitoring guidelines

The microemulsion formulation is available in 25-mg, 50-mg, and 100-mg capsules. The recommended starting dose [189] for patients with stable, generalized psoriasis or for patients whose disease severity lies between moderate and severe is 2.5 mg/kg per day in one or two divided doses. If improvement is not noted within 2 to 4 weeks, the cyclosporine dose can then be increased in increments of 0.5 to 1.0 mg/kg per day every 2 weeks to a maximum of 5 mg/kg per day. For patients in whom a rapid improvement is critical (ie, those with severe, inflammatory flares of psoriasis or the presence of other diseases that have failed previous therapies), the starting dose should be 5 mg/kg per day. (Note: the US Food and Drug Administration [FDA] has decreased the upper-limit dose for cyclosporine treatment of psoriasis to 4 mg/kg/d.) In this scenario, as soon as the patient has a significant response, the dose can be decreased by 0.5 to 1 mg/kg per day every week until the minimum effective maintenance dose is attained. Monitoring guidelines are presented in Table 2. In either the high- or low-dose scheme, dosage adjustments should be made in response to adverse effects. If, for instance, the serum creatinine level increases by more than 30% above baseline, and a repeat creatinine level 2 weeks later still shows the increase, the dose of cyclosporine should be decreased by at least 1 mg/kg per day, with the creatinine level to be rechecked in 1 month. If, at that point, serum creatinine decreases to less than 30% above the patient's baseline, treatment can be continued, and if not, then therapy should be discontinued and not resumed until the creatinine levels return to within 10% of the patient's baseline. Another adverse effect is an increase in blood pressure. When this occurs, the physician can either attempt to control this through antihypertensive therapy or by decreasing the cyclosporine dose by 25% to 50% [189].

Mycophenolate mofetil

Mycophenolate mofetil (MMF) is a morpholino-ethyl ester of mycophenolic acid (MPA) [190], which, on biotransformation after absorption, converts to MPA, the active metabolite. As an immune suppressant, MMF has been widely applied in organ transplantation medicine since the early 1990s. More recently, it has found other clinical applications in dermatology, rheumatology, and gastroenterology.

Pharmacology

MMF, or 2-morpholinoethyl (E)-6-(1,3-dihydro-4-hydroxy-6-methoxy-7-methyl-3-oxo-5-isobenzo-furanyl)-4-methyl-4-hexenoate, is the 2-morpho-linoethyl ester of MPA. It is rapidly absorbed following oral administration and then undergoes ester hydrolysis in the liver to form mycophenolic acid, the active metabolite [191,192]. Its oral bio-availability is high at 94.1% in healthy volunteers [193]. The active metabolite MPA is a noncompeti-tive inhibitor of the cellular inosine monophosphate dehydrogenase required for de novo purine biosyn-thesis [190,194,195]. As a result, it blocks RNA and DNA synthesis, which is critical for the immune response. Because the lymphocytes rely predomi-nantly on de novo purine biosynthesis rather than the salvage pathway for purine synthesis (HGPRT), the T- and B-cell proliferative response is inhibited [196,197]. Therefore, MMF inhibits antibody pro-duction and the formation of cytotoxic T lympho-cytes [190,195]. The selectivity for lymphocytes has another mechanism. MPA is 5 times more active against the type 2 isoform of inosine monophospha-tase dehydrogenase (IMPDH), which is activated in activated lymphocytes, than against the type 1 IMPDH, which is active in most cell types [198]. Once ingested, MPA has a half-life of 17.9 hours in healthy volunteers, and as part of its metabolism, it undergoes glucuronidation to form phenolic glucuro-nide of MPA, which is not pharmacologically active. Most of the metabolite (93%) is excreted in the urine, with 6% excreted in the feces.

Adverse effects

The reported side effects of MMF are mainly related to gastrointestinal and hematologic systems, with little effect on hepatic and renal function [199,200]. The side-effect profile makes MMF highly complementary to many other immune suppressants used for dermatologic diseases, such as cyclosporine, methotrexate, cyclophosphamide, and azathioprine, which have renal or hepatic toxicities [1].

Gastrointestinal

The most common side effects of MMF include nausea, vomiting, diarrhea, and abdominal cramps, with an incidence of 12% to 36% [201]. In a recent study of MMF in 54 patients with systemic lupus, 39% of patients had gastrointestinal adverse events [202]. Recently, it has been suggested that MMF caused erosive enterocolitis in renal transplant patients receiving the drug; however, a direct, causal link has not been established [203]. If gastrointestinal symptoms develop, the daily dose can often be spread over more than two daily doses. If adverse effects persist for a longer period of time and seem more serious, MMF may have to be withdrawn while a comprehensive invasive diagnostic process is per-formed to rule out any opportunistic infections. Severe gastrointestinal complications with MMF are rare, but when they do occur they may require extensive diagnosis and treatment [204].

Hematologic

For 11% to 34% of patients, the most serious hematologic side effect is leukopenia. Severe leuko-penia is only present in 0.5%–2.0% of patients. These effects are generally reversible on drug discontinuation [201,205]. In a study of 57 patients who underwent liver transplants, approximately half received MMF, and the rest received azathioprine [206]. Of the MMF-treated patients, 21% had thrombocytopenia, whereas leukopenia was seen in 7% of MMF-treated patients. Both of these adverse effects occurred less frequently with MMF than with azathioprine.

Oncogenic potential

In a clinical trial involving 1483 patients enrolled for the prevention of renal transplant rejection, there was a slight increase of lymphoproliferative malig-nancies in the MMF group after more than 1 year (incidence, 0.6%–1.0%) on therapy compared with placebo or azathioprine (incidence, 0.3%) [201]. The 3-year safety data showed no unexpected changes in malignancy incidences compared with the 1-year data

[207]. In a recent retrospective examination of 106 renal transplant patients receiving azathioprine and 106 receiving MMF, four patients using azathioprine were diagnosed with a malignancy (three post-transplant lymphoproliferative disorders, one SCC) compared with two MMF patients (prostate cancer, basal skin cell carcinoma) [208]. In a more recent 3-year safety study of 128 renal transplant patients, there were slightly more malignancies (predominantly cutaneous) in patients given MMF (14.2%) versus those patients on azathioprine (10.2%) [209]. In the previously described studies involving transplant patients, however, the different patient groups in these studies were all taking cyclophosphamide as well, so the above numbers are relevant only in that they convey the risk of neoplasm from MMF relative to azathioprine.

Infections

Because MMF is an immune suppressant, it has been associated with increased infection rates in patients, primarily herpetic viral infections, with a relative risk of 2 to 3 times normal rates [205]. The studies that showed an increased risk of infection primarily reported on transplant patients. A recent retrospective study of 23 transplant patients on 2 g of MMF per day of MMF showed 10 patients developing 22 opportunistic or serious viral or bacterial infections [210]. The link of MMF specifically to cytomegalovirus (CMV) infection is more controversial. One study on transplant patients found that the addition of MMF to the cyclosporine-prednisone combination did not result in an increase in primary CMV infections, but CMV infections led more often to CMV disease in patients treated with MMF than in those not receiving MMF [211]. In a similar study, MMF did not increase the overall incidence of CMV infection in renal transplant patients but increased the severity of CMV infection in terms of the frequency of organ involvement and number of organs involved [212]. More recently, however, a study of 48 patients showed that MMF puts transplant patients at a significant increased risk (with a calculated relative risk of 19) of a CMV infection [213].

Clinical use in dermatology

The primary indication for MMF is for the prophylaxis of organ transplant rejection, in combination with cyclosporine and corticosteroids [201]. Since the report of the successful treatment of bullous pemphigoid and phemphigus vulgaris with MMF in 1997 [214,215], however, dermatologic applications of this new immune suppressant have been expanded to many other bullous and inflammatory conditions. Also since this initial report, other reports have confirmed the usefulness of MMF for treating bullous pemphigoid [216–219]. Similarly, other bullous disorders have been reported to be responsive to MMF, including pemphigus vulgaris [214,217,220,221], pemphigus foliaceous [222], bullous and hypertrophic lichen planus [223], linear IgA bullous dermatosis [224], cicatricial pemphigoid [225], and paraneoplastic pemphigus [226,227]. Epidermolysis bullosa acquisita failed to respond to a combination treatment of MMF and prednisone in one report [227],but succeeded in another [228]. A recent case series of 17 patents with pemphigus (12 with pemphigus vulgaris, 4 with pemphigus foliaceous, and 1 with paraneoplastic pemphigus) treated with MMF showed improvement in 12 patients [229]. In general, most of the reports are on combinations of MMF and glucocorticoids. One exception is the report of successful treatment with MMF monotherapy of a patient who had pemphigus vulgaris [220]. The dosages in these reports ranged from 2 to 3 g per day, and patients generally tolerated the treatment well. In addition, MPA was used in the 1970s for the successful treatment of psoriasis [230].

Since MMF became available clinically in the early 1990s, Haufs et al [231] reported that one patient responded to MMF at a dosage of 1 to 1.5 g twice daily in 6 weeks, with a 50% reduction in Psoriasis Area and Severity Index (PASI) score. Subsequently, Nousari et al [218] reported on another patient with plaque psoriasis who responded to MMF plus topical steroid and calcipotriol. In a series of five patients with plaque-type psoriasis taking 1 g of MMF twice daily for 10 weeks, two patients with mild to moderate disease showed improvement, whereas those with severe psoriasis did not respond [232]. In a study of 11 patients with severe, stable plaque-type psoriasis, it was shown that MMF at dosages of 1 g twice daily for 3 weeks was an effective and seemingly safe treatment option [233]. In a more recent study, 23 patients with moderate to severe psoriasis were treated with MMF at a dosage of 2 to 3 g per day for 12 weeks in an open-label uncontrolled trial; approximately three fourths of the patients were observed to have a significant reduction in symptom scores, with only few adverse events [234]. MMF (2–3 g/d) has been used in combination with cyclosporine for the treatment of recalcitrant pyoderma gangrenosum [235–238]. Grundmann–Kollmann et al [239] reported on two patients with severe atopic dermatitis who dramatically responded to MMF monotherapy after 2 to 3 weeks, with no side effects. The effectiveness of MMF for atopic dermatitis was supported in two separate pilot studies, each involving 10 patients with moderate-to-severe or severe atopic dermatitis [240,241]. In another report, however, none of the five patients with atopic dermatitis responded to MMF [242]. Pickenacker et al [243] reported on a patient with severe dyshidrotic eczema who responded to MMF at a dosage of 3 g per day, but in another report, a patient apparently developed dyshidrotic eczema while on MMF therapy [244]. Clinical experiences have been reported for successful treatment of systemic [245–248], subacute cutaneous [249], and discoid [250] lupus erythematosus, and other dermatologic diseases, including vasculitis [251–255], sarcoidosis [256], ulcerated necrobiosis lipoidica [257], and dermatomyositis [258]. Almost all of the reports of the effectiveness of MMF in patients with dermatologic diseases are case reports, case series, or small-scale, uncontrolled clinical trials.

Usage guidelines

MMF is contraindicated in patients with hypersensitivity to MMF, MPA, or any component of the drug product [201,207]. It is also contraindicated in pregnancy. Caution should be exercised in patients with gastrointestinal disorders because rare gastrointestinal bleeding has been reported. Patients with severe renal function impairment (glomerular filtration rate of < 25 mL/min/1.73 m^3) should not receive more than 2 g of MMF per day [201].

Drug interactions

No major drug interactions have been reported. Although there is some evidence to suggest that glucocorticoids interfere with the bioavailability of MMF [259], it is unclear as to the clinical significance of this phenomenon. The coadministration of MMF with antacids, iron, and cholestyramine causes a reduction of MMF absorption [201,260]. One case report attempted to ascribe the cause of a patient's neutropenia to an interaction between MMF and valacyclovir [261]. Also, because of its similar effects on purine metabolism and bone marrow suppression, MMF should not be used concomitantly with azathioprine.

Dosage and monitoring

MMF is available as 250- and 500-mg tablets. Typical daily dosages are 2 to 3 g per day in twice-daily dosing. Although MMF has been used in dermatologic conditions, official approval for its use in the treatment of such diseases is still not available. There are therefore no formal consensus guidelines

for monitoring MMF when used for dermatologic indications. The current authors' recommendations have been adapted from previous guidelines [207] and are presented in Table 2. Recent literature has suggested a possible benefit in monitoring serum levels of MMF in transplant patients, but the relationship between pharmacokinetic parameters and adverse events remains unclear [262].

The use of systemic immunobiologic agents

Alefacept, efalizumab, etanercept, and infliximab are currently the immunobiologic agents most commonly used in dermatology. At present, within the dermatologic therapeutic armamentarium, these therapies are used mainly for the treatment of psoriasis and psoriatic arthritis; however, their utility has been shown in several other cutaneous disorders as well. A focus on the use of these agents for the treatment of psoriasis, with anecdotal commentary on other disease-specific clinical applications of these medications, and the pharmacology, mechanism of action, dosages, and side-effect profiles of these drugs will allow for a more thorough understanding of these agents for the treatment of cutaneous disease.

A greater understanding of the role that T lymphocytes play in the pathogenesis of cutaneous inflammatory disease has transformed physicians' understanding of the mechanism of these disorders and resulted in a therapeutic revolution. It is now understood that psoriasis, for example, is an autoimmune disease, with an unknown antigenic stimulus. The epidermal hyperplasia of psoriasis is a CD8$^+$ and CD4$^+$ T-lymphocyte–mediated reaction that occurs within focal skin regions [263]. Much of the current understanding of this process has come from experiments using the severe combined immunodeficiency, or SCID, mouse model of psoriasis in which clinically normal skin from a patient with psoriasis is transplanted onto an immunodeficient mouse. When syngeneic T cells are activated in vitro and injected into the transplanted skin, the skin develops a phenotypic expression nearly identical to psoriatic skin [264,265]. These experiments have confirmed the paramount role of activated T cells in the induction of the psoriasis plaque. Furthermore, studies using monoclonal antibodies have elucidated the specific subsets of T cells involved in the formation and maintenance of the psoriasis plaque and their roles at precise sites within psoriatic skin. For example, CD8$^+$ T cells (mainly cytotoxic or "killer lymphocytes") are found in high concentrations in the epidermis, whereas CD4$^+$ T cells predominate in the dermis [266,267]. Psoriasis is

Table 3
Summary of the common immunobiologic agents used in dermatology

Features	Alefacept (Amevive)	Efalizumab (Raptiva)	Etanercept (Enbrel)	Infliximab (Remicade)
Type of agent	Fusion protein	Humanized monoclonal antibody	Fusion protein	Chimeric monoclonal antibody
Mechanism of action	Blocks T-cell activation. Selective reduction of memory effector T cells	Anti CD11a blocks T-cell activation and reduces trafficking of T cells to inflamed skin	TNF-α inhibitor	TNF-α inhibitor
Route of administration	IM	SC	SC	IV
Approval status	Psoriasis: FDA approved for chronic moderate to severe plaque-type psoriasis, January 2003	Psoriasis: FDA approved for chronic moderate to severe plaque-type psoriasis, October 2003	Psoriasis: FDA approved for chronic moderate to severe plaque-type psoriasis, April 2004	Psoriasis: Phase 3

Abbreviation: IM, intramuscular.

considered to be a Th1 immune disease because in psoriasis both $CD4^+$ and $CD8^+$ T cells produce mainly type 1 cytokines. The understanding of the Th1 phenotype has facilitated the creation of therapies that target specific steps within the Th1 pathway. Many now recognize psoriasis to be one of the most prevalent T-cell–mediated inflammatory diseases in humans, and it is considered to be the model Th1 immune disorder by many researchers [263,268].

The understanding of the T-cell–mediated pathogenesis of psoriasis has resulted in an explosive research effort toward the development of biologic therapies designed to target the immunologic process at specific points along the inflammatory cascade. The biologics can be divided into three classes of agents: (1) recombinant human cytokines or growth factors, (2) monoclonal antibodies, and (3) fusion proteins. The classes and mechanism of action of the four most commonly used immunobiologic agents used in dermatology are outlined in Table 3. Alefacept, efalizumbab, etanercept, and infliximab, examples of the latter two kinds of biologic agents, target highly specific steps in the aforementioned T-cell–mediated inflammatory cascade. These therapies therefore are able to control psoriatic disease with minimal impairment of immune function and significantly fewer side effects than traditional immunosuppressive agents.

Alefacept

Pharmacology/Mechanism of action

Alefacept is given as an intramuscular injection in a dose containing 15 mg of alefacept per 0.5 mL of reconstituted solution. In patients who received alefacept as a 7.5-mg IV administration, the mean volume of distribution was 94 mL/kg, the mean clearance was 0.25 mL/kg per hour, and the mean elimination half-life was approximately 270 hours. Bioavailability was found to be 63% post-intramuscular injection [269]. The pharmacokinetics of alefacept in pediatric patients has not been studied. The effects of renal or hepatic impairment on the pharmacokinetics of alefacept also have not been studied.

Alefacept is a fusion protein consisting of the first extracellular domain of human leukocyte function antigen-3 (LFA-3) fused to the hinge Ch2 and Ch3 sequences of human IgG1 [268]. The drug is produced by recombinant DNA technology in a Chinese hamster ovary mammalian cell expression system [269]. Alefacept acts as an immunosuppressive agent by inhibiting T-cell activation and proliferation by binding to CD2 on T cells and blocking the LFA-3–CD2 interaction [270–272]. Alefacept also engages FcγRIII IgG receptors (on NKCs and macrophages), resulting in the apoptosis of T cells that express high levels of CD2 [264]. Because CD2 expression is higher on activated memory ($CD4^+$ $CD45RO^+$ and $CD8^+$ $CD45RO^+$) than on naive ($CD45RA^+$) T cells, alefacept produces a selective reduction in memory T cells [268,273–276].

Because the targeting of memory T cells is selective, naive ($CD45RA^+$) populations are minimally affected. This situation allows patients to maintain the ability to mount appropriate immune responses to infectious agents [277]. This result was shown when alefacept-treated patients and controls were able to mount comparable antibody responses to immunization with a novel T-cell–dependent antigen (bacteriophage phiX174) and a recall antigen (tetanus toxoid) [278].

The T-cell reductive effect observed in the circulation has been shown in the skin. Patients with psoriasis who were treated with alefacept showed decreased activation of T cells and memory T cells and a reduction in IFN-γ production in lesional skin [279,280]. Because the skin takes time to repopulate, by selectively targeting the epidermal T cells, alefacept is able to induce longer lasting remissions than many other biologic agents.

Adverse effects

Oncogenic potential

The package insert for alefacept warns that the drug may increase the risk of acquiring a malignancy. No statistically significant increased incidence of malignancy has been observed in any studies to date, however. In a study that looked at repeat courses of alefacept, five cases of malignancies (two systemic, three cutaneous) were reported [281]. In each case, the patient had additional potential risk factors for developing a malignancy, and the overall incidence of cancers in the study was similar to what would be statistically expected in untreated individuals of the same age. As is true of all of the biologic agents, alefacept is a novel therapy, and the adverse effect profile may not be established until after years of clinical experience. Patients with a history of systemic malignancy should not be treated with alefacept.

Infections

One or two 12-week courses of intramuscular alefacept were shown in phase 3 studies to have safety and tolerability profiles similar to placebo [281]. No increase in the incidence of opportunistic infections was noted [282]. No association between infections and CD4+ T-cell counts was observed. In the largest phase 3 trial, the only adverse event that occurred with an incidence of 5% or more in the alefacept group versus the placebo group in course 1 was chills (10% versus 1%) [283]. The incidence of chills was temporally related to dosing. Chills tended to occur soon after dosing, and the frequency of chills was lower in the second course. Of note, chills were not a side effect in the other large-scale phase 3 study [282] that examined the efficacy and tolerability of intramuscular alefacept, and this side effect can therefore most likely be attributed to the IV route of administration, which is no longer available. In course 2 of the aforementioned phase 3 trial, accidental injury and pharyngitis were the only adverse events that occurred with an incidence of 5% or more in the alefacept group versus the placebo group (20% versus 15%, and 16% versus 11%, respectively) [283].

Alefacept is an immunosuppressive agent and therefore should not be administered to patients with clinically significant infections. To avoid clinically significant immunosuppression, other immunosuppressive agents should be avoided or used with caution in patients receiving alefacept. If a patient develops a serious infection, alefacept should be discontinued and the patient should be closely monitored. Therapy can be reinitiated on resolution of infection at the physician's clinical discretion.

Effects on the immune system

The biologic agents, as with any exogenous protein molecule administered as therapy, have the potential for immunogenicity. Antibody titers were low (< 1:40) in both of the largest phase 3 trials, and no immune hypersensitivity reactions occurred [282,283].

Injection site reactions

In the largest phase 3 clinical trial that evaluated the intramuscular route of administration, injection site pain and injection site inflammation were adverse events that occurred at least 5% more frequently in alefacept-treated patients than in those taking a placebo. Injection site reactions were typically classified as mild, were usually single episodes, and did not result in any patient discontinuing the study [282].

Summary of efficacy data from important clinical trials

Two important randomized, double-blind, placebo-controlled phase 3 trials were conducted to evaluate the efficacy and tolerability of alefacept. In the first trial, two 12-week courses of once-weekly 7.5-mg IV alefacept versus placebo were given in a randomized double-blind study, and patients were followed up for 12 weeks after each treatment course [283]. Clinical outcomes were measured as follows: a 75% or more reduction in the PASI, a 50% or more PASI reduction, or a Physician Global Assessment (PGA) of "clear" or "almost clear" [283]. Because many patients show continued clinical improvement after cessation of therapy as shown by phase 2 data [276], the overall response rate was evaluated during both the 12-week treatment period and during the 12-week follow-up period.

Of patients treated during course 1, 28% achieved a 75% or greater reduction in PASI as compared with 8% of placebo-treated patients ($P < 0.001$); of those who achieved a 75% or greater reduction in PASI, 23% achieved a PGA of clear/almost clear as compared with 6% of placebo-treated patients (P < 0.001). Of patients treated during course 1, 56% achieved a 50% or greater reduction in PASI as compared with 24% of placebo-treated patients (P < 0.001).

A second course of alefacept provided additional benefit. Of patients who received two 12-week courses of alefacept, 40% achieved a 75% or greater reduction in PASI, 71% achieved a 50% or greater reduction in PASI, and 32% achieved a PGA of clear/almost clear. Patients who were treated with two courses of alefacept had a maximum mean reduction of 54% from baseline PASI at 6 weeks post treatment [283].

The data showing that alefacept produced durable clinical improvements among patients who responded were significant. Those patients, who received a single course of alefacept and achieved 75% or greater overall PASI reduction, were able to maintain a 50% or greater reduction in PASI for a median duration of more than 7 months. Patients who achieved a PGA of clear or almost clear maintained a 50% or greater reduction in PASI for a median duration of approximately 8 months. Two courses of alefacept resulted in a greater duration of response than a single course. This durable response makes alefacept the only psoriasis therapy besides PUVA [284], the Goeckerman regimen [285,286], and possibly UVB [287] that can be considered a remittive treatment. Psoriasis therapies can be either suppressive, where symptoms of disease recur shortly after withdrawal of therapy, or remittive. Remittive therapies, such as alefacept, provide long-lasting remission by mechanisms that reduce T cells in the skin.

In the other pivotal phase 3 trial, the first randomized controlled trial of weekly intramuscular doses of alefacept, 507 patients were randomized to one of three treatment groups (10 mg, 15 mg, or placebo) of intramuscular alefacept administered once weekly for 12 weeks with a 12-week follow-up [282]. To assess overall response rate, the clinical outcome was measured throughout both the treatment and follow-up periods as follows: a 75% or greater PASI reduction, a 50% or greater PASI reduction, or a PGA of clear/almost clear. Response rates were compared among dosage groups.

The percentage of patients who achieved a 75% or greater reduction in PASI was significantly higher (P < 0.001) in patients who received 15 mg of alefacept (33%) or 10 mg of alefacept (28%) as compared with the placebo group (13%). Of patients who achieved a 50% or greater PASI reduction throughout the study period, 57% were in the 15-mg alefacept group (P < 0.001 versus placebo), 53% were in the 10-mg alefacept group (P = 0.002 versus placebo), and 35% were in the placebo group (P < 0.001). Overall response rates for a PGA of clear or almost clear were 24%, 22%, and 8% of patients in the 15-mg, 10-mg, and placebo groups, respectively (P < 0.001 for comparisons of both doses of alefacept versus placebo). Again, the clinical response was durable and attributed to the drug's mechanism of action. Of patients in the 15-mg group who had achieved at least a 75% reduction from baseline 2 weeks after the last dose, 74% maintained at least a 50% reduction in PASI during the 12-week follow-up period. Of patients in the 15-mg group who achieved between a 50% and 75% PASI reduction, 79% maintained at least a 25% reduction in PASI from baseline during the 12-week follow-up period [282].

Clinical use in dermatology

Alefacept is indicated for the treatment of adult patients with moderate to severe plaque-type psoriasis (~1.5 million in the United States) [288] who are candidates for systemic therapy or phototherapy. Patients who have comorbidities, such as liver and renal disease, for whom systemic immunosuppressive therapies are not options, represent an additional potential patient population that can benefit from biologic therapies like alefacept. As mentioned previously, alefacept is considered to be a remittive therapy that allows patients to enjoy long periods of treatment-free, disease-free living. It is therefore advantageous for the patient who needs a reprieve from chronic therapy.

Unlike most biologic agents that require the patient to self-inject subcutaneously, alefacept is a physician-administered intramuscular injection. This mode of administration represents a clear advantage for patients who, for either psychologic or physical reasons, are not able to self-inject.

Usage guidelines

Alefacept is contraindicated in patients with a known hypersensitivity to the drug or any of its components [269]. Alefacept has not been formally studied in women who are pregnant or nursing. It is not known whether alefacept is excreted in human milk. The drug has been labeled pregnancy category B and should therefore only be used during pregnancy when clinically necessary. Reproductive toxicology studies were performed in cynomolgus

Table 4
Monitoring guidelines for use of immunobiologic agents

Drug	Monitoring tests	Frequency	Guidelines for dosage modification
Alefacept	CBC and platelets, including total lymphocytes and $CD4^+$ T-cell counts (both must be within normal limits to begin therapy)	Baseline	Hold therapy if $CD4^+$ T-lymphocyte counts are below < 250 cells/μL
	$CD4^+$ T-cell counts	Weekly	Discontinue drug if $CD4^+$ counts remain below 250 cells/μL for 1 mo
Efalizumab	Platelet counts	Baseline and once per month for the initial 3-mo treatment period; periodic testing should be done throughout the treatment period	Discontinue if thrombocytopenia develops
Etanercept	None required	—	—
Infliximab	Tuberculin skin test	Baseline	—

monkeys with alefacept in doses of up to 5 mg/kg per week (~62 times the human dose based on body weight) and revealed no evidence of impaired fertility or harm to the fetus. Weekly IV bolus injections of alefacept administered to cynomolgus monkeys from organogenesis to gestation did not cause abortifacient or teratogenic effects [269]. Caution should be used when treating elderly individuals because of the higher incidence of infections and malignancies in this population. Alefacept is not indicated for the treatment of pediatric patients.

Drug interactions

No formal interaction studies have been performed [269].

Dosage and monitoring

Alefacept is approved by the FDA as a single 15-mg intramuscular dose given weekly for 12 weeks. The IV formulation is no longer available. After a 12-week rest period off the drug, patients can be treated with a second 12-week course. The drug is supplied as a sterile, preservative-free, lyophilized powder to be reconstituted with 0.6 mL of sterile water before injection. Monitoring guidelines are presented in Table 4.

Efalizumab

Pharmacology/Mechanism of action

Efalizumab is administered as a weekly subcutaneous (SC) injection. Patients (n = 26) with moderate to severe plaque psoriasis who received a starting (SC) dose of 0.7 mg/kg followed by 11 weekly SC doses of 1 mg/kg per week reached steady-state

serum concentrations at 4 weeks, with a mean trough concentration of approximately 9 μg/mL. The mean steady-state clearance was 24 mL/kg per day (range, 5–76 mL/kg/d; n = 25). After the last steady-state dose, the mean elimination time of efalizumab was 25 days (range, 13–35 d; n = 17). Mean efalizumab SC bioavailability was estimated to be 50%. Body weight was found to be the most significant covariate affecting clearance of the drug. Patients who received weekly SC doses of 1 mg/kg of efalizumab had similar exposure across body weight quartiles [289].

Efalizumab is a humanized monoclonal antibody directed against CDlla, the α subunit of LFA-1. This binding reversibly blocks the interaction between LFA-1 and intracellular adhesion molecule 1 (ICAM-1). LFA-1 expression is increased on memory T cells, and ICAM-1 is expressed on vascular endothelial cells at sites of inflammation and on keratinoctyes in various T-cell–mediated disorders [290–293]. Thus, the mechanism of efalizumab prevents the binding of T cells to endothelial cells and blocks T-cell movement into the skin without depleting memory effector T lymphocytes.

Adverse effects

Oncogenic potential

Of 2762 patients who received efalizumab at various doses for a median duration of 8 months [289], 31 patients were diagnosed with 37 malignancies. Efalizumab-treated patients had a 1.8 per 100 patient-years incidence of malignancies compared with 1.6 per 100 patient-years in placebo-treated patients. Most malignancies were nonmelanoma skin cancers. The incidence of noncutaneous solid tumors and malignant melanoma were within the range that would be expected in the general, non–efalizumab-treated population. Efalizumab, like alefacept, is a novel immunosuppressive agent without long-term safety and efficacy data. Therefore, the role of efalizumab in the long-term development of malignancies will require longer follow-up before any role in the development of malignancy can be excluded.

Infections

In a pivotal phase 3 multicenter, randomized, placebo-controlled, double-blind study [294] that evaluated the efficacy and safety of efalizumab in dosages of 1 or 2 mg/kg per week, subjects (N = 597) were treated with efalizumab for a maximum of 24 weeks with no increased rate of infection observed among efalizumab-treated patients [294]. The package insert for efalizumab states that the overall incidence of hospitalization for infections was 1.6 per 100 patient-years for efalizumab-treated patients compared with 1.2 per 100 patient-years for placebo-treated patients [289].

Effects on the immune system

In the previously described large-scale phase 3 study of 597 patients, 5% of the subjects who were treated with efalizumab developed antiefalizumab antibodies [294]. These effects were not believed to be clinically significant.

Thrombocytopenia

During clinical trials, thrombocytopenia, as defined as platelet counts at or below 52,000 cells per μL, was observed in eight (0.3%) of efalizumab-treated patients and no placebo-treated patients [289]. Five of the eight patients were treated with systemic steroids. The thrombocytopenia resolved in seven of the eight patients (the eighth patient was lost to follow-up).

Miscellaneous

First-dose reactions are sometimes associated with the administration of monoclonal antibodies. An analysis of the pooled adverse events from the efficacy and safety data for 1095 patients who were treated with efalizumab showed a higher incidence of acute adverse events (defined as headache, chills, fever, nausea, vomiting, or myalgia that occurred on the day of injection or 2 days post injection) than placebo controls (43% versus 27%) [295]. These events were generally mild to moderate in severity and tended to occur after the initial injection, and decreased with each subsequent injection. By the third dose, the incidence of acute adverse events was similar to the placebo-treated group.

Summary of efficacy data from important clinical trials

Data on efalizumab pooled from two phase 3 clinical trials from 1095 patients with moderate to severe psoriasis showed an improvement of 75% or greater in PASI relative to baseline on day 84 in 29.2% of patients who received efalizumab in dosages of 1.0 mg/kg per week and in 27.6% of patients who received dosages of 2.0 mg/kg per week compared with 3.4% of placebo-treated patients [296]. Of patients who achieved an improvement of 50% or more in PASI, 55.6% had been treated with efalizumab in dosages of 1.0 mg/kg per week and 54.5% had been treated with efalizumab in dosages of 2.0 mg/kg per week compared with 15.1% of patients who were treated with placebo. An extended treatment trial (ACD2059g) was conducted in responders ($\geq$ 75% PASI improvement from baseline) and partial responders ($\geq$ 50% PASI improvement from baseline) to examine the effects of continued treatment with the same weekly dosing schedule versus a potentially more convenient every-other-week dosing schedule versus discontinuation of therapy to assess time to relapse. Results showed that every-other-week dosing was sufficient to maintain an improvement of 75% or more in PASI in responders, but weekly dosing resulted in a better clinical response rate among partial responders. After cessation of therapy, psoriasis relapsed at a loss of 50% of the original PASI improvement, with a median time to relapse of 60 to 80 days [295]. Of note, the patients who "rebounded" were discontinued from efalizumab therapy abruptly, without taper or transition to other therapeutic modalities. Currently, there are several ongoing phase 3 trials designed to establish more optimal strategies for cessation of efalizumab therapy, to determine optimal dosing schedules, and to further support efalizumab as a potential long-term therapy.

Clinical use in dermatology

Efalizumab was FDA-approved in October 2003 for the treatment of chronic moderate to severe plaque psoriasis. Efalizumab can be compared favorably with the current systemic antipsoriasis agents in that it is associated with rapid onset and continued clinical improvement in patients with moderate to severe plaque-type psoriasis. It is also similar in that on cessation of therapy, some patients in clinical trials have shown relapse or exacerbation of disease. Of 2589 clinical trial patients treated with efalizumab, 19 (0.7%) experienced worsening of their psoriasis (n = 5) or worsening past baseline after discontinuation of efalizumab (n = 14) [289]. Some of these patients developed pustular or erythrodermic psoriasis. In comparison to systemic immunosuppressive agents, however, efalizumab's mechanism of action is highly specific, and clinical trial data have shown its potential role as a safe and effective long-term therapy without the dose-limiting side effects of the systemic agents. To date, although the long-term safety and efficacy data supporting efalizumab as a chronic therapy have not been established, the favorable side-effect profile and the convenience of a weekly self-administered SC injection make the long-term administration of efalizumab feasible. Trials are currently being conducted to evaluate efalizumab as a potential therapeutic agent for chronic psoriasis.

Usage guidelines

Efalizumab is contraindicated in patients with a known hypersensitivity to the drug or any of its components. No reproductive toxicity studies have been conducted in pregnant women. Efalizumab has been labeled pregnancy category C. It is not known whether efalizumab is excreted in human milk. The drug should not be used in pregnancy unless the clinical benefits clearly outweigh the risks.

In a developmental toxicity study that used antimouse CD11a antibody at up to 30 times the recommended clinical dose of efalizumab, there was no evidence of maternal toxicity, embryotoxicity, or teratogenicity observed during organogenesis [289].

Caution should be used when treating elderly individuals because of the higher incidence of infections and malignancies in this population. Efalizumab has not been studied in pediatric patients.

Drug interactions

Drug interaction studies have not been performed. Efalizumab should not be used concomitantly with other immunosuppressive agents [289].

Dosage and monitoring

Efalizumab is administered as a single 0.7-mg/kg, SC conditioning dose followed by a weekly SC dosage of 1 mg/kg. The maximum dosage should not exceed 200 mg weekly [289]. The drug is supplied as a lyophilized, sterile powder to be reconstituted with

1.3 mL of sterile water before injection. Monitoring guidelines are presented in Table 2.

Etanercept

Pharmacology/Mechanism of action

Etanercept is a dimeric fusion protein that competitively inhibits the action of TNF-α, rendering it biologically inactive. Etanercept is created with two identical p75 TNF-α receptor peptides fused to the Fc region of IgG1 [297]. It is this dimeric property of the drug that enables it to bind to two receptors on TNF-α with greater affinity than natural monomeric receptors [298].

TNF-α is produced by type 1 helper T cells within psoriatic plaques. TNF-α has an integral role in the amplification and maintenance of the inflammatory cascade within psoriatic plaques by stimulating the production of chemokines and the expression of adhesion molecules by keratinocytes and vascular endothelial cells [299]. The importance of TNF-α in the inflammatory process has been demonstrated by showing that levels of TNF-α in the serum [300] and blister fluids [301] of involved psoriatic skin are higher than in those of controlled nonpsoriatic skin. In addition, TNF-α levels have been significantly correlated with PASI scores, and decreased levels are associated with clinical improvement after treatment [300].

Pharmacokinetic studies of 25 patients with RA showed that administration of 25 mg of etanercept by a single SC injection resulted in a mean (± standard deviation) half-life of 102 (±30) hours with a clearance of 160 (±80) mL per hour [302]. Pharmacokinetic studies have not been conducted to study the effects of renal or hepatic impairment in patients taking etanercept.

Adverse effects

Oncogenic potential

The incidence of malignancies in the etanercept-treated population is best evaluated using data from RA studies because these studies represent the longest experience available and published phase 3 data evaluating etanercept in psoriasis clinical trials are currently limited. Moreland et al [303] examined the safety of etanercept therapy in a population of 1272 patients with RA 5 years after they had been treated and found the incidence of malignancies to be 35 in the treatment group. This number was what would be expected according to the National Cancer Institute, Surveillance, Epidemiology, and End Results database.

Infections

Similar to data on oncogenic potential, data concerning the incidence of infections are also best gleaned from RA studies that have longer clinical experience with the drug. Safety data from 5 years of clinical experience with etanercept therapy in a population of 1272 patients with RA showed the frequency of infections requiring hospitalization or IV antibiotics to be 0.04 per patient-year in the total population [303]. This rate was the same as the rate in the control group.

More recent short-term data from placebo-controlled trials investigating etanercept for the treatment of psoriasis also have examined rates of infection. In a double-blind, placebo-controlled 24-week study that examined the safety and efficacy of etanercept as monotherapy in 672 patients with moderate to severe psoriasis, rates of infection were similar across all treatment groups [304]. The study reported that 11% of placebo-treated patients, 10% of low-dose (25-mg 1×/wk) etanercept-treated patients, 9% of medium-dose (25-mg 2×/wk) etanercept-treated patients, and 5% of high-dose (50-mg 2×/wk) etanercept-treated patients developed an upper respiratory tract infection during the first 12 weeks of therapy. There were no cases of opportunistic infections or tuberculosis (TB) reported during the study. Similarly, in a randomized, double-blind, placebo-controlled 12-week study [305] that looked at the efficacy and safety of etanercept in dosages of 25 mg twice weekly, versus placebo in 60 patients with psoriasis and psoriatic arthritis, the safety profile of etanercept-treated patients was similar to the profiles previously reported in the RA population [306,307]. Upper respiratory tract infections were one of the most common adverse events, but no adverse event occurred in a significantly greater proportion in the treatment group relative to the placebo group.

Postmarketing reports have reported serious infections and sepsis, including fatalities, associated with the use of etanercept. Many of these serious infections occurred in patients using concomitant immunosuppressive therapy [302]. Usage guidelines concerning infections are discussed in the "Usage guidelines" section.

The reactivation of latent TB has been observed in patients treated with etanercept and infliximab, the other biologic agent that targets TNF. TB also has been reported in much lower numbers in etanercept-treated patients. Thirteen patients (eight in the United States and five in Europe) of approximately 102,000 patients with RA developed TB [299]. The etanercept-related cases occurred sporadically and later during the course of therapy than the infliximab cases. Currently, TB screening is required by the FDA before starting infliximab but not before the initiation of therapy with etanercept. Some experts believe that testing should be done before the initiation of etanercept as well.

Effects on the immune system

Data from clinical trials showed that 11% of etanercept-treated patients developed a new positive antinuclear antibody (ANA) titer of 1:40 or greater compared with 5% of placebo-treated patients [299]. Anti-dsDNA antibodies occurred in 15% of etanercept-treated patients compared with 4% of placebo-treated patients [299]. In addition, cases of drug-induced systemic lupus and subacute cutaneous lupus have been reported [308,309]. These conditions resolved after therapy with etanercept was discontinued, and in one case after corticosteroid treatment was initiated without withdrawal of etanercept therapy [308]. Full cases of systemic lupus erythematosus associated with etanercept therapy are rare [310].

Demyelinating disease

In a review of the Adverse Events Reporting System of the FDA, Mohan et al [311] identified 19 patients who developed neurologic symptoms, 17 following etanercept therapy and 2 following infliximab therapy. The neurologic symptoms were in most cases associated with demyelinating lesions of the CNS and were all temporally related to anti–TNF-α therapy. Symptoms improved in all patients after discontinuation of anti–TNF-α therapy. One patient's symptoms returned on rechallenge with etanercept. It is important to note that 4 of the 19 patients had a prior history of MS or MS-like symptoms. The authors suggested avoiding anti–TNF-α therapy in patients with MS or in patients with a family history of MS. An outline of the clinical approach to patients receiving anti–TNF-α therapy who develop new neurologic signs suggestive of demyelination is also provided in this study [311].

Injection site reactions

In controlled clinical trials, injection site reactions were the only adverse event that occurred significantly more often in etanercept-treated patients than in placebo-treated patients. Approximately between 42% and 49% of etanercept-treated patients in controlled clinical trials experienced injection site reactions [306,307]. In a study that retrospectively reviewed medical records of patients who had received etanercept injections and who were still being actively treated with etanercept, 21 (20%) of 103 patients reported injection site reactions [312]. The reactions occurred within the first months of therapy, within 1 to 2 days of injecting, and resolved within a few days. The lower incidence of injection site reactions found in this study compared with the 42% to 49% incidence in controlled clinical trials was attributed to the retrospective nature of the study. The authors of this study performed a histologic and immunophenotypic analysis of skin biopsy specimens and concluded that the reactions may be an example of a T-lymphocyte–mediated delayed-type hypersensitivity reaction. Injection site reactions can be treated with cool compresses and 1% hydrocortisone ointment. Rotating sites of injection is also recommended.

Summary of efficacy data from important clinical trials

Several clinical trials have investigated etanercept as monotherapy for the treatment of psoriasis. A 24-week phase 2, multicenter, double-blind, placebo-controlled trial of 112 patients with chronic moderate to severe plaque-type psoriasis who were treated with etanercept in SC dosages of 25 mg twice weekly found that, at week 12, 30% of etanercept-treated patients achieved at least a 75% improvement in PASI, compared with 2% of placebo-treated patients ($P < 0.001$) [313]. By week 24, 56% of etanercept-treated patients and 5% of placebo-treated patients achieved an improvement of 75% or greater in PASI ($P < 0.001$).

A phase 3, placebo-controlled, double-blind, parallel-group study assessed the safety and efficacy of a 24-week course of etanercept in SC dosages of 25 mg once weekly (low dose), 25 mg twice weekly (medium dose), 50 mg twice weekly (high dose), or placebo in 672 patients with moderate to severe plaque-type psoriasis [304]. At week 12, 14%, 34%, 49%, and 4% of the patients in the low, medium, high, and placebo groups, respectively, achieved a PASI improvement of at least 75% ($P < 0.001$ for all three comparisons with the placebo group). As early as week 2 of the study, the mean percentages of PASI improvements were statistically significant for all three etanercept-treatment groups compared with baseline. At week 12, mean levels of improvement were 40.9%, 52.6%, 64.2%, and 14% in the low-dose, medium-dose, high-dose, and placebo groups, respectively. Results at week 24 showed an improve-

ment of 75% or greater in 25%, 44%, and 59% of the patients in the low-, medium-, and high-dose groups, respectively. There was no placebo comparison group at this point in the study.

Clinical use in dermatology

Etanercept has more than 130,000 patient-years of treatment experience (mostly in the RA population) in both controlled clinical trials and postmarketing experience [299]. Etanercept was FDA-approved in April 2004 for the treatment of adult patients with chronic moderate to severe plaque-type psoriasis. Etanercept was previously granted FDA approval for the treatment of psoriatic arthritis. It is also indicated for reducing signs and symptoms of moderate to severe active polyarticular-course juvenile RA. Because between 5% and 42% of patients with psoriasis also have concomitant psoriatic arthritis [314], etanercept represents an ideal biologic agent in physicians' current armamentarium for the treatment of both of these disorders. In addition, similar to efalizumab, etanercept can be administered with methotrexate, a benefit that has numerous favorable clinical implications when treating patients with psoriasis or psoriatic arthritis. Like other SC self-administered biologics, etanercept can be administered by the patient at home, a feature that offers tremendous patient independence. Unlike many biologics, etanercept requires no laboratory monitoring during treatment. Data extrapolated from RA studies suggest that etanercept therapy may (similar to efalizumab) have a role as a therapeutic agent in chronic conditions administered on a long-term continuous basis.

Etanercept has been reported to be clinically effective in several other cutaneous disorders, including the following: scleroderma [315]; cicatricial pemphigoid [316]; in a patient with common variable immunodeficiency who presented with scarring alopecia, arthritis, diarrhea, and recurrent infections [317]; and for recurrent apthous stomatitis [318].

Usage guidelines

Etanercept is contraindicated in patients with a known hypersensitivity to the drug or any of its components and should not be administered to patients with sepsis. Treatment with etanercept should not be initiated in patients with active or chronic localized infections. The manufacturer of etanercept cautions that the drug should not be administered to patients who develop serious infections or sepsis and caution should be taken when considering treating patients with conditions that may predispose to infections, such as poorly controlled or advanced diabetes. Caution should also be exercised when considering using etanercept in patients with pre-existing or recent-onset CNS demyelinating disorders [302].

Developmental toxicity studies of etanercept performed in rats and rabbits in doses between 60- to 100-fold higher than the human dose have not resulted in harm to the fetus [303]. Whether etanercept can impair fertility in humans is unknown. The drug should not be used during pregnancy unless the clinical benefits clearly outweigh the risks. Etanercept has been labeled as pregnancy category B. It is not known whether etanercept is excreted in human milk. Caution should be used when treating elderly individuals because of the higher incidence of infections and malignancies in this population. Etanercept is indicated for the treatment of poly-articular-course juvenile RA, but it has not been studied in children younger than 4 years [302].

Drug interactions

No formal interaction studies have been performed. In a study of patients with RA who were treated with etanercept and anakinra therapy for up to 24 weeks, however, the rate of serious infections was 7% in the dual-treatment group compared with 0% in those with etanercept alone [302].

Dosage and monitoring

Etanercept is indicated for adult patients with moderate to severe plaque-type psoriasis as a step-down dosing regimen of 50 mg administered twice weekly for 3 months, followed by a 50-mg weekly maintenance dose. Etanercept is also indicated for adults with psoriatic arthritis or RA as a 25-mg twice-weekly SC injection administered 72 to 96 hours apart [302]. The drug is supplied as a sterile, preservative-free, lyophilized powder to be reconstituted with 1 mL of bacteriostatic water before injection. Monitoring guidelines are presented in Table 4.

Infliximab

Pharmacology/Mechanism of action

Pharmacokinetic study data from 17 patients with moderate to severe psoriasis treated with either 5 mg/kg or 10 mg/kg doses of infliximab showed maximum infliximab concentrations at day 14 [319]. For the 5- and 10-mg/kg–dose groups, the concen-trations were 158.14 mg/mL and 298.89 mg/mL, respectively—concentrations that were directly proportional to the administered doses. The median elimination half-life for infliximab was 7.62 (inter-quartile range, 6.62–10.15) and 9.97(interquartile range, 6.17–10.1432) days for the 5 mg/kg and 10 mg/kg doses, respectively. The half-life and maximum infliximab concentrations in the 10-mg/kg psoriasis group were similar to those seen in patients with Crohn's disease who were treated with 5 mg/kg of infliximab.

Infliximab is a monoclonal antibody that targets TNF-α. It is composed of a human constant region and a murine variable region, factors that make infliximab chimeric in nature. By binding to both soluble and transmembrane forms of TNF-α, infliximab can trigger complement-mediated lysis of cells expressing TNF-α [320]. As previously described, TNF-α is an important inflammatory cytokine to target because it is central to the pathogenesis of psoriasis. TNF-α fuels the synthesis of many key cytokines involved in the inflammatory cascade, such as IL-1, IL-6, and IL-8, and stimulates Langerhans' cell maturation and migration from the skin to lymph nodes [321]. TNF-α activates nuclear factor κB, a transcription factor that is central to the inflammatory process leading to psoriasis [322]. TNF-α also has been shown to increase keratinocyte proliferation in vitro [319]. In addition, both psoriatic lesional skin and the plasma of patients with psoriasis have shown increased levels of TNF-α [323].

Adverse effects

Oncogenic potential

The long-term risks of development of infliximab-associated malignancies remain unknown. Nahar et al's [324] review of the use of infliximab for the treatment of Crohn's disease and RA reported that 18 of 1372 infliximab-treated patients developed 19 new or recurrent malignancies over 1430 patient-years of follow-up [324]. The authors concluded that it could not be determined whether these malignancies were induced by infliximab treatment. There are several factors that complicate the ability to determine whether the reported occurrences of lymphoma and other malignancies are related to infliximab treatment. Although controversial, rates of lymphoproliferative disease have been shown to be higher among RA, Crohn's disease, and psoriasis populations [325–333]. In addition, lymphoproliferative disorders tend to occur at an increased rate in patients who are immunosuppressed [332,333]. Many patients who have chronic inflammatory diseases, such as RA, Crohn's disease, or psoriasis, have long exposure histories to immunosuppressive agents, complicating the ability to analyze the potential causal relationship even further. Last, because Epstein-Barr virus is a well-known cause of lymphoma in organ transplant patients [334,335], the virus may also have an integral role in the development of malignancies in patient populations where immunosuppressive agents are commonly used.

Infections

Infections, and especially reactivation of TB, have been a major issue of concern associated with the use of infliximab. Keane et al [336] performed an analysis of all reports as of May 29, 2001, of TB cases that occurred after infliximab therapy through the FDA's MedWatch system. Details of this system are available at http://www.fda.gov/cder/aers/. At the time of the analysis, approximately 147,000 patients worldwide had received infliximab. The analysis showed 70 reported cases of TB that occurred after treatment with infliximab for a median of 12 weeks. TB developed in 48 of the patients after three or fewer infusions of infliximab. Of the 70 cases, 40 were extrapulmonary disease. Most cases (64) occurred in countries with a low incidence of TB. The reported frequency of TB associated with infliximab therapy was much higher than the reported frequency of other opportunistic infections. Several cases of histoplasmosis also have been reported, however. Although the authors were not able to completely assess the TB status of the patients pretreated with infliximab, they concluded that the TB was likely reactivation TB.

As mentioned previously, histoplasmosis is another potentially life-threatening infection that has been reported to the FDA as a possible complication associated with infliximab therapy. In a review of the FDA's passive surveillance database for monitoring postlicensure adverse events, Lee et al [337] identified all cases of histoplasmosis received through July 2001 in patients who had been treated with either infliximab or etanercept, the two licensed anti–TNF-α biologic agents. Ten cases of *Histoplasma capsulatum* (HC) infection were reported. Nine of these cases were associated with infliximab therapy, and one case was associated with etanercept therapy. Clinical manifestations of histoplasmosis, including fever, malaise, cough, dyspnea, and interstitial pneumonitis, occurred within 1 week to 6 months of the first dose. It is important to note that all of the patients had been treated with concomitant immunosuppressive agents during infliximab therapy, and all of the patients resided in HC-endemic areas. A

detailed discussion of the clinical implications of the association of infliximab with reactivation TB and histoplasmosis will be addressed in the "Usage guidelines" section.

In a review of the published literature and presentations at scientific meetings from a search of Medline and pre-Medline English-language articles published from 1966 to June 2002 of infliximab for the treatment of RA and Crohn's disease, Nahar et al [324] found that treated infections were reported in 36% of patients receiving infliximab compared with 26% of placebo-treated patients. Respiratory and urinary tract infections were the most frequently reported type of infection. In addition, several serious infections were reported, including pneumonia, abscess, cellulites, skin ulceration, pyelonephritis, sepsis, two cases of TB, and one case of disseminated coccidioidomycosis. The authors pointed out that most of the patients were on concomitant immunosuppressive therapies in two of the large clinical trials in the review, A Crohn's Disease Clinical Trial Evaluating Infliximab in a New Long-Term Treatment Regimen (ACCENT) [338] and Anti-TNF Trial in Rheumatoid Arthritis with Concomitant Therapy (ATTRACT) [339].

Chaudhari et al [340] assessed the clinical benefit and safety of infliximab for the treatment of moderate to severe plaque psoriasis in a double-blind randomized trial of 33 patients. In contrast to the aforementioned data from the literature, the investigators did not observe any serious adverse events during the 10-week study period where patients were randomized to receive 5 mg/kg, 10 mg/kg, or placebo in a 1:1:1 ratio. Patients enrolled in the study did not use any other treatments for their psoriasis during the study and had stopped taking systemic therapy (including cyclosporine, methotrexate, acitretin, and UVB and PUVA) at least 4 weeks before the first dose of study medication. Therefore, unlike many of the patients in previous clinical trials who were receiving concomitant immunosuppressive agents, the patients in this trial were not, a factor that may explain the lack of serious adverse event occurrences. In addition, all patients had a clear chest radiograph within 1 month of receiving the first dose of the study medication.

Effects on the immune system

In the review of the literature of patients with RA and Crohn's disease treated with infliximab, Nahar et al [324] found that approximately 10% of all patients in clinical trials developed antibodies to infliximab. The development of antibodies to the drug was associated with an increased likelihood of developing infusion reactions. Approximately 44% of patients with Crohn's disease treated with infliximab developed ANAs between screening and the last clinical evaluation [324].

In the ATTRACT study [339], a multicenter, randomized, double-blind, placebo-controlled phase 3 trial, 428 patients with active RA were treated with continuous methotrexate and randomized to one of four infliximab treatment regimens. Of 342 exposed patients, 16% (54) developed anti-dsDNA antibodies using the Farr assay of 10 units/mL compared with 0% of placebo-treated patients. Of the 54 patients, 15 (4%) had titers greater than 25 units/mL.

Infusion reactions

Infusion reactions, defined as any adverse event occurring during an infusion or within 1 to 2 hours after an infusion, occurred in approximately 20% of infliximab-treated patients compared with 10% of placebo-treated patients in clinical trials [341]. Less than 1% were considered serious reactions characterized by clinical symptoms of anaphylaxis, convulsions, erythematous rash, or hypotension. Of the patients who experienced infusion reactions, approximately 3% discontinued infliximab therapy because of the reactions. Infusion reactions can be avoided by slowing down the infusion, premedicating with antihistamines, and, in some cases, administering systemic corticosteroids [310]. It is therefore recommended that medications such as antihistamines, corticosteroids, and epinephrine be available at the infusion site.

There have been reports of patients experiencing delayed infusion reactions in instances where infliximab was restarted [324]. In a study in which 37 of 41 patients with Crohn's disease were retreated after a 2- to 4-year lapse between treatments, 10 of the patients experienced adverse events that occurred 3 to 12 days following the infusion. Clinical signs and symptoms included myalgia or arthralgia, with fever or rash, pruritus, edema of the face, hand, or lip, dysphagia, urticaria, sore throat, and headache. None of the patients had experienced an infusion-related adverse event previously. Approximately 39% (9 of 23) of the patients had received a liquid formulation, which is no longer available, and 7% (1 of 14) had received the lyophilized formulation. The makers of the drug do not know if occurrences of these reactions were caused by differences in formulation [341].

Congestive heart failure

Infliximab has been associated with adverse outcomes in patients with congestive heart failure.

In a randomized study of 150 patients with stable New York Heart Association class 3 or 4 heart failure and left ventricular ejection fraction of 35% or less, patients were randomized to receive either placebo (n = 49), infliximab doses of 5 mg/kg (n = 50), or infliximab doses of 10 mg/kg (n = 51) [342]. The results suggested that infliximab therapy over a 6-week period was associated with an increased risk of worsening heart failure in patients in the high-dose (10 mg/kg) group. The authors concluded that although a similar risk was not observed in the low-dose (5 mg/kg) group, longer term treatment with infliximab at this dose could result in more severe adverse events.

Postmarketing reports of worsening heart failure in patients being treated with infliximab have been reported. These reports have occurred in patients with and without precipitating factors. In addition, there have been rare postmarketing reports of new-onset heart failure in patients without diagnosed cardiac disease. There is a detailed discussion of the clinical implications of treating patients who have heart failure with infliximab in the "Usage guidelines" section.

Demyelinating disease

As mentioned previously, neurologic symptoms associated with demyelination of the CNS have been reported to be associated with the anti–TNF-α therapies.

Summary of efficacy data from important clinical trials

The first case documenting the efficacy of infliximab for the treatment of psoriasis was described in a case report of a patient with Crohn's disease and severe psoriasis who was treated with a single 5-mg/kg infusion of infliximab and achieved an improvement in PASI of 22 points within 4 weeks [343]. Subsequent to that case, several reports have attested to the efficacy of infliximab for the treatment of moderate to severe psoriasis [344,345].

A small-scale study was conducted to garner information about the efficacy of infliximab for the treatment of psoriasis in patients with concomitant psoriatic arthritis [346]. Six patients with psoriasis and psoriatic arthritis unresponsive to methotrexate therapy were treated with 5-mg/kg doses of infliximab at weeks 0, 2, and 6, and PASI evaluations were performed at baseline and 10 weeks after therapy started. At week 10, all six patients achieved improvement in psoriasis as measured by PASI score.

In a randomized, double-blind, placebo-controlled clinical trial designed to assess the clinical benefit and safety of infliximab as monotherapy for patients with moderate to severe psoriasis, 33 patients were assigned to receive placebo (n = 11), infliximab doses of 5 mg/kg (n = 11), or infliximab doses of 10 mg/kg (n = 11) at weeks 0, 2, and 6 [340]. Assessments were performed at week 10 using the PGA as the primary endpoint and the PASI score as the secondary endpoint. Nine of 11 (82%) of patients in the 5-mg/kg treatment group and 10 of 11 (91%) of patients in the 10-mg/kg group achieved the primary endpoint on the PGA at week 10 of good, excellent, or clear. This finding was in comparison to 11 (18%) of patients in the placebo group. The difference between infliximab doses of 5 mg/kg and placebo was 64% (95% confidence interval [CI], 20–89; $P = 0.0089$). The difference between infliximab doses of 10 mg/kg and placebo was 73% (CI, 30–94; $P = 0.0019$). Data regarding the secondary endpoint of the study, change in PASI score, were also significant. Nine of 11 (82%) of patients in the 5-mg/kg group and 8 of 11 (73%) of patients in the 10-mg/kg group showed an improvement of 75% or more in PASI score compared with 11 (18%) patients in the placebo group. The difference between infliximab doses of 5 mg/kg and placebo was 64% (CI, 20–90; $P = 0.0089$); and the difference between infliximab doses of 10 mg/kg and placebo was 55% (CI, 9–85; $P = 0.03$). The mean percentage improvements in PASI scores were significantly higher among the infliximab-treated patients as early as week 2 of therapy ($P < 0.0003$). The median time to response in both treatment arms was 4 weeks.

Clinical use in dermatology

Infliximab is currently approved for treatment of RA and Crohn's disease and has been reported to have clinical efficacy in several cutaneous disorders, including the following: psoriasis [340,344–346]; psoriatic arthritis [346]; pustular psoriasis [347]; hidradenitis suppurativa [348]; pyoderma gangrenosum [344,349–352]; Behçet's syndrome [353–355]; synovitis, acne, pustulosis, hyperostosis, and osteitis, or SAPHO, syndrome [356]; subcorneal pustular dermatosis [357]; and toxic epidermal necrolysis [358]. Similar to the clinical response to cyclosporine, high percentages of patients respond to infliximab, and response rates tend to be rapid. Unlike cyclosporine therapy, however, infliximab is not associated with the concerning cumulative dose-related side effects of decreased renal function and hypertension. Another advantage of infliximab is that, similar to efalizumab

and etanercept, infliximab has shown clinical efficacy for both psoriasis and psoriatic arthritis, although it is not yet FDA-approved for either indication. In addition, psoriasis is more prevalent in patients who have inflammatory bowel disease [359]. Infliximab therapy could be beneficial therefore for patients with concomitant inflammatory bowel disease and psoriasis. Although both etanercept and infliximab inhibit TNF-α, infliximab has shown superior clinical efficacy for the treatment of psoriasis. Chaudhari et al [340] offered some explanations for this discrepancy. They asserted that differences may be from the route of administration (IV for infliximab versus SC for etanercept), differences in the patient populations in clinical trials, or differences in the mechanism by which the drugs work. The different mechanisms have been shown by in vitro data, which have shown that, unlike etanercept, infliximab is able to trigger complement-mediated lysis of TNF-α–expressing cells [320]. If this mechanism is accurate, then the implications are that inflximab is able to abolish activated T cells and antigen-presenting cells, a potential explanation for the rapidity and thoroughness of the clinical responses observed in trials.

Usage guidelines

A black box warning has been issued by the manufacturer of infliximab cautioning that the drug should not be given to patients with clinically important active infections. Caution should also be taken when considering the use of infliximab for patients with chronic or recurrent infections. If a patient develops a serious infection while being treated with infliximab, the treatment should be discontinued. TB (frequently disseminated or extrapulmonary at clinical presentation), invasive fungal infections, and other opportunistic infections have been observed in patients being treated with infliximab [341]. Some infections have been fatal. Patients should be evaluated for latent TB infection with a tuberculin skin test, and treatment of latent TB infections should be started before infliximab therapy. For patients who have resided in regions where histoplasmosis or coccidioidomycosis is endemic, the benefits and risks of infliximab therapy should be carefully considered before initiation of therapy.

Infliximab should only be used in patients with heart failure after other treatment options have been considered. If a decision is made to administer infliximab to these patients, the patients should be closely monitored during therapy and treatment should be discontinued if new or worsening symptoms of heart failure appear [341].

Physicians should exercise caution when considering the use of infliximab for the treatment of patients with pre-existing or recent-onset CNS demyelinating or seizure disorders [341].

Infliximab should not be administered to patients with known hypersensitivity to any murine proteins or other component of the drug. To date, no animal reproduction studies have been performed. It is therefore advised that infliximab only be used in pregnancy when clearly clinically necessary [341].

Infliximab only cross-reacts with TNF-α in humans and chimpanzees. In a developmental toxicity study using cV1q antimouse TNF-α, an analogous antibody that inhibits mouse TNF-α, no evidence of carcinogenesis, mutagenesis, or impairment of fertility was observed [341]. Doses of up to 40 mg/kg did not produce any adverse effects in animal reproduction studies. It is not known whether infliximab can cause harm to the fetus, if it can affect reproductive capacity, or if it is excreted in human milk or absorbed systemically post ingestion. Infliximab has been labeled pregnancy category B.

Because of the higher incidence of infections in the elderly population, caution should be used when treating elderly patients. Infliximab is currently not indicated for pediatric use.

Drug interactions

Drug interaction studies with infliximab have not been conducted. In RA and Crohn's disease clinical trials, most patients were treated with one or more concomitant medications. Patients with RA were treated with concomitant methotrexate, NSAIDs, folic acid, corticosteroids, or narcotics. Patients with Crohn's disease in clinical trials were treated with concomitant antibiotics, antiviral medications, corticosteroids, 6-MP/azathioprine, and aminosalicylates. Patients with Crohn's disease who received immunosuppressants tended to have fewer infusion reactions. As previously mentioned, Nahar et al [324] reported that concomitant treatment with immunosuppressants may have predisposed patients in the ACCENT [338] and ATTRACT [339] clinical trials to increased rates of serious infections.

Dosage and monitoring

Infliximab is indicated for the treatment of RA and Crohn's disease. Infliximab is administered as an IV drip over the course of several hours. The mode of administration of infliximab is a potential drawback for both patients and physicians because of the time commitment involved, increased need for skilled health care workers in the office at the time of administration, and potential physical burden for arthritic patients who may have difficulty sitting in one position for the length of the infusion. For the treatment of RA, infliximab is given as a 3-mg/kg IV infusion followed by infusions at weeks 2 and 6, and then every 8 weeks thereafter. Infliximab should be administered in combination with methotrexate for the treatment of RA. Doses of up to 10 mg/kg may be used for patients with RA who have incomplete clinical responses to lower doses. For treatment of patients with Crohn's disease, the recommended dose of infliximab is 5 mg/kg as an induction dose at baseline and weeks 2 and 6. Maintenance doses of 5 mg/kg every 8 weeks after induction can be used to treat moderate to severe active Crohn's disease or fistulizing disease. Doses of up to 10 mg/kg may be used for the treatment of Crohn's disease. For treatment of psoriasis and Crohn's disease, the lower 5-mg/kg dose of infliximab has shown greater efficacy than the 10-mg/kg dose [340,360].

The drug is supplied as a sterile, white, lyophilized powder for IV infusion. Infliximab vials do not contain preservatives and must therefore be used immediately after reconstitution. Monitoring guidelines are presented in Table 4.

Summary

Azathioprine, cyclophosphamide, methotrexate, cyclosporine, and MMF are the nonsteroidal immunosuppressive agents most commonly used by dermatologists. Azathioprine has a relatively good safety profile and is therefore often preferred for the treatment of chronic eczematous dermatitides and bullous disorders. Awareness of the role of genetic polymorphisms in its metabolism can increase the efficacy and safety of this drug. Cyclophosphamide is an antimetabolite that has a more rapid onset of immunosuppressive effect than azathioprine but has significant short- and long-term toxicity. It is of use in fulminant, life-threatening cutaneous disease. Methotrexate is an antimetabolite that has significant anti-inflammatory activity. Despite its hepatotoxicity, its role in inflammatory dermatoses is broadening. Cyclosporine has potent T-cell inhibitory effects secondary to interference with intracellular signal transduction, and its use in dermatology is rapidly expanding. Given the evidence for cumulative renal toxicity, it currently has a role in the short-term treatment of refractory psoriasis and atopic dermatitis, and in select inflammatory dermatoses. MMF is an immune suppressant with wide potential dermatologic applications, especially for bullous disorders, pyoderma gangrenosum, and psoriasis. It has a mechanism of action similar to azathioprine, and it is generally well tolerated. Although some studies found a slightly higher incidence of lymphoproliferative malignancies, MMF has a better overall safety profile than azathioprine. It is more expensive, however. Both mycophenolate and azathioprine should be used in conjunction with oral corticosteroids because they are "steroid sparing" but not "steroid replacing." They are usually required when it is impossible to reduce steroids to an acceptably low level. When they are added, as they become effective, the corticosteroid taper is resumed toward the target maintenance dose.

Alefacept, efalizumab, etanercept, and infliximab are the immunobiologic agents currently most commonly used by dermatologists. Alefacept, the first immunobiologic agent to be approved for the treatment of adult patients with moderate to severe plaque-type psoriasis, is a fusion protein that blocks T-cell activation and selectively reduces memory T cells. Because of its unique mechanism of action, alefacept is considered to be the only remittive biologic agent. Therefore, patients who respond effectively to alefacept can enjoy long-lasting therapy-free reprieves for more than 7 months. Alefacept is also safe; safety and tolerability profiles were shown to be similar to placebo in phase 3 clinical trials. Similar to all of the immunobiologic agents, data on the potential for the development of malignancies require longer follow-up periods before a possible role of these agents in the development of malignancy can be excluded. The intramuscular route of administration, and the need for weekly CD4$^+$ T-cell counts, also distinguishes alefacept, because it requires the patient to make weekly visits to a physician's office. Efalizumab, a humanized monoclonal antibody directed against CD11a, is indicated for the treatment of chronic moderate to severe plaque-type psoriasis. Unlike alefacept, efalizumab is administered as a weekly SC injection. Thrombocytopenia was reported in a small percentage of clinical trial patients; therefore, platelet counts must be monitored throughout treatment. Efalizumab is generally well tolerated but, similar to many of the systemic immunomodulators previously discussed, on cessation of therapy, some patients have experienced clinically significant relapse or exacerbation of psoriasis. Although long-term safety data have not been established for any of the immunobiologic agents, efalizumab has been shown to have a favorable side-effect profile and potential as a long-term therapeutic agent for chronic psoriasis. Etanercept is a dimeric fusion protein that inhibits TNF-α. Etanercept is FDA-approved for the treatment of

psoriasis, psoriatic arthritis, and RA, and for reducing signs and symptoms of moderate to severe active polyarticular-course juvenile RA. Etanercept has a favorable safety profile. It is the only immunobiologic agent of the four discussed that does not require laboratory monitoring. Infliximab is a chimeric monoclonal antibody that targets TNF-α. It is currently indicated for the treatment of RA and Crohn's disease but has shown efficacy for a wide array of dermatologic conditions, especially psoriasis and psoriatic arthritis, pyoderma gangrenosum, and the cutaneous manifestations of Behçet's syndrome. High percentages of patients with psoriasis respond to infliximab, and response rates tend to be rapid and long-lasting. Infliximab has several potential drawbacks, however, including its route of administration, which is by means of an IV drip over the course of several hours. Infusion reactions also have been a concern, although less than 1% of infusion reactions in clinical trials were considered serious. Other issues have been postmarketing reports of worsening heart failure, reactivation TB, and other opportunistic infections. In addition, some patients have developed neutralizing antibodies. Unlike methotrexate and cyclosporine, for example, infliximab is neither hepatotoxic nor nephrotoxic; it therefore represents a useful therapeutic agent for patients with severe psoriasis who have contraindications to other immunosuppressive agents or who are recalcitrant to other therapies.

References

[1] Dutz J, Ho V. Immunosuppressive agents in skin disorders. Clin Immunother 1996;5:268–93.

[2] Ho VC, Zloty DM. Immunosuppressive agents in dermatology. Dermatol Clin 1993;11:73–85.

[3] Dutz JP, Ho VC. Immunosuppressive agents in dermatology. An update. Dermatol Clin 1998;16: 235–51.

[4] Zhou Y, Dutz JP, Ho VC. Mycophenolate mofetil (CellCept (R)) for dermatological diseases. J Cutan Med Surg 2001;5:26–9.

[5] Lebwohl M. Future psoriasis therapy. Dermatol Clin 1985;13:415–23.

[6] Lebwohl M. Advances in psoriasis therapy. Dermatol Clin 2000;18:13–21.

[7] Lennard L, Rees C, Lilleyman J, Maddocks JL. Childhood leukemia: a relationship between intracellular 6-mercaptopurine metabolism and neutropenia. Br J Clin Pharmacol 1983;16:359–63.

[8] Holme SA, Duley JA, Sanderson J, Routledge PA, Anstey AV. Erythrocyte thiopurine methyl transferase assessment prior to azathioprine use in the UK. QJM 2002;95:439–44.

[9] Chocair P, Duley J, Simmonds H, Cameron JS. The importance of thiopurine methyltransferase activity for the use of azathioprine in transplant patients. Transplantation 1992;53:1051–6.

[10] Lennard L, Harrington C, Wood M, Maddocks JL. Metabolism of azathioprine to 6-thioguanine nucleotides in patients with pemphigus vulgaris. Br J Clin Pharmacol 1987;23:229–33.

[11] Snow J, Gibson L. A pharmacogenetic basis for the safe and effective use of azathioprine and other thiopurine drugs in dermatology patients. J Am Acad Dermatol 1995;32:114–6.

[12] Yates C, Krynetski E, Loennechen T, et al. Molecular diagnosis of thiopurine S-methyltransferase deficiency: genetic basis for azathioprine and mercaptopurine intolerance. Ann Intern Med 1997;126: 608–14.

[13] Anstey A. Management of immunobullous disorders: the clinical significance of interindividual variation in azathioprine metabolism. Clin Exp Dermatol 1997; 21:244–51.

[14] Marra CA, Esdaile JM, Anis AH. Practical pharmacogenetics: the cost effectiveness of screening for thiopurine s-methyltransferase polymorphisms in patients with rheumatological conditions treated with azathioprine. J Rheumatol 2002;29:2507–12.

[15] Vesell E. Therapeutic lessons from pharmacogenetics [editorial]. Ann Intern Med 1997;126:653–5.

[16] Aberer W, Wolff-Schreiner EC, Stingl G, Wolff K. Azathioprine in the treatment of pemphigus vulgaris. J Am Acad Dermatol 1987;16:527–33.

[17] Tan BB, Lear JT, Gawkrodger DJ, English JS. Azathioprine in dermatology: a survey of current practice in the UK. Br J Dermatol 1997;136:351–5.

[18] Singh G, Fries JF, Spitz P, Williams CA. Toxic effects of azathioprine in rheumatoid arthritis: a national post-marketing perspective. Arthritis Rheum 1989; 32:837–43.

[19] Schwab M, Schaffeler E, Marx C, et al. Azathioprine therapy and adverse drug reactions in patients with inflammatory bowel disease: impact of thiopurine S-methyltransferase polymorphism. Pharmacogenetics 2002;12:429–36.

[20] Guillaume JC, Vaillant L, Bernard P, et al. Controlled trial of azathioprine and plasma exchange in addition to prednisolone in the treatment of bullous pemphigoid. Arch Dermatol 1993;129:49–53.

[21] Penn I. Cancers in cyclosporine-treated versus azathioprine-treated patients. Transplant Proc 1996;28: 876–8.

[22] Bouwes Bavinck JN, Hardie DR, Green A, et al. The risk of skin cancer in renal transplant recipients in Queensland, Australia. A follow-up study. Transplantation 1996;61:715–21.

[23] Confavreux C, Saddier P, Grimaud J, Moreau T, Adeleine P, Aimard G. Risk of cancer from azathioprine therapy in multiple sclerosis: a case-control study. Neurology 1996;46:1607–12.

[24] Fraser AG, Orchard TR, Robinson EM, Jewell DP. Long-term risk of malignancy after treatment of inflammatory bowel disease with azathioprine. Aliment Pharmacol Ther 2002;16:1225–32.

[25] Beckett CG, Hill P, Hine KR. Leucocytoclastic vasculitis in a patient with azathioprine hypersensitivity [review]. Postgrad Med J 1996;72:437–8.

[26] Compton MR, Crosby DL. Rhabdomyolysis associated with azathioprine hypersensitivity syndrome [letter]. Arch Dermatol 1996;132:1254–5.

[27] Knowles S, Gupta A, Shear N, Sauder D. Azathioprine hypersensitivity-like reactions—a case report and review of the literature. Clin Exp Dermatol 1995; 20:353–6.

[28] Corbett M, Schlup M. Azathioprine hypersensitivity mimicking underlying inflammatory bowel disease. Intern Med J 2001;31:366–7.

[29] Saway PA, Heck LW, Bonner JR, Kirklin JK. Azathioprine hypersensitivity. Am J Med 1988;84: 960–4.

[30] Blanco R, Martinez-Taboada VM, Gonzalez-Gay MA, et al. Acute febrile toxic reaction in patients with refractory rheumatoid arthritis who are receiving combined therapy with methotrexate and azathioprine [review]. Arthritis Rheum 1996;39:1016–20.

[31] van der Pijl JW, Bavinck JN, de Fijter JW. Isotretinoin and azathioprine: a synergy that makes hair curl [letter]? Lancet 1996;348:622–3.

[32] Sudhir RR, Rao SK, Shanmugam MP, Padmanabhan P. Bilateral macular hemorrhage caused by azathioprine-induced aplastic anemia in a corneal graft recipient. Cornea 2002;21:712–4.

[33] Bystryn JC, Steinman NM. The adjuvant therapy of pemphigus. An update [review]. Arch Dermatol 1996;132:203–12.

[34] Villalba L, Adams EM. Update on therapy for refractory dermatomyositis and polymyositis [review]. Curr Opin Rheumatol 1996;8:544–51.

[35] Lear JT, English JS, Jones P, Smith AG. Retrospective review of the use of azathioprine in severe atopic dermatitis. J Am Acad Dermatol 1996;35:642–3.

[36] Berth-Jones J, Takwale A, Tan E, et al. Azathioprine in severe adult atopic dermatitis: a double-blind, placebo-controlled, crossover trial. Br J Dermatol 2002;147:324–30.

[37] Lear JT, English JS, Smith AG. Nodular prurigo responsive to azathioprine [letter]. Br J Dermatol 1996;134:1151.

[38] Yazici H, Pazarli H, Barnes CG, et al. A controlled trial of azathioprine in Behcet's syndrome. N Engl J Med 1990;322:281–5.

[39] Hamuryudan V, Ozyazgan Y, Hizli N, et al. Azathioprine in Behcet's syndrome: effects on long-term prognosis. Arthritis Rheum 1997;40:769–74.

[40] Klein LR, Callen JP. Azathioprine: effective steroid-sparing therapy for generalized lichen planus. South Med J 1992;85:198–201.

[41] Lear JT, English JS. Erosive and generalized lichen planus responsive to azathioprine. Clin Exp Dermatol 1996;21:56–7.

[42] Briggs GG, Freeman RK, Yaffe SJ, editors. Drugs in pregnancy and lactation, a reference guide to fetal and neonatal risk. 4th edition. Baltimore, MD: Williams & Wilkins; 1994. p. 79a–82a.

[43] Friedman JM, Polifka JE. In: Teratogenic effects of drugs, a resource for clinicians. Baltimore, MD: John Hopkins University Press; 1994. p. 53–5.

[44] Cummins D, Sekar M, Halil O, Banner N. Myelosuppression associated with azathioprine-allopurinol interaction after heart and lung transplantation. Transplantation 1996;61:1661–2.

[45] Schutz E, Gummert J, Mohr F, Armstrong VH, Oellerich M. Should 6-thioguanine nucleotides be monitored in heart transplant recipients given azathioprine? Ther Drug Monit 1996;18:228–33.

[46] Gossmann J, Kachel HG, Schoeppe W, Scheuermann EH. Anemia in renal transplant recipients caused by concomitant therapy with azathioprine and angiotensin-converting enzyme inhibitors. Transplantation 1993;56:585–9.

[47] Gossmann J, Thurmann P, Bachmann T, et al. Mechanism of angiotensin converting enzyme inhibitor-related anemia in renal transplant recipients. Kidney Int 1996;50:973–8.

[48] American College of Rheumatology Ad Hoc Committee on Clinical Guidelines. Guidelines for monitoring drug therapy in rheumatoid arthritis. Arthritis Rheum 1996;39:723–31.

[49] Bradley PP, Warden GD, Maxwell JG, Rothstein G. Neutropenia and thrombocytopenia in renal allograft recipients treated with trimethoprim-sulfamethoxazole. Ann Intern Med 1980;93:560–2.

[50] Olsen SL, Renlund DG, O'Connell JB, et al. Prevention of Pneumocystis carinii pneumonia in cardiac transplant recipients by trimethoprim sulfamethoxazole. Transplantation 1993;56:359–62.

[51] Rivier G, Khamashta MA, Hughes GR. Warfarin and azathioprine: a drug interaction does exist [letter]. Am J Med 1993;95:342.

[52] Havrda DE, Rathbun S, Scheid D. A case report of warfarin resistance due to azathioprine and review of the literature. Pharmacotherapy 2001;21:355–7.

[53] Murphy LA, Atherton D. A retrospective evaluation of azathioprine in severe childhood atopic eczema, using thiopurine methyltransferase levels to exclude patients at high risk of myelosuppression. Br J Dermatol 2002;147:308–15.

[54] McDonald CJ. Cytotoxic agents for use in dermatology I. J Am Acad Dermatol 1985;12:753–75.

[55] Moore MJ. Clinical pharmacokinetics of cyclophosphamide. Clin Pharmacokinet 1991;20:194–208.

[56] Hemendinger RA, Bloom SE. Selective mitomycin C and cyclophosphamide induction of apoptosis in differentiating B lymphocytes compared to T lymphocytes in vivo. Immunopharmacology 1996;35:71–82.

[57] Rothe H, Burkart V, Faust A, Kolb H. Interleukin-12 gene expression mediates the accelerating effect of cyclophosphamide in autoimmune disease. Ann N Y Acad Sci 1996;795:397–9.

[58] Marcinkiewicz J, Bryniarski K, Ptak W. Cyclophosphamide uncovers two separate macrophage subpopulations with opposite immunogenic potential and different patterns of monokine production. Cytokine 1994;6:472–7.

[59] Yarboro CH, Wesley R, Amantea MA, Klippel JH, Pucino F. Modified oral ondansetron regimen for cyclophosphamide-induced emesis in lupus nephritis. Ann Pharmacother 1996;30:752–5.

[60] Aapro MS, Thuerlimann B, Sessa C, De Pree C, Bernhard J, Maibach R. A randomized double-blind trial to compare the clinical efficacy of granisetron with metoclopramide, both combined with dexamethasone in the prophylaxis of chemotherapy-induced delayed emesis. Ann Oncol 2003;14:291–7.

[61] Fraiser L, Kanekal S, Kehrer J. Cyclophosphamide toxicity. Characterising and avoiding the problem. Drugs 1991;42:781–91.

[62] Stillwell TJ, Benson Jr RC. Cyclophosphamide-induced hemorrhagic cystitis—a review of 100 patients. Cancer 1988;61:451–7.

[63] Talar-Williams C, Hijazi YM, Walther MM, et al. Cyclophosphamide-induced cystitis and bladder cancer in patients with Wegener granulomatosis. Ann Intern Med 1996;124:477–84.

[64] Haselberger M, Schwinghammer T. Efficacy of mesna for the prevention of hemorrhagic cystitis after high-dose cyclophosphamide therapy. Ann Pharmacother 1995;29:918–20.

[65] Fairchild WV, Spence CR, Soloman HD. The incidence of bladder cancer after cyclophosphamide therapy. J Urol 1979;122:163–4.

[66] Baker GL, Kahl LE, Zee BC. Malignancy following treatment of rheumatoid arthritis with cyclophosphamide; long-term case-control follow-up study. Am J Med 1987;83:1–9.

[67] Baltus JA. The occurrence of malignancies in patients with rheumatoid arthritis treated with cyclophosphamide: a controlled retrospective follow up. Ann Rheum Dis 1983;42:368–73.

[68] Radis CD, Kahl LE, Baker GL, et al. Effects of cyclophosphamide on the development of malignancy and on long-term survival of patients with rheumatoid arthritis. A 20-year follow-up study. Arthritis Rheum 1995;38:1120–7.

[69] Volm T, Pfaff P, Gnann R, Kreienberg R. Bladder carcinoma associated with cyclophosphamide therapy for ovarian cancer occurring with a latency of 20 years. Gynecol Oncol 2001;82:197–9.

[70] Masala A, Faedda R, Alagna S, et al. Use of testosterone to prevent cyclophosphamide-induced azoospermia. Ann Intern Med 1997;126:292–5.

[71] Blumenfeld Z, Haim N. Prevention of gonadal damage during cytotoxic therapy. Ann Med 1997;29:199–206.

[72] Pryor BD, Bologna SG, Kahl LE. Risk factors for serious infection during treatment with cyclophos-

phamide and high-dose corticosteroids for systemic lupus erythematosus. Arthritis Rheum 1996;39: 1475–82.

[73] Cohen MA, Cohen JJ, Kerdel FA. Immunoablative high-dose cyclophosphamide without stem cell rescue in pemphigus foliaceus. Int J Dermatol 2002;41: 340–4.

[74] Hayag MV, Cohen JA, Kerdel FA. Immunoablative high-dose cyclophosphamide without stem cell rescue in a patient with pemphigus vulgaris. J Am Acad Dermatol 2000;43:1065–9.

[75] Werth VP. Pulse intravenous cyclophosphamide for treatment of autoimmune blistering disease. Is there an advantage over oral routes [editorial]? Arch Dermatol 1997;133:229–30.

[76] Pasricha JS, Khaitan BK. Curative treatment for pemphigus [letter]. Arch Dermatol 1996;132:1518–9.

[77] Pandya AG, Warren KJ, Bergstresser PR. Cicatricial pemphigoid successfully treated with pulse intravenous cyclophosphamide [letter]. Arch Dermatol 1997;133:245–7.

[78] Itoh T, Hosokawa H, Shirai Y, Horio T. Successful treatment of bullous pemphigoid with pulsed intravenous cyclophosphamide. Br J Dermatol 1996;134: 931–3.

[79] Castle SP, Mather-Mondrey M, Bennion S, David-Bajar K, Huff C. Chronic herpes gestationis and antiphospholipid antibody syndrome successfully treated with cyclophosphamide. J Am Acad Dermatol 1996;34:333–6.

[80] Frangogiannis NG, Boridy I, Mazhar M, Mathews R, Gangopadhyay S, Cate T. Cyclophosphamide in the treatment of toxic epidermal necrolysis. South Med J 1996;89:1001–3.

[81] Heng MCY, Allen SG. Efficacy of cyclophosphamide in toxic epidermal necrolysis. J Am Acad Dermatol 1991;25:778–86.

[82] Dawisha SM, Yarboro CH, Vaughan EM, Austin III HA, Balow JE, Klippel JH. Out-patient monthly oral bolus cyclophosphamide therapy in systemic lupus erythematosus. J Rheumatol 1996;23:273–8.

[83] Craig NM, Putterman AM, Roenigk RK, Wang TD, Roenigk HH. Multiple periorbital cutaneous myxomas progressing to scleromyxedema. J Am Acad Dermatol 1996;34:928–30.

[84] Liang GC, Granston AS. Complete remission of multicentric reticulohistiocytosis with combination therapy of steroid, cyclophosphamide, and low-dose pulse methotrexate. Case report, review of the literature, and proposal for treatment [review]. Arthritis Rheum 1996;39:171–4.

[85] Bhagat R, Sporn TA, Long GD, Folz RJ. Amiodarone and cyclophosphamide: potential for enhanced lung toxicity. Bone Marrow Transplant 2001;27:1109–11.

[86] Balis FM, Mirro J, Reaman GH, et al. Pharmacokinetics of subcutaneous methotrexate. J Clin Oncol 1988;6:1882–6.

[87] Bannwarth B, Pehourcq F, Schaeverbeke T, Dehais J. Clinical pharmacokinetics of low-dose pulse methotrexate in rheumatoid arthritis [review]. Clin Pharmacokinet 1996;30:194–210.

[88] Bannwarth B, Labat L, Moride Y, Schaeverbeke T. Methotrexate in rheumatoid arthritis, an update. Drugs 1994;47:25–50.

[89] Olsen EA. The pharmacology of methotrexate. J Am Acad Dermatol 1991;25:306–18.

[90] Cronstein BN. Molecular therapeutics. Methotrexate and its mechanism of action [review]. Arthritis Rheum 1996;39:1951–60.

[91] Jeffes III EWB, McCullough JL, Pittelkow MR, et al. Methotrexate therapy of psorisas: differential sensitivity of proliferating lymphoid and epithelial cells to the cytotoxic and growth-inhibitory effects of methotrexate. J Invest Dermatol 1995;104:183–8.

[92] Phillips DC, Woollard KJ, Griffiths HR. The anti-inflammatory actions of methotrexate are critically dependent upon the production of reactive oxygen species. Br J Pharmacol 2003;138:501–11.

[93] Cronstein BN. Molecular therapeutics. Methotrexate and its mechanism of action [review]. Arthritis Rheum 1996;39:1951–60.

[94] Andersson SE, Johansson LH, Lexmuller K, Ekstrom GM. Anti-arthritic effect of methotrexate: is it really mediated by adenosine? Eur J Pharm Sci 2000;9: 333–43.

[95] Cronstein BN, Naime D, Ostad E. The antiinflammatory mechanism of methotrexate. J Clin Invest 1993; 92:2675–82.

[96] Van Dooren-Greebe RJ, Kuijpers AL, Mulder J, De Boo T, Van de Kerkhof PC. Methotrexate revisited: effects of long-term treatment in psoriasis. Br J Dermatol 1994;130:204–10.

[97] Al-Awadhi A, Dale P, McKendry RJ. Pancytopenia associated with low dose methotrexate therapy. A regional survey. J Rheumatol 1993;20:1121–5.

[98] Guzzo C. Folic acid supplementation with methotrexate therapy: what benefit if any? J Am Acad Dermatol 1994;31:689.

[99] Kirby B, Lyon CC, Griffiths CE, Chalmers RJ. The use of folic acid supplementation in psoriasis patients receiving methotrexate: a survey in the United Kingdom. Clin Exp Dermatol 2000;25:265–8.

[100] Duhra P. Treatment of gastrointestinal symptoms associated with methotrexate therapy for psoriasis. J Am Acad Dermatol 1993;28:466–9.

[101] Kremer JM, Alarcon GS, Lightfoot Jr RW, et al. Methotrexate for rheumatoid arthritis: suggested guidelines for monitoring liver toxicity. Arthritis Rheum 1994;37:316–28.

[102] Whiting-O'Keefe Q, Fye KH, Sack KD. Methotrexate and histologic hepatic abnormalities: a meta-analysis. Am J Med 1991;90:711–6.

[103] Auerbach R. Psoriasis symposium. Methotrexate. Semin Dermatol 1992;11:23–9.

[104] Zachariae H, Sogaard H, Heickendorff L. Methotrexate-induced liver cirrhosis. Clinical, histological and serological studies—a further 10-year followup. Dermatology 1996;192:343–6.

[105] Roenigk Jr HH, Auerbach R, Maibach HI, Wein-
      stein G, Lebwohl M. Methotrexate in psoriasis: con-
      sensus conference. J Am Acad Dermatol 1998;38:
      478–85.

[106] Rothe MJ, Grin-Jorgensen C, Ramsey WH, Grant-
      Kels JM. Monitoring patients taking methotrexate.
      J Am Acad Dermatol 1995;32:680.

[107] Petrazzuoli M, Rothe MJ, Grin-Jorgensen C, Ramsey
      WH, Grant-Kels JM. Monitoring patients taking
      methotrexate for hepatotoxicity. J Am Acad Dermatol
      1994;31:969–77.

[108] Rosenthal D, Guenther L, Kelly J. Current thoughts
      on the use of methotrexate in patients with psoriasis.
      J Cutan Med Surg 1997;2:41–6.

[109] Boffa M, Chalmers R, Haboubi N, Shomaf M,
      Mitchell DM. Sequential liver biopsies during long-
      term methotrexate treatment for psoriasis: a reap-
      praisal. Br J Dermatol 1995;133:774–8.

[110] Kumar B, Saraswat A, Kaur I. Short-term methotrex-
      ate therapy in psoriasis: a study of 197 patients. Int J
      Dermatol 2002;41:444–8.

[111] Boffa MJ, Smith A, Chalmers RJ, et al. Serum type III
      procollagen aminopeptide for assessing liver damage
      in methotrexate-treated psoriatic patients. Br J Der-
      matol 1996;135:538–44.

[112] Zachariae H, Heickendorff L, Sogaard H. The value
      of amino-terminal propeptide of type III procollagen
      in routine screening for methotrexate-induced liver
      fibrosis: a 10-year follow-up. Br J Dermatol 2001;
      144:100–3.

[113] Stern RS, Laird N. The carcinogenic risk of treat-
      ments for severe psoriasis. Cancer 1994;73:2759–64.

[114] Zumtobel U, Schwarze HP, Favre M, Taieb A,
      Delaunay M. Widespread cutaneous carcinomas
      associated with human papillomaviruses 5, 14 and
      20 after introduction of methotrexate in two long-
      term PUVA-treated patients. Dermatology 2001;202:
      127–30.

[115] Kamel OW, Weiss LM, van de Rijn M, Colby TV,
      Kingma DW, Jaffe ES. Hodgkin's disease and
      lymphoproliferations resembling Hodgkin's disease
      in patients receiving long-term low-dose methotrexate
      therapy. Am J Surg Pathol 1996;20:1279–87.

[116] Paul C, LeTourneau A, Cayuela JM, et al. Epstein-
      Barr virus-associated lymphoproliferative disease
      during methotrexate therapy for psoriasis. Arch
      Dermatol 1997;133:867–71.

[117] Ebeo CT, Girish MR, Byrd RP, Roy TM, Mehta JB.
      Methotrexate-induced pulmonary lymphoma. Chest
      2003;123:2150–3.

[118] Hirose Y, Masaki Y, Okada J, et al. Epstein-Barr
      virus-associated B-cell type non-Hodgkin's lym-
      phoma with concurrent p53 protein expression in a
      rheumatoid arthritis patient treated with methotrexate.
      Int J Hematol 2002;75:412–5.

[119] Moder KG, Tefferi A, Cohen MD, Menke DM,
      Luthra HS. Hematologic malignancies and the use of
      methotrexate in rheumatoid arthritis: a retrospective
      study. Am J Med 1995;99:276–81.

[120] Donnenfeld AE, Pastuszak A, Noah JS, Schick B,
      Rose NC, Koren G. Methotrexate exposure prior and
      during pregnancy [letter]. Teratology 1994;49:79–81.

[121] Boerbooms AMT, Kerstens PJ, van Loenhout JW,
      Mulder J, van de Putte LB. Infections during low-
      dose methotrexate treatment in rheumatoid arthritis.
      Semin Arthritis Rheum 1995;24:411–21.

[122] Alkins SA, Byrd JC, Morgan SK, Ward FT, Weiss
      RB. Anaphylactoid reactions to methotrexate
      [review]. Cancer 1996;77:2123–6.

[123] Pearce HP, Wilson BB. Erosion of psoriatic plaques:
      an early sign of methotrexate toxicity [review]. J Am
      Acad Dermatol 1996;35:835–8.

[124] Ben-Amitai D, Hodak E, David M. Cutaneous ulcer-
      ation: an unusual sign of methotrexate toxicity—first
      report in a patient without psoriasis. Ann Pharma-
      cother 1998;32:651–3.

[125] Zonneveld IM, Bakker WK, Dijkstra PF, Bos JD, van
      Soesbergen RM, Dinant HJ. Methotrexate osteopathy
      in long-term, low-dose methotrexate treatment for
      psoriasis and rheumatoid arthritis. Arch Dermatol
      1996;132:184–7.

[126] Pigatto PD, Gibelli E, Ranza R, Rossetti A. Metho-
      trexate in psoriatic polyarthritis. Acta Derm Venereol
      1994;74:114–5.

[127] Clayton BD, Jorizzo JL, Hitchcock MG, et al. Adult
      pityriasis rubra pilaris: a 10 year case series. J Am
      Acad Dermatol 1997;36:959–64.

[128] Andersen WK, Feingold DS. Adverse drug interac-
      tions clinically important for the dermatologist. Arch
      Dermatol 1995;131:468–73.

[129] Vonderheid EC, Sajjadian A, Kadin ME. Methotrex-
      ate is effective therapy for lymphomatoid papulosis
      and other primary cutaneous CD30-positive lympho-
      proliferative disorders. J Am Acad Dermatol 1996;
      34:470–81.

[130] Kasteler JS, Callen JP. Low-dose methotrexate
      administered weekly is an effective corticosteroid-
      sparing agent for the treatment of the cutaneous
      manifestations of dermatomyositis. J Am Acad
      Dermatol 1997;36:67–71.

[131] Carson PJ, Hameed A, Ahmed AR. Influence of
      treatment on the clinical course of pemphigus
      vulgaris. J Am Acad Dermatol 1996;34:645–52.

[132] Paul MA, Jorizzo JL, Fleischer AJ, White WL. Low-
      dose methotrexate treatment in elderly patients with
      bullous pemphigoid. J Am Acad Dermatol 1994;31:
      620–5.

[133] Teitel AD. Treatment of pyoderma gangrenosum with
      methotrexate. Cutis 1996;57:326–8.

[134] Seyger MM, van den Hoogen FH, de Boo T, de Jong
      EM. Low-dose methotrexate in the treatment of
      widespread morphea. J Am Acad Dermatol 1998;
      39:220–5.

[135] Franck N, Amor B, Ayral X, et al. Multicentric
      reticulohistiocytosis and methotrexate. J Am Acad
      Dermatol 1995;33:524–5.

[136] Faulds D, Goa KL, Benfield P. Cyclosporin: a review
      of its pharmacodynamic and pharmacokinetic proper-

ties, and therapeutic use in immunoregulatory disorders. Drugs 1993;45:953–1040.

[137] Erkko P, Granlund H, Nuutinen M, Reitamo S. Comparison of cyclosporin A pharmacokinetics of a new microemulsion formulation and standard oral preparation in patients with psoriasis. Br J Dermatol 1997;136:82–8.

[138] Bourke JF, Berth-Jones J, Holder J, Graham-Brown RA. A new microemulsion formulation of cyclosporin (Neoral) is effective in the treatment of cyclosporin-resistant dermatoses. Br J Dermatol 1996;134:777–9.

[139] Ho V, Cloutier MAR, Gratton D, et al. Neoral in the treatment of psoriasis: consensus treatment guidelines. J Cutan Med Surg 1997;1:209–15.

[140] Gulliver WP, Murphy GF, Hannaford VA, Primmett DR. Increased bioavailability and improved efficacy, in severe psoriasis, of a new microemulsion formulation of cyclosporin. Br J Dermatol 1996;48:35–9.

[141] Liu J. FK506 and cyclosporin, molecular probes for studying intracellular signal transduction. Immunol Today 1993;14:290–5.

[142] Wong RL, Winslow CM, Cooper KD. The mechanisms of action of cyclosporin A in the treatment of psoriasis [review]. Immunol Today 1993;14:69–74.

[143] Pei Y. Chronic cyclosporine nephrotoxicity in rheumatoid arthritis. J Rheumatol 1996;23:4–5.

[144] Sheikh-Hamad D, Nadkarni V, Choi YJ, et al. Cyclosporine A inhibits the adaptive responses to hypertonicity: a potential mechanism of nephrotoxicity. J Am Soc Nephrol 2001;12:2732–41.

[145] Feutren G, Mihatsch M. Risk factors for cyclosporine-induced nephropathy in patients with autoimmune diseases. N Engl J Med 1992;326:1654–60.

[146] Lowe NJ, Wieder JM, Rosenbach A, et al. Long-term low-dose cyclosporine therapy for psoriasis: effects on renal function and structure. J Am Acad Dermatol 1996;35:710–9.

[147] Pei Y, Scholey JW, Katz A, Schachter R, Murphy GF, Cattran D. Chronic nephrotoxicity in psoriatic patients treated with low-dose cyclosporine. Am J Kidney Dis 1994;23:528–36.

[148] Powles AV, Cook T, Hulme B, et al. Renal function and biopsy findings after 5 years' treatment with low-dose cyclosporin for psoriasis. Br J Dermatol 1993;128:159–65.

[149] Feutren G, Abeywickrama K, Friend D, von Graffenried B. Renal function and blood pressure in psoriatic patients treated with cyclosporin A. Br J Dermatol 1990;122(Suppl 36):57–69.

[150] Rodicio JL. Calcium antagonists and renal protection from cyclosporine nephrotoxicity: long-term trial in renal transplantation patients. J Cardiovasc Pharmacol 2000;35:S7–11.

[151] Asai T, Nakatani T, Yamanaka S, et al. Magnesium supplementation prevents experimental chronic cyclosporine a nephrotoxicity via renin-angiotensin system independent mechanism. Transplantation 2002;74:784–91.

[152] Thurman RG, Zhong Z, von Frankenberg M, Stachlewitz RF, Bunzendahl H. Prevention of cyclosporine-induced nephrotoxicity with dietary glycine. Transplantation 1997;63:1661–7.

[153] Andoh TF, Gardner MP, Bennett WM. Protective effects of dietary L-arginine supplementation on chronic cyclosporine nephrotoxicity. Transplantation 1997;64:1236–40.

[154] Zackheim HS. Cyclosporine-associated lymphoma [letter]. J Am Acad Dermatol 1999;40:1015–6.

[155] Koo J, Lebwohl M. Reply. J Am Acad Dermatol 1999;40:1016.

[156] Paul CF, Ho VC, McGeown C, et al. Risk of malignancies in psoriasis patients treated with cyclosporine: a 5 y cohort study. J Invest Dermatol 2003; 120:211–6.

[157] van de Kerhof PCM, de Rooij MJM. Multiple squamous cell carcinomas in a psoriatic patient following high-dose photochemotherapy and cyclosporin treatment: response to long-term acitretin maintenance. Br J Dermatol 1997;136:275–8.

[158] Shupack J, Abel E, Bauer E, et al. Cyclosporine as maintenance therapy in patients with severe psoriasis. J Am Acad Dermatol 1997;36:423–32.

[159] Laburte C, Grossman R, Abi-Rached J, Abeywickrama KH, Dubertret L. Efficacy and safety of oral cyclosporin A (CyA; Sandimmun) for long-term treatment of chronic severe plaque psoriasis. Br J Dermatol 1994;130:366–75.

[160] Mahrle G, Schulze HJ, Brautigam M, et al. Anti-inflammatory efficacy of low-dose cyclosporin A in psoriatic arthritis. A prospective multicentre study. Br J Dermatol 1996;135:752–7.

[161] Ho VC, Griffiths CE, Berth-Jones J, et al. Intermittent short courses of cyclosporine microemulsion for the long-term management of psoriasis: a 2-year cohort study. J Am Acad Dermatol 2001;44:643–51.

[162] Camp RD, Reitamo S, Friedmann PS, Ho V, Heule F. Cyclosporin A in severe, therapy-resistant atopic dermatitis: report of an international workshop. Br J Dermatol 1993;129:127–220.

[163] Berth-Jones J, Graham-Brown RA, Marks R, et al. Long-term efficacy and safety of cyclosporin in severe adult atopic dermatitis. Br J Dermatol 1997; 136:76–81.

[164] Czech W, Brautigam M, Weidinger G, Schopf E. A body-weight-independent dosing regimen of cyclosporine microemulsion is effective in severe atopic dermatitis and improves the quality of life. J Am Acad Dermatol 2000;42:653–9.

[165] Granlund H, Erkko P, Sinisalo M, Reitamo S. Cyclosporin in atopic dermatitis: time to relapse and effect of intermittent therapy. Br J Dermatol 1995; 132:106–12.

[166] Granlund H, Erkko P, Eriksson E, Reitamo S. Comparison of cyclosporine and topical betamethasone-17, 21-diproprionate in the treatment of severe chronic hand eczema. Acta Derm Venereol 1996; 76:371–6.

[167] Lim KK, Su WP, Schroeter AL, Sabers CJ, Abraham RT, Pittelkow MR. Cyclosporine in the treatment of dermatologic disease: an update. Mayo Clin Proc 1996;71:1182–91.

[168] Ruzicka T. Cyclosporin in less common immune-mediated skin diseases [review]. Br J Dermatol 1996; 48:40–2.

[169] Capella GL, Casa-Alberighi OD, Finzi AF. Therapeutic concepts in clinical dermatology: cyclosporine A in immunomediated and other dermatoses. Int J Dermatol 2001;40:551–61.

[170] Levell NJ, Munro CS, Marks JM. Severe lichen planus clears with very low-dose cyclosporin [letter]. Br J Dermatol 1992;127:66–7.

[171] Mobini N, Padilla Jr T, Ahmed AR. Long-term remission in selected patients with pemphigus vulgaris treated with cyclosporine. J Am Acad Dermatol 1997;36:264–6.

[172] Chrysomallis F, Ioannides D, Teknetzis A, Panagiotidou D, Minas A. Treatment of oral pemphigus vulgaris. Int J Dermatol 1994;33:803–7.

[173] Ioannides D, Chrysomallis F, Bystryn JC. Ineffectiveness of cyclosporine as an adjuvant to corticosteroids in the treatment of pemphigus. Arch Dermatol 2000; 136:868–72.

[174] Vardy DA, Cohen AD. Cyclosporine therapy should be considered for maintenance of remission in patients with pemphigus [letter]. Arch Dermatol 2001;137:505–6.

[175] Zeller V, Cohen P, Prieur AM, Guillevin L. Cyclosporin a therapy in refractory juvenile dermatomyositis. Experience and longterm follow-up of 6 cases. J Rheumatol 1996;23:1424–7.

[176] Shapiro J, Lui H, Tron V, Ho V. Systemic cyclosporine and low-dose prednisone in the treatment of chronic severe alopecia areata: a clinical and immunopathologic evaluation. J Am Acad Dermatol 1997; 36:114–7.

[177] Ostrov BE, Athreya BH, Eichenfield AH, Goldsmith DP. Successful treatment of severe cytophagic histiocytic panniculitis with cyclosporine A. Semin Arthritis Rheum 1996;25:404–13.

[178] Zaki I, Patel S, Reed R, Dalziel KL. Toxic epidermal necrolysis associated with severe hypocalcemia, and treated with cyclosporin [letter]. Br J Dermatol 1995; 133:337–8.

[179] Buckley DA, Rogers S. Cyclosporin-responsive hidradenitis suppurativa. J R Soc Med 1995;88: 289P–90P.

[180] Berth-Jones J, Smith SG, Graham-Brown RAC. Nodular prurigo responds to cyclosporin. Br J Dermatol 1995;132:795–9.

[181] Berth-Jones J, Smith SG, Graham-Brown RAC. Benign familial chronic pemphigus (Hailey-Hailey disease) responds to cyclosporin. Clin Exp Dermatol 1995;20:70–2.

[182] Filotico R, Vena GA, Coviello C, Angelini G. Cyclosporine in the treatment of generalized granuloma annulare. J Am Acad Dermatol 1994;30:487–8.

[183] Ho V. Cyclosporine in the treatment of generalized granuloma annulare [letter]. J Am Acad Dermatol 1995;33:298.

[184] Stinco G, Codutti R, Frattasio A, De Francesco V, Patrone P. Chronic actinic dermatitis treated with cyclosporine-A. Eur J Dermatol 2002;12:455–7.

[185] Kiyohara A, Takamori K, Niizuma N, Ogawa H. Successful treatment of severe recurrent Reiter's syndrome with cyclosporine. J Am Acad Dermatol 1997;36:482–3.

[186] Herr H, Koh JK. Eosinophilic cellulitis (Wells' syndrome) successfully treated with low-dose cyclosporine. J Korean Med Sci 2001;16:664–8.

[187] von den Driesch P, Steffan C, Zobe A, Hornstein OP. Sweet's syndrome—therapy with cyclosporin. Clin Exp Dermatol 1994;19:274–7.

[188] Berth-Jones J, Voorhees JJ. Consensus conference on cyclosporin A microemulsion for psoriasis. Br J Dermatol 1996;135:775–7.

[189] Lebwohl M, Ellis C, Gottlieb A, et al. Cyclosporine consensus conference: with emphasis on the treatment of psoriasis. J Am Acad Dermatol 1998;39:464–75.

[190] Ransom JT. Mechanism of action of mycophenolate mofetil. Ther Drug Monit 1995;17:681–4.

[191] Parker G, Bullingham R, Kamm B, Hale M. Pharmacokinetics of oral mycophenolate mofetil in volunteer subjects with varying degrees of hepatic oxidative impairment. J Clin Pharmacol 1996;36: 332–44.

[192] Langman LJ, Shapiro AM, Lakey JR, LeGatt DF, Kneteman NM, Yatscoff RW. Pharmacodynamic assessment of mycophenolic acid-induced immunosuppression by measurement of inosine monophosphate dehydrogenase activity in a canine model. Transplantation 1996;61:87–92.

[193] Bullingham R, Monroe S, Nicholls A, Hale M. Pharmacokinetics and bioavailability of mycophenolate mofetil in healthy subjects after single-dose oral and intravenous administration. J Clin Pharmacol 1996;36:315–24.

[194] Kitchin JE, Pomeranz MK, Pak G, Washenik K, Shupack JL. Rediscovering mycophenolic acid: a review of its mechanism, side effects, and potential uses. J Am Acad Dermatol 1997;37:445–9.

[195] Morris RE. Mechanisms of action of new immunosuppressive drugs. Ther Drug Monit 1995;17:564–9.

[196] Allison AC, Eugui EM. Immunosuppressive and other effects of mycophenolic acid and an ester prodrug, mycophenolate mofetil. Immunol Rev 1993;136:5–28.

[197] Eugui EM, Allison AC. Immunosuppressive activity of mycophenolate mofetil. Ann N Y Acad Sci 1993; 685:309–29.

[198] Allison AC, Eugui EM. Mycophenolate mofetil and its mechanisms of action. Immunopharmacology 2000;47:85–118.

[199] Lipsky JJ. Mycophenolate mofetil. Lancet 1996; 348:1357–9.

[200] Yamani MH, Starling RC, Goormastic M, et al. The

impact of routine mycophenolate mofetil drug monitoring on the treatment of cardiac allograft rejection. Transplantation 2000;69:2326–30.

[201] CellCept (mycophenolate mofetil) [package insert]. Mississauga (Canada): Hoffmann–La Roche Ltd; 1997.

[202] Riskalla MM, Somers EC, Fatica RA, McCune WJ. Tolerability of mycophenolate mofetil in patients with systemic lupus erythematosus. J Rheumatol 2003; 30:1508–12.

[203] Maes BD, Dalle I, Geboes K, et al. Erosive enterocolitis in mycophenolate mofetil-treated renal-transplant recipients with persistent afebrile diarrhea. Transplantation 2003;75:665–72.

[204] Behrend M. Adverse gastrointestinal effects of mycophenolate mofetil: aetiology, incidence and management. Drug Saf 2001;24:645–63.

[205] Simmons WD. Preliminary risk–benefit assessment of mycophenolate mofetil in transplant rejection. Drug Saf 1997;17:75–92.

[206] Sterneck M, Fischer L, Gahlemann C, Gundlach M, Rogiers X, Broelsch C. Mycophenolate mofetil for prevention of liver allograft rejection: initial results of a controlled clinical trial. Ann Transplant 2000;5: 43–6.

[207] CellCept (mycophenolate mofetil). Hoffmann–La Roche Ltd; 2003.

[208] Triemer HL, Pearson TC, Odom KL, Larsen CP. Analysis of a single-center experience with mycophenolate mofetil based immunosuppression in renal transplantation. Clin Transplant 2000;14:413–20.

[209] Mycophenolate Mofetil Acute Renal Rejection Study Group. Mycophenolate mofetil for the treatment of a first acute renal allograft rejection: three-year followup. Transplantation 2001;71:1091–7.

[210] Baudard M, Vincent A, Moreau P, Kergueris MF, Harousseau JL, Milpied N. Mycophenolate mofetil for the treatment of acute and chronic GVHD is effective and well tolerated but induces a high risk of infectious complications: a series of 21 BM or PBSC transplant patients. Bone Marrow Transplant 2002; 30:287–95.

[211] ter Meulen CG, Wetzels JF, Hilbrands LB. The influence of mycophenolate mofetil on the incidence and severity of primary cytomegalovirus infections and disease after renal transplantation. Nephrol Dial Transplant 2000;15:711–4.

[212] Sarmiento JM, Dockrell DH, Schwab TR, Munn SR, Paya CV. Mycophenolate mofetil increases cytomegalovirus invasive organ disease in renal transplant patients. Clin Transplant 2000;14:136–8.

[213] Hambach L, Stadler M, Dammann E, Ganser A, Hertenstein B. Increased risk of complicated CMV infection with the use of mycophenolate mofetil in allogeneic stem cell transplantation. Bone Marrow Transplant 2002;29:903–6.

[214] Enk AH, Knop J. Treatment of pemphigus vulgaris with mycophenolate mofetil [letter]. Lancet 1997; 350:494.

[215] Bohm M, Beissert S, Schwarz T, Metze D, Luger T. Bullous pemphigoid treated with mycophenolate mofetil [letter]. Lancet 1997;349:541.

[216] Popovsky JL, Camisa C. New and emerging therapies for diseases of the oral cavity. Dermatol Clin 2000; 18:113–25.

[217] Grundmann-Kollmann M, Kaskel P, Leiter U, et al. Treatment of pemphigus vulgaris and bullous pemphigoid with mycophenolate mofetil monotherapy [letter]. Arch Dermatol 1999;135:724–5.

[218] Nousari HC, Sragovich A, Kimyai-Asadi A, Orlinsky D, Anhalt GJ. Mycophenolate mofetil in autoimmune and inflammatory skin disorders. J Am Acad Dermatol 1999;40:265–8.

[219] Nousari HC, Griffin WA, Anhalt GJ. Successful therapy for bullous pemphigoid with mycophenolate mofetil. J Am Acad Dermatol 1998;39:497–8.

[220] Bredlich RO, Grundmann-Kollmann M, Behrens S, Kerscher M, Peter RU. Mycophenolate mofetil monotherapy for pemphigus vulgaris [letter]. Br J Dermatol 1999;141:934.

[221] Enk AH, Knop J. Mycophenolate is effective in the treatment of pemphigus vulgaris. Arch Dermatol 1999;135:54–6.

[222] Katz KH, Marks Jr JG, Helm KF. Pemphigus foliaceus successfully treated with mycophenolate mofetil as a steroid-sparing agent. J Am Acad Dermatol 2000;42:514–5.

[223] Nousari HC, Goyal S, Anhalt GJ. Successful treatment of resistant hypertrophic and bullous lichen planus with mycophenolate mofetil [letter, comment]. Arch Dermatol 1999;135:1420–1.

[224] Glaser R, Sticherlin M. Successful treatment of linear IgA bullous dermatosis with mycophenolate mofetil [letter]. Acta Derm Venereol 2002;82:308–9.

[225] Megahed M, Schmiedeberg S, Becker J, Ruzicka T. Treatment of cicatricial pemphigoid with mycophenolate mofetil as a steroid-sparing agent. J Am Acad Dermatol 2001;45:256–9.

[226] Williams JV, Marks Jr JG, Billingsley EM. Use of mycophenolate mofetil in the treatment of paraneoplastic pemphigus. Br J Dermatol 2000;142:506–8.

[227] Schattenkirchner S, Eming S, Hunzelmann N, Krieg T, Smola H. Treatment of epidermolysis bullosa acquisita with mycophenolate mofetil and autologous keratinocyte grafting [letter]. Br J Dermatol 1999; 141:932–3.

[228] Trebing D, Ziemer A. [Acquired epidermolysis bullosa with a highly varied clinical picture and successful treatment with mycophenolate mofetil]. Hautarzt 2001;52:717–21.

[229] Powell AM, Albert S, Al Fares S, et al. An evaluation of the usefulness of mycophenolate mofetil in pemphigus. Br J Dermatol 2003;149:138–45.

[230] Lynch W, Roenigk HHJ. Mycophenolic acid in psoriasis. Arch Dermatol 1977;113:1203–8.

[231] Haufs MG, Beissert S, Grabbe S, Shutte B, Luger TA. Psoriasis vulgaris treated successfully with mycophenolate mofetil. Br J Dermatol 1998;138:179–81.

[232] Grundmann-Kollmann M, Mooser G, Schraeder P,

et al. Treatment of chronic plaque-stage psoriasis and psoriatic arthritis with mycophenolate mofetil. J Am Acad Dermatol 2000;42:835–7.

[233] Geilen CC, Arnold M, Orfanos CE. Mycophenolate mofetil as a systemic antipsoriatic agent: positive experience in 11 patients. Br J Dermatol 2001;144: 583–6.

[234] Zhou Y, Rosenthal D, Dutz J, Ho V. Mycophenolate mofetil (CellCept(R)) for psoriasis: a two-center, prospective, open-label clinical trial. J Cutan Med Surg 2003;7:193–7.

[235] Michel S, Hohenleutner U, Mohr V, Landthaler M. [Therapy-resistant pyoderma gangrenosum—treatment with mycophenolate mofetil and cyclosporine A]. Hautarzt 1999;50:428–31 [in German].

[236] Hohenleutner U, Mohr VD, Michel S, Landthaler M. Mycophenolate mofetil and cyclosporin treatment for recalcitrant pyoderma gangrenosum [letter]. Lancet 1997;350:1748.

[237] Nousari HC, Lynch W, Anhalt GJ, Petri M. The effectiveness of mycophenolate mofetil in refractory pyoderma gangrenosum. Arch Dermatol 1998;134: 1509–11.

[238] Gilmour E, Stewart DG. Severe recalcitrant pyoderma gangrenosum responding to a combination of mycophenolate mofetil with cyclosporin and complicated by a mononeuritis. Br J Dermatol 2001;144: 397–400.

[239] Grundmann-Kollmann M, Korting HC, Behrens S, et al. Successful treatment of severe refractory atopic dermatitis with mycophenolate mofetil [letter]. Br J Dermatol 1999;141:175–6.

[240] Neuber K, Schwartz I, Itschert G, Dieck AT. Treatment of atopic eczema with oral mycophenolate mofetil. Br J Dermatol 2000;143:385–91.

[241] Grundmann-Kollmann M, Podda M, Ochsendorf F, Boehncke WH, Kaufmann R, Zollner TM. Mycophenolate mofetil is effective in the treatment of atopic dermatitis. Arch Dermatol 2001;137:870–3.

[242] Hansen ER, Buus S, Deleuran M, Andersen KE. Treatment of atopic dermatitis with mycophenolate mofetil. Br J Dermatol 2000;143:1324–6.

[243] Pickenacker A, Luger TA, Schwarz T. Dyshidrotic eczema treated with mycophenolate mofetil [letter]. Arch Dermatol 1998;134:378–9.

[244] Semhoun-Ducloux S, Ducloux D, Miguet JP. Mycophenolate mofetil-induced dyshidrotic eczema [letter]. Ann Intern Med 2000;132:417.

[245] Ruiz-Irastorza G, Khamashta MA, Hughes GR. Therapy of systemic lupus erythematosus: new agents and new evidence. Expert Opin Invest Drugs 2000; 9:1581–93.

[246] Chan TM, Li FK, Tang CS, et al. Efficacy of mycophenolate mofetil in patients with diffuse proliferative lupus nephritis. Hong Kong–Guangzhou Nephrology Study Group. N Engl J Med 2000;343: 1156–62.

[247] Austin HA, Balow JE. Treatment of lupus nephritis. Semin Nephrol 2000;20:265–76.

[248] Gaubitz M, Schorat A, Schotte H, Kern P, Domschke W. Mycophenolate mofetil for the treatment of systemic lupus erythematosus: an open pilot trial. Lupus 1999;8:731–6.

[249] Schanz S, Ulmer A, Rassner G, Fierlbeck G. Successful treatment of subacute cutaneous lupus erythematosus with mycophenolate mofetil. Br J Dermatol 2002;147:174–8.

[250] Goyal S, Nousari HC. Treatment of resistant discoid lupus erythematosus of the palms and soles with mycophenolate mofetil. J Am Acad Dermatol 2001; 45:142–4.

[251] Worm M, Sterry W, Kolde G. Mycophenolate mofetil is effective for maintenance therapy of hypocomplementaemic urticarial vasculitis. Br J Dermatol 2000; 143:1324.

[252] Nowack R, Gobel U, Klooker P, Hergesell O, Andrassy K, van der Woude FJ. Mycophenolate mofetil for maintenance therapy of Wegener's granulomatosis and microscopic polyangiitis: a pilot study in 11 patients with renal involvement. J Am Soc Nephrol 1999;10:1965–71.

[253] Waiser J, Budde K, Braasch E, Neumayer HH. Treatment of acute c-ANCA-positive vasculitis with mycophenolate mofetil. Am J Kidney Dis 1999; 34:e9.

[254] Gross WL. New concepts in treatment protocols for severe systemic vasculitis. Curr Opin Rheumatol 1999;11:41–6.

[255] Nowack R, Birck R, van der Woude FJ. Mycophenolate mofetil for systemic vasculitis and IgA nephropathy [letter]. Lancet 1997;349:774.

[256] Kouba DJ, Mimouni D, Rencic A, Nousari HC. Mycophenolate mofetil may serve as a steroid-sparing agent for sarcoidosis. Br J Dermatol 2003; 148:147–8.

[257] Reinhard G, Lohmann F, Uerlich M, Bauer R, Bieber T. Successful treatment of ulcerated necrobiosis lipoidica with mycophenolate mofetil [letter]. Acta Derm Venereol 2000;80:312–3.

[258] Gelber AC, Nousari HC, Wigley FM. Mycophenolate mofetil in the treatment of severe skin manifestations of dermatomyositis: a series of 4 cases. J Rheumatol 2000;27:1542–5.

[259] Cattaneo D, Perico N, Gaspari F, Gotti E, Remuzzi G. Glucocorticoids interfere with mycophenolate mofetil bioavailability in kidney transplantation. Kidney Int 2002;62:1060–7.

[260] Morii M, Ueno K, Ogawa A, et al. Impairment of mycophenolate mofetil absorption by iron ion. Clin Pharmacol Ther 2000;68:613–6.

[261] Royer B, Zanetta G, Berard M, et al. A neutropenia suggesting an interaction between valacyclovir and mycophenolate mofetil. Clin Transplant 2003;17: 158–61.

[262] Cox VC, Ensom MH. Mycophenolate mofetil for solid organ transplantation: does the evidence support the need for clinical pharmacokinetic monitoring? Ther Drug Monit 2003;25:137–57.

[263] Krueger JG. The immunologic basis for the treatment of psoriasis with new biologic agents. J Am Acad Dermatol 2002;46:1–23.

[264] Nickoloff BJ. Characterization of lymphocyte-dependent angiogenesis using a SCID mouse: human skin model of psoriasis. J Investig Dermatol Symp Proc 2000;5:67–73.

[265] Nickoloff BJ, Kunkel SL, Burdick M, Strieter RM. Severe combined immunodeficiency mouse and human psoriatic skin chimeras. Validation of a new animal model. Am J Pathol 1995;146:580–8.

[266] Bos JD, Hagenaars C, Das PK, Krieg SR, Voorn WJ, Kapsenberg ML. Predominance of "memory" T cells (CD4+ CDw29+) over "naïve" T cells (CD4+, CD45R+) in both normal and diseased skin. Arch Dermatol Res 1989;281:24–30.

[267] Austin LM, Coven TR, Bhardwaj N, Steinman R, Krueger JG. Intraepidermal lymphocytes in psoriatic lesions are activated GMP-17(TIA-1)+ CD8+ CD3+ CTLs as determined by phenotypic analysis. J Cutan Pathol 1998;25:79–88.

[268] Gottlieb AB. Psoriasis. Immunopathology and immunomodulation. Dermatol Clin 2001;19:1–13.

[269] Alefacept [package insert]. Cambridge (MA): Biogen Idec; 2003. Available at: http://www.fda.gov/cder/foi/label/2003/alefbio013003LB.htm. Accessed November 2003.

[270] Chisholm PL, Williams CA, Jones WE, et al. The effects of an immunomodulatory LFA3-IgG1 fusion protein on nonhuman primates. Ther Immunol 1994; 1:205–16.

[271] Miller GT, Hochman PS, Meier W, et al. Specific interaction of lymphocyte function-associated antigen 3 with CD2 can inhibit T-cell responses. J Exp Med 1993;178:211–22.

[272] Meier W, Gill A, Rogge M, et al. Immunomodulation by LFA3TIP, and LFA-3/IgG1 fusion protein: cell line dependent glycosylation effects on pharmacokinetics and pharmacodynamic markers. Ther Immunol 1995;2:159–71.

[273] Majeau GR, Meier W, Jimmo B, Kioussis D, Hochman PS. Mechanism of lymphocyte function-associated molecule 3-Ig fusion proteins inhibition of T cell responses. Structure/function analysis in vitro and in human CD2 transgenic mice. J Immunol 1994;152: 2753–67.

[274] Sanders MW, Makgoba MW, Sharrow SO, et al. Human memory T lymphocytes express increased levels of three cell adhesion molecules (LFA-3, CD2, and LFA-1) and three other molecules (UCHL1, CDw29, and Pgp-1) and have enhanced IFN-γ production. J Immunol 1988;140:1401–7.

[275] Majeau GR, Whitty A, Yim K, Meier W, Hochman PS. Low affinity binding of an LFA-3/IgG1 fusion protein to CD2+ T cells is independent of cell activation. Cell Adhes Commun 1999;7:267–9.

[276] Ellis CN, Krueger GG. Treatment of chronic plaque psoriasis by selective targeting of memory effector T lymphocytes. N Engl J Med 2001;345:248–55.

[277] Gottlieb AB, Bos JD. Recombinantly engineered human proteins: transforming the treatment of psoriasis. Clin Immunol 2002;105:105–16.

[278] Gottlieb AB, Casale T, Frankel E, et al. CD4+ T-cell-directed antibody responses are maintained in patients with psoriasis receiving alefacept: results of a randomized study. J Am Acad Dermatol 2003;49: 816–25.

[279] Krueger JG, Gilleaudeau P, Kikuchi T, Lee E. Psoriasis-related subpopulations of memory CD4+ and CD8+ T cells are selectively reduced by alefacept. J Invest Dermatol 2002;119:823.

[280] Lowe N, Gonzalez J, Bagel J, Caro I, Ellis C, Menter A. Repeat courses of intravenous alefacept in patients with chronic plaque psoriasis provide consistent safety and efficacy. Int J Dermatol 2003;42:224–30.

[281] Akhavan A, Lebwohl M. Systemic psoriasis treatment with alefacept. Psoriasis Forum 2003;9:4–5.

[282] Lebwohl M, Enno C, Langley R, et al. An international, randomized, double-blind, placebo-controlled phase 3 trial of intramuscular alefacept in patients with chronic plaque psoriasis. Arch Dermatol 2003; 139:719–27.

[283] Krueger GG, Papp KA, Stough DB, Loven KH, Gulliver WP, Ellis CN. A randomized, double-blind, placebo-controlled phase III study evaluating efficacy and tolerability of 2 courses of alefacept in patients with chronic plaque psoriasis. J Am Acad Dermatol 2002;47:821–33.

[284] Spuls PI, Witkamp L, Bossuyt PM, Bos JD. A systematic review of five systemic treatments for severe psoriasis. Br J Dermatol 1997;137:943–9.

[285] Koo J, Lebwohl M. Duration of remission of psoriasis therapies. J Am Acad Dermatol 1999;41:51–9.

[286] Menter A, Cram DL. The Goeckerman regimen in two psoriasis day care centers. J Am Acad Dermatol 1983;9:59–65.

[287] Krueger GG, Ellis CN. Alefacept therapy produces remission for patients with chronic plaque psoriasis. Br J Dermatol 2003;148:784–8.

[288] Krueger GG, Callis KP. Development and use of alefacept to treat psoriasis. J Am Acad Dermatol 2003;49:S87–97.

[289] Efalizumab [package insert]. South San Francisco (CA): Genentech, Inc; 2003. Available at: http://www.google.com/search?q=cache:fCZgcnAKE6IJ:www.bbriefings.com/pdf/790/genentech.pdf+efalizumab+package+insert&hl=en&ie=UTF-8. Accessed October 2003.

[290] Grakoui A, Bromley SK, Sumen C, et al. The immunological synapse: a molecular machine controlling T cell activation. Science 1999;285:221–7.

[291] Sanders ME, Makgoba MW, Sharrow SO, et al. Human memory T lymphocytes express increased levels of three cell adhesion molecules (LFA-3, CD2, and LFA-1) and three other molecules (UCHL1, CDw29, and Pgp-1) and have enhanced IFN-γ production. J Immunol 1988;140:1401–7.

[292] Van Seventer GA, Shimizu Y, Horgan KJ, Ginter

Luce GE, Webb D, Shaw S. Remote T cell costimulation via LFA-1/ICAM-1 and CD2/LFA-3: demonstration with immobilized ligand/mAb and in monocyte-mediated costimulation. Eur J Immunol 1991;21:1711.

[293] Nickoloff BJ, Mitra RS, Green J, et al. Accessory cell function of keratinocytes for superantigens. J Immunol 1993;150:2148–59.

[294] Lebwohl M, Tyring SK, Hamilton TK, et al. A novel targeted T-cell modulator, efalizumab, for plaque psoriasis. N Engl J Med 2003;349:2004–13.

[295] Leonardi CL. Efalizumab: an overview. J Am Acad Dermatol 2003;49:S98–104.

[296] Lebwohl M, Papp KA, Tyring S, et al. Continued treatment with subcutaneous efalizumab is safe: pooled results from two phase III trials. Presented at the American Academy of Dermatology. New York, July 31–August 4, 2002.

[297] Nussbaum R, Krueger JG. Treatment of inflammatory dermatoses with novel biologic agents: a primer. Adv Dermatol 2002;18:45–89.

[298] Weinberg JM, Saini R. Biologic therapy for psoriasis: the tumor necrosis factor inhibitors—infliximab and etanercept. Cutis 2003;71:25–9.

[299] Goffe B, Cather JC. Etanercept: an overview. J Am Acad Dermatol 2003;49:S105–11.

[300] Mussi A, Bonifati C, Carducci M, et al. Serum TNF-alpha levels correlate with disease severity and are reduced by effective therapy in plaque-type psoriasis. J Biol Regul Homeost Agents 1997;11:115–8.

[301] Bonifati C, Carducci M, Cordiali FP, et al. Correlated increases of tumour necrosis factor-alpha, interleukin-6 and granulocyte monocyte-colony stimulating factor levels in suction blister fluids and sera of psoriatic patients—relationships with disease severity. Clin Exp Dermatol 1994;19:383–7.

[302] Etanercept [package insert]. Thousand Oaks (CA): Amgen; 2003. Available at: http://www.google.com/search?q=cache:6CgATD0-sNEJ:www.fda.gov/cder/foi/label/2003/etanimm060503LB.pdf+Etanercept+package+insert&hl=en&ie=UTF-8. Accessed December 2003.

[303] Moreland L, Cohen S, Fleischmann RM, et al. Safety and efficacy of up to five years etanercept (Enbrel) therapy in rheumatoid arthritis. Presented at European League Against Rheumatism. June 12–15, 2002, Stockholm, Sweden.

[304] Leonardi CL, Powers JL, Matheson RT, et al. Etanercept as monotherapy in patients with psoriasis. N Engl J Med 2003;349:2014–22.

[305] Mease PJ, Goffe BS, Metz J, VanderStoep A, Finck B, Burge DJ. Etanercept in the treatment of psoriatic arthritis and psoriasis: a randomized trial. Lancet 2000;356:385–90.

[306] Weinblatt ME, Kremer JM, Bankhurst AD, et al. Trial of etanercept, a recombinant tumor necrosis factor receptor: Fc fusion protein, in patients with rheumatoid arthritis receiving methotrexate. N Engl J Med 1999;340:253–9.

[307] Moreland LW, Schiff MH, Baumgartner SW, Tindall EA, Fleischmann RM, Bulpitt KJ. Etanercept theapy in rheumatoid arthritis: a randomized, controlled trial. Ann Intern Med 1999;130:478–86.

[308] Shakoor N, Michalska M, Harris CA, Block JA. Drug-induced systemic lupus erythematosus associated with etanercept therapy. Lancet 2002;359:579–80.

[309] Bleumink GS, ter Borg EJ, Ramselaar CG, Stricker BH. Etanercept induced subacute cuatneous lupus erythematosus. Rheumatology [Oxford] 2001;40:1317–9.

[310] Lebwohl M. Psoriasis. Lancet 2003;361:1197–204.

[311] Mohan N, Edwards ET, Cupps TR, et al. Demyelination occurring during anti-tumor necrosis factor α therapy for inflammatory arthritides. Arthritis Rheum 2001;44:2862–9.

[312] Zeltser R, Valle L, Tanck C, Holyst MM, Ritchlin C, Gaspari AA. Clinical, histological, and immunophenotypic characteristics of injection site reactions associated with etanercept. Arch Dermatol 2001;137:893–9.

[313] Gottlieb AB, Matheson RT, Lowe N, et al. A randomized trial of etanercept as monotherapy for psoriasis. Arch Dermatol 2003;139:1627–32.

[314] Brockbank J, Gladman DD. Psoriatic arthritis. Expert Opin Investig Drugs 2000;9:1511–22.

[315] Ellman MII, MacDonald PA, Hayes FA. Etanercept as treatment for diffuse scleroderma: a pilot study. Arthritis Rhem 2000;43:S392.

[316] Sacher C, Rubbert A, König C, Scharffetter-Kochanek K, Krieg T, Hunzelmann N. Treatment of recalcitrant cicatricial pemphigoid with tumor necrosis factor α antagonist etanercept. J Am Acad Dermatol 2002;46:113–5.

[317] Smith KJ, Skelton H. Common variable immunodeficiency treated with a recombinant human IgG, tumour necrosis factor-α receptor fusion protein. Br J Dermatol 2001;144:597–600.

[318] Robinson ND, Guitart J. Recalcitrant, recurrent aphthous stomatitis treated with etanercept. Arch Dermatol 2003;139:1259–61.

[319] Gottlieb AB, Masud S, Ramamurthi R, et al. Pharmacodynamic and pharmacokinetic response to anti-tumor necrosis factor-α monoclonal antibody (infliximab) treatment of moderate to severe psoriasis vulgaris. J Am Acad Dermatol 2003;48:1–11.

[320] Scallon BJ, Arevalo Moore M, Trinh H, Knight DM, Ghrayeb J. Chimeric anti-TNF-α monoclonal antibody cA2 binds recombinant transmembrane TNF-α and activates immune effector functions. Cytokine 1995;7:251–9.

[321] Gottlieb AB. Infliximab for psoriasis. J Am Acad Dermatol 2003;49:S112–7.

[322] Barnes PJ, Karin M. Nuclear factor-kappaB: a pivotal transcription factor in chronic inflammatory disease. N Engl J Med 1997;336:1066–72.

[323] Ettehadi P, Greaves MW, Wallach D, Aderka D, Camp RDR. Elevated tumor necrosis factor-alpha

(TNF-alpha) biological activity in psoriatic skin lesions. Clin Exp Immunol 1994;96:146–51.

[324] Nahar IK, Shojania K, Marra CA, Alamgir AH, Anis AH. Infliximab treatment of rheumatoid arthritis and Crohn's disease. Ann Pharmacother 2003; 37:1256–65.

[325] Bernstein CN, Blanchard JF, Kliewer E, Wajda A. Cancer risk in patients with inflammatory bowel disease: a population-based study. Cancer 2001;91: 854–62.

[326] Greenstein AJ, Gennuso R, Sachar DB, Heimann T, Janowitz HD, Aufses Jr AH. Extraintestinal cancers in inflammatory bowel disease. Cancer 1985;56: 2914–21.

[327] Baecklund E, Sundstrom C, Ekbom A, et al. Lymphoma subtypes in patients with rheumatoid arthritis: increased proportion of diffuse large B cell lymphoma. Arthritis Rheum 2003;48:1543–50.

[328] Kamel OW, Holly EA, van de Rijn M, Lele C, Sah A. A population based, case-control study of non-Hodgkin's lymphoma in patients with rheumatoid arthritis. J Rheumatol 1999;26:1676–80.

[329] Gridley G, McLaughlin JK, Ekbom A, et al. Incidence of cancer among patients with rheumatoid arthritis. J Natl Cancer Inst 1993;85:307–11.

[330] Thomas E, Brewster DH, Black RJ, Macfarlane GJ. Risk of malignancy among patients with rheumatic conditions. Int J Cancer 2000;88:497–502.

[331] Hannuksela-Svahn A, Pukkala E, Läärä E, Poikolainen K, Karonen J. Psoriasis, its treatment, and cancer in a cohort of Finnish patients. J Invest Dermatol 2000;114:587–90.

[332] Margolis D, Bilker W, Hennessy S, Vittorio C, Santanna J, Strom BL. The risk of malignancy associated with psoriasis. Arch Dermatol 2001;137:778–83.

[333] Gelfand JM, Berlin J, Voorhees AV, Margolis DJ. Lymphoma rates are low but increased in patients with psoriasis. Arch Dermatol 2003;139:1425–9.

[334] Gross TG, Steinbuch M, DeFor T, et al. B cell lymphoproliferative disorders following hematopoietic stem cell transplantation: risk factors, treatment and outcome. Bone Marrow Transplant 1999;23: 251–8.

[335] Okano M, Gross TG. A review of Epstein-Barr virus infection in patients with immunodeficiency disorders. Am J Med Sci 2000;319:392–6.

[336] Keane J, Gershon S, Wise RP, et al. Tuberculosis associated with infliximab, a tumor necrosis factor α-neutralizing agent. N Engl J Med 2001;345: 1098–104.

[337] Lee J-H, Slifman NR, Gershon SK, et al. Life-threatening histoplasmosis complicating immunotherapy with tumor necrosis factor α antagonists infliximab and etanercept. Arthritis Rheum 2002;46: 2565–70.

[338] Hanauer SB, Feagan BG, Lichtenstein GR, et al. Maintenance infliximab for Crohn's disease: the ACCENT I randomized trial. Lancet 2002;359: 1541–9.

[339] Maini R, St. Clair EW, Breedveld F, et al, for the ATTRACT Study Group. Infliximab (chimeric anti-tumor necrosis factor alpha monoclonal antibody) versus placebo in rheumatoid arthritis patients receiving concomitant methotrexate: a randomized phase III trial. Lancet 1999;354:1932–9.

[340] Chaudhari U, Romano P, Mulcahy LD, Dooley LT, Baker DG, Gottlieb AB. Efficacy and safety of infliximab monotherapy for plaque-type psoriasis: a randomised trial. Lancet 2001;357:1842–7.

[341] Infliximab [package insert]. Malvern (PA): Centocor, Inc; 2003. Available at: http://www.remicade.com/PI/interactive_PI.jsp. Accessed 2003.

[342] Chung ES, Packer M, Lo KH, Fasanmade AA, Willerson JT. Randomized, double-blind, placebo-controlled, pilot trial of infliximab, a chimeric monoclonal antibody to tumor necrosis factor-α, in patients with moderate-to severe heart failure. Circulation 2003;107:3133–40.

[343] Oh CJ, Das KM, Gottlieb AB. Treatment with anti-tumor necrosis factor α (TNF-α) monoclonal antibody dramatically decreases the clinical activity of psoriasis lesions. J Am Acad Dermatol 2000;42: 829–30.

[344] Tan M-H, Gordon M, Lebwohl O, George J, Lebwohl M. Improvement of pyoderma gangrenosum and psoriasis associated with Crohn disease with anti-tumor necrosis factor α monoclonal antibody. Arch Dermatol 2001;137:930–3.

[345] O'Quinn RP, Miller JL. The effectiveness of tumor necrosis factor α antibody (infliximab) in treating recalcitrant psoriasis. Arch Dermatol 2002;138: 644–8.

[346] Ogilvie ALJ, Antoni C, Dechant C, et al. Treatment of psoriatic arthritis with antitumour necrosis factor-α antibody clears skin lesions of psoriasis resistant to treatment with methotrexate. Br J Dermatol 2001; 144:587–9.

[347] Newland MR, Weinstein A, Kerdel F. Rapid response to infliximab in severe pustular psoriasis, von Zumbusch type. Int J Dermatol 2002;41:449–52.

[348] Sullivan TP, Welsh E, Kerdel FA, Burdick AE, Kirsner RS. Infliximab for hidradenitis suppurativa. Br J Dermatol 2003;149:1046–9.

[349] Zaccagna A, Bertone A, Puiatti P, et al. Anti-tumor necrosis factor alpha monoclonal antibody (infliximab) for the treatment of pyoderma gangrenosum associated with Crohn's disease. Eur J Dermatol 2003;13:258–60.

[350] Kugathasan S, Miranda A, Nocton J, Drolet BA, Raasch C, Binion DG. Dermatologic manifestations of Crohn disease in children: response to infliximab. J Pediatr Gastroenterol Nutr 2003;37:150–4.

[351] Romero-Gomez M, Sanchez-Munoz D. Infliximab induces remission of pyoderma gangrenosum. Eur J Gastroenterol Hepatol 2002;14:907.

[352] Triantafillidis JK, Cheracakis P, Sklavaina M, Apostolopoulou K. Favorable response to infliximab treatment in a patient with active Crohn disease and

pyoderma gangrenosum. Scand J Gastroenterol 2002;
37:863 – 5.

[353] Estrach C, Mpofu S, Moots RJ. Behcet's syndrome: response to infliximab after failure of etanercept. Rheumatology [Oxford] 2002;41:1213 – 4.

[354] Saulsbury FT, Mann JA. Treatment with infliximab for a child with Behcet's disease. Arthritis Rheum 2003;49:599 – 600.

[355] Katsiari CG, Theodossiadis PG, Kaklamanis PG, Markomicheiakis NN. Successful long-term treatment of refractory Adamantiades-Behcet's disease (ABD) with infliximab: report of two patients. Adv Exp Med Biol 2003;528:551 – 5.

[356] Olivieri I, Padula A, Ciancio G, Salvarani C, Niccoli L, Cantini F. Successful treatment of SAPHO syndrome with infliximab: report of two cases. Ann Rheum Dis 2002;61:375 – 6.

[357] Voigtlander C, Luftl M, Schuler G, Hertl M. Infliximab (anti-tumor necrosis factor alpha antibody): a novel, highly effective treatment of recalcitrant subcorneal pustular dermatosis (Sneddon-Wilkinson disease). Arch Dermatol 2001;137:1571 – 4.

[358] Fischer M, Fiedler E, Marsch WC, Wolhlrab J. Antitumour necrosis factor-α antibodies (infliximab) in the treatment of a patient with toxic epidermal necrolysis. Br J Dermatol 2002;146:707 – 8.

[359] Yates VM, Watkinson G, Kelman A. Further evidence for an association between psoriasis, Crohn's disease, and ulcerative colitis. Br J Dermatol 1982; 106:323.

[360] Targan SR, Hanauer SB, van Deventer SJ, et al. A short-term study of chimeric monoclonal antibody cA2 to tumor necrosis factor-alpha for Crohn's disease. N Engl J Med 1997;337:1029 – 35.

ELSEVIER
SAUNDERS

Dermatol Clin 23 (2005) 301 – 312

DERMATOLOGIC
CLINICS

What's New in Antibiotics?

Ravindran A. Padmanabhan, MD, MRCP[a],*, Steven P. LaRosa, MD[a,1],
Kenneth J. Tomecki, MD[b]

[a]Department of Infectious Diseases, Cleveland Clinic Foundation, 9500 Euclid Avenue Cleveland, OH 44195, USA
[b]Department of Dermatology, Cleveland Clinic Foundation, 9500 Euclid Avenue Cleveland, OH 44195, USA

Antibiotics are important agents in dermatologic practice. New, important drugs have expanded the therapeutic approach to uncomplicated skin infections, such as simple abscesses, impetigo, furuncles, erysipelas, folliculitis, and cellulitis, and complicated infections involving deeper soft tissue or infections that require surgical intervention, such as infected ulcers, burns, and major abscesses, including significant underlying diseases that complicate the response to treatment [1]. New antibiotics of dermatologic importance include daptomycin (cyclic lipopeptide), linezolid (oxazolidinone), quinupristin-dalfopristin (streptogramins), moxifloxacin and gatifloxacin (fluoroquinolones), and dalbavancin and oritavancin, which are under investigation.

Daptomycin (Cubicin)

Historical perspective

Daptomycin, the first antibiotic of the cyclic lipopeptides, a new structural class, was discovered at Eli Lilly in the early 1980s through the classic approach of screening bacterial fermentation extracts for antibiotic activity [2].

* Corresponding author.
E-mail address: padmanr@ccf.org (R.A. Padmanabhan).
[1] *Present address:* Division of Infectious Diseases, Rhode Island Hospital, 593 Eddy Street, Gerry House 113, Providence, RI 02903.

Mechanism of action

Daptomycin is derived from the fermentation of *Streptomyces roseosporus* [3]. Its mode of action is unique in that it rapidly kills gram-positive bacteria by disrupting many aspects of bacterial membrane function. The drug binds to components of the cell membranes of susceptible organisms and causes rapid depolarization [4–6], which in turn inhibits intracellular synthesis of DNA, RNA, and protein. Although gross morphologic changes occurred in both a methicillin-sensitive and a methicillin-resistant strain of *Staphylococcus aureus* and in a strain of *Enterococcus faecalis*, the bacteria were not lysed when observed under electron microscopy [7]. Daptomycin is bactericidal, and bacterial killing is concentration-dependent.

Indications

Daptomycin is indicated for the treatment of complicated infections of skin and skin structures caused by susceptible strains of the gram-positive organisms *Staphylococcus aureus* (including methicillin-resistant strains), *Streptococcus pyogenes*, *Streptococcus agalactiae*, *Streptococcus dysgalactiae* subsp *equisimilis*, and *E faecalis* (vancomycin-susceptible strains only) [3,8].

Clinical data

In two randomized, multinational, multicenter, investigator-blinded trials [8,9] involving adult patients with clinically documented complicated infections of skin and skin structures (cSSSI) caused by a range of gram- positive bacteria, the efficacy of daptomycin (4 mg/kg intravenously [IV] once daily) was compared with the current standard treatments for cSSSI, either vancomycin (1 g IV twice daily) or a semisynthetic penicillin (4–12 g/day IV). Patients were switched to oral therapy after 4 days if a clinical improvement occurred [8]. One study (no. 9801) was conducted in the United States and South Africa, and the other (no. 9901) was conducted in Europe and Australia, and the efficacy was equivalent [8]. Clinical success rates in the evaluable population were 76.3% for daptomycin and 76.7% for comparator drugs in study no. 9801 [8]. Two multicenter, randomized phase II trials evaluated the clinical efficacy of daptomycin versus conventional therapy (β-lactam agents or vancomycin) in 285 patients [3,9]. Daptomycin had activity against a variety of causative organisms, including *Staphylococcus aureus*, and its efficacy against skin and soft tissue infections was comparable to conventional therapy. Clinical cure or improvement occurred in 29 of 30 (96.6%) evaluable patients treated with daptomycin (2 mg/kg once daily) compared with 37 of 39 (94.9%) evaluable patients treated with conventional therapy. The number of evaluable patients was low because many enrolled patients did not have a bacteriologically confirmed infection and because of the high numbers of heroin users among the enrollees who did not complete follow-up. A favorable bacteriological outcome (ie, in which the pathogen was eliminated) occurred with daptomycin and conventional therapy in 96.1% and 93.9% of evaluable patients, respectively.

Two separate phase III trials evaluated daptomycin as the treatment for community-acquired pneumonia. One study enrolled patients from North America, western and Eastern Europe, and Russia, and the other study enrolled patients from South and Central America. Contradictory results were obtained in a subset analysis and negated the use of daptomycin in the treatment of pneumonia [10]. When daptomycin was administered to patients with bacteremia, it produced a favorable clinical outcome and bacteriological cure in 17 of 19 (89.5%) evaluable patients, but the number of patients treated conventionally was too small for meaningful comparison [10].

Pharmacokinetics and dosing

Daptomycin is 92% protein-bound and is predominantly excreted in the urine (78% is excreted primarily as unchanged drug) and the feces (6%). Pharmacodynamic studies in mice have suggested that its bactericidal activity is concentration-dependent

[11–13]. Plasma clearance is low, resulting in part from high protein binding [14]. Interference with hepatically metabolized drugs is low [3], although daptomycin may displace other protein-bound drugs.

The recommended dosage for adults is 4 mg/kg once daily [15], infused intravenously over 30 minutes for 7 to 14 days. In patients for whom the creatinine clearance is less than 30 mL/minute and for those who are undergoing hemodialysis or continuous ambulatory peritoneal dialysis, the dosage should be 4 mg/kg every 48 hours. Daptomycin should be discontinued in patients who develop an unexplained myopathy with creatine phosphokinase (CPK) levels higher than five times the upper limit of normal or more than 1000 U/L or in any patient with an isolated increase in CPK of more than 10 times the upper limit of normal. As such, the CPK level should be monitored weekly during therapy [8].

Drug interactions

No clinically significant interactions have been identified, although caution is warranted when daptomycin and tobramycin are coadministered. Theoretically, the concurrent use of drugs that may cause myopathy may increase the risk of these reactions. Limited clinical studies with β-hydroxy-β-methylglutaryl-CoA reductase inhibitors have not demonstrated an increase in adverse effects.

Adverse effects

In laboratory animals, daptomycin has produced adverse effects primarily on skeletal muscle and less so on the kidneys, the gastrointestinal tract, and the nervous system [3]. Myopathy was easily predicted and monitored by measuring CPK concentrations and was reversible on cessation of therapy.

Axonal degeneration of peripheral nerves occurred at higher dose levels. Skeletal muscle effects were dependent on dosing frequency and dose level. In dog studies [15], skeletal muscle effects were greater with fractionated versus once-daily administration of the same daily dose. As such, once-daily dosing may increase the therapeutic efficacy and decrease skeletal muscle adverse effects. With once-daily administration, daptomycin exhibits linear pharmacokinetics and minimal accumulation at doses of up to 6 mg/kg in healthy volunteers [3]. Intravenous daptomycin administered to healthy men in phase I studies was well tolerated at single doses of up to 6 mg/kg and at multiple doses of up to 3 mg/kg every 12 hours [3]. In the phase II trials, the adverse events and rates of discontinuation caused by adverse events were comparable between patients who received daptomycin and those who received conventional treatment, and no serious adverse effects were related to either daptomycin or conventional therapy. Daptomycin was not associated with neurotoxicity at any dose level tested. Transient muscle weakness and myalgia occurred in two of five phase I study subjects who received daptomycin at 4 mg/kg every 12 hours after 6 and 11 days of administration, respectively. Elevations in CPK concentrations preceded these events by 2 to 3 days. CPK levels rose rapidly, and weakness occurred with moderate to severe myalgia of the hands, wrists, or forearms. Mobility was not affected, and there were no changes in vibratory sensation or electromyographic studies. CPK levels peaked at 10,000 to 20,000 U/L 1 day after daptomycin was discontinued and approached baseline approximately 1 week later. All signs of muscle toxicity subsided as CPK concentrations returned to normal. No effects on cardiac or smooth muscle were detected, consistent with the results in volunteers.

A broad spectrum of antibacterial activity, rapid concentration-dependent bactericidal activity, a low frequency of resistance, linear pharmacokinetics, and once-daily dosing regimen are factors that suggest that daptomycin may be a useful antibiotic for the treatment of gram-positive infections. The potential efficacy of the drug against resistant pathogens adds to its appeal, and the results of clinical trials will provide more data on its safety and efficacy against infections caused by such strains.

Linezolid (Zyvox)

Historical perspective

The oxazolidinones are a unique class of synthetic antimicrobial agents originally developed as monoamine oxidase inhibitors for the treatment of depression. The DuPont Company developed the first oxazolidinone antimicrobial agents in the late 1970s for the control of bacterial and fungal diseases of plants [16]. Further chemical modification of these agents by scientists at DuPont led to compounds (DuP-105 and DuP-721) that showed activity when given orally or parenterally to experimental animals and had a broad in vitro spectrum of activity against most gram-positive bacteria, several anaerobes, and *Mycobacterium tuberculosis* [17]. The animal toxicity of DuP-721 negated further study [16], but scientists at Upjohn Laboratories discovered two oxazolidinones, eprezolide and linezolid, which had excellent in vitro activity and reduced toxicity

compared with DuP-721. Linezolid (PNU-100766) was the better drug because of its bioavailability and serum levels [18].

Mechanism of action

The oxazolidinones have a unique mechanism of action: they stop the first step in which bacteria assemble ribosomes from their dissociated subunits [19–21] by binding to a site on the 50S ribosomal subunit near its interface with the 30S unit, thus preventing the formation of a 70S initiation complex [19–21].

Spectrum of activity

Linezolid has excellent in vitro activity against all of the major gram-positive pathogens in humans, including activity against the gram-negative bacteria *Neisseria gonorrhoeae* and *N meningitidis*. It has only borderline activity against *Haemophilus influenzae* and is inactive against both *Enterobacteriaceae* and *Pseudomonas* species [22,23]. Although linezolid possesses activity against "atypical organisms," including *Legionella pneumophila*, *M pneumoniae*, and *Chlamydia pneumoniae*, in vitro data to date are inconclusive [22]. Linezolid has good activity against many gram-positive anaerobes. Its activity against *Bacteroides fragilis* is borderline, but it provides bactericidal activity against these organisms [22]. Linezolid exhibits relatively good in vitro activity against many strains of *M tuberculosis* [22] and has activity against the *M avium* complex and several rapidly growing mycobacteria, including *M fortuitum*, *M chelonae*, and *M abscessus* [24,25]. Linezolid also has excellent in vitro activity against *Nocardia* species (including *N asteroides*, *N farcinica*, *N brasiliensa*, and four other species) [26].

Indications

The US Food and Drug Administration (FDA) has approved linezolid for the treatment of complicated infections of skin and soft tissue caused by *Staphylococcus aureus* (methicillin-resistant and -susceptible strains), *Streptococcus pyogenes*, or *Streptococcus agalactiae* and for treating uncomplicated infections of skin and soft tissue caused by *Staphylococcus aureus* (methicillin-susceptible strains only) or *Streptococcus pyogenes* [27]. The FDA has also approved linezolid for the treatment of vancomycin-resistant *E faecium* infections (including cases with concurrent bacteremia), community-acquired pneumonia caused by *Streptococcus pneumoniae* (penicillin-susceptible strains only) or *Staphylococcus aureus*, and nosocomial pneumonia caused by *Staphylococcus aureus* (methicillin-susceptible and -resistant strains) or *Streptococcus pneumoniae* (penicillin-susceptible strains). Linezolid has poor activity against *H influenzae*, which mitigates its use a first-line treatment for community-acquired pneumonia [27,28].

Clinical data

In a multinational, randomized, double blind study [29,30], the effect of linezolid (400 mg twice daily) was compared with clarithromycin (250 mg twice daily) as the treatment for 332 adult patients with uncomplicated infections of skin and skin structures. The most common diagnoses in both groups were cellulitis, skin abscesses, and furuncle. Treatment continued for 7 to 14 days, with follow-up on 7 to 21 days after the end of treatment. Of 124 clinically evaluable patients who received linezolid, 113 (91%) showed a clinical cure, compared with 114 (93%) of 123 patients who received clarithromycin [29,30]. For microbiologically evaluable patients, the microbiological success rate was 98% in linezolid-treated patients and 97% in clarithromycin-treated patients [29,30]. The rate of eradication of *Staphylococcus aureus* was 97% (38 of 39) for the linezolid group and 96% (51 of 53) for the clarithromycin group [29,30]. Adverse events were generally mild to moderate, including primarily nausea and diarrhea in both groups [29,30]. No deaths occurred in either treatment group [29,30].

A randomized, double blind study compared the activity of linezolid (600 mg IV twice daily initially, followed by a switch to oral therapy) with oxacillin (2 g IV four times daily) followed by dicloxacillin (500 mg four times daily) for the treatment of complicated infections of the skin and skin structure in 800 patients [30–32]. Patients received therapy for 10 to 21 days, plus aztreonam for those patients who required gram-negative coverage, with follow-up 12 to 21 days after the end of therapy. The most common baseline diagnoses in both groups were cellulitis and skin abscesses [30–32]. Of 291 clinically evaluable patients who received linezolid, 91% (264) showed a clinical cure, and of 300 clinically evaluable patients who received oxacillin-dicloxacillin, 86% (259) showed a clinical cure.

The rates of eradication of *Staphylococcus aureus, Streptococcus agalactiae,* and *Streptococcus pneumoniae* were 88% (73 of 83), 100% (6 of 6), and 69% (18 of 26), respectively, for linezolid-treated patients and 86% (72 of 84), 50% (3 of 6), and 75% (21 of 28), respectively, for oxacillin-dicloxacillin-

treated patients [30–32]. Adverse events were generally mild to moderate, with nausea and headache most commonly described in both groups. Three deaths occurred in the linezolid-treated group and one in the oxacillin-dicloxacillin-treated group, but none of the deaths were considered drug-related [30–32]. Linezolid should not be used as a first- or second-line agent for the treatment of community-acquired pneumonia [28,33].

Pharmacokinetics

Linezolid is 100% bioavailable when the drug is administered orally or intravenously. Maximum plasma concentrations occur 1 to 2 hours after ingestion of the drug. Concomitant food delays uptake slightly, but the total amount of drug absorbed is unchanged. Serum plasma protein binding is low (approximately 31%). Linezolid is metabolized by the oxidation of its morpholino ring, resulting in two metabolites, an aminoethoxyacetic acid metabolite, and a hydroxyethyl glycine metabolite. The drug does not induce cytochrome P-450 enzymes and does not seem to be metabolized by cytochrome P-450 in humans, and it does not inhibit the activity of human P-450 isoforms [27]. Approximately 30% to 35% of the parent compound is excreted in the urine, and none is found in feces [27]. The pharmacokinetic characteristics of linezolid are unaltered in patients with renal insufficiency, and no dosage adjustment is necessary for patients with renal or hepatic insufficiency. Both linezolid and its metabolites are eliminated by dialysis [27]. In patients receiving hemodialysis, supplemental or postdialysis dosing is necessary [34].

Dosing

A standard dosage of 600 mg every 12 hours is recommended for the treatment of most serious infections. In uncomplicated infections of skin and skin structures, an oral dosage of 400 mg every 12 hours is officially recommended [27], with no need for alteration based on weight or gender.

Drug interactions

Surveillance after marketing revealed 18 cases of thrombocytopenia or reversible anemia associated with the use of linezolid, including five patients with anemia, nine with thrombocytopenia, and four with neutropenia or anemia and thrombocytopenia. Many of these patients had received concomitant medications known to cause bone marrow suppression, and many had complex illnesses [28]. A prospective study by Rao et al [35] showed an equal incidence of thrombocytopenia in patients treated with vancomycin or linezolid. Patients with the highest rate of thrombocytopenia received vancomycin for 2 weeks, followed by linezolid [35].

Oxazolidinones are known to be monoamine oxidase inhibitors, which raises the possibility of monoamine oxidase inhibition in patients treated with linezolid. An enhanced pressor response has been seen in patients taking certain adrenergic agents, including phenylpropanolamine and pseudoephedrine, and it is specifically noted that the doses of these drugs should be reduced in patients receiving linezolid [27] and that serotonergic agents (eg, tricyclic antidepressants, venlafaxine, trazodone, sibutramine, meperidine, dextromethorphan, and selective serotonin reuptake inhibitors) may cause a serotonin syndrome (hyperpyrexia, cognitive dysfunction) when used concomitantly. Thus far, it appears that the potential for significant adverse effects resulting from monoamine oxidation inhibition by linezolid is low [28].

Hendershot et al [36] evaluated the pharmacokinetic and pharmacodynamic responses to the coadministration of oral linezolid and sympathomimetic agents (pseudoephedrine and phenylpropanolamine) and a serotonin reuptake inhibitor (dextromethorphan). Following coadministration, minimal but statistically significant increases in pseudoephedrine and phenylpropanolamine plasma concentrations occurred, and a minimal but statistically significant decrease in dextrorphan (the primary metabolite of dextromethorphan) plasma concentrations occurred. Increased blood pressure occurred after the coadministration of linezolid and either pseudoephedrine or phenylpropanolamine, but no significant effects occurred with dextromethorphan. None of these drugs had a significant effect on linezolid pharmacokinetics. Minimal adverse events occurred. The potentiation of sympathomimetic activity by linezolid was clinically insignificant. Linezolid used concurrently with tramadol may increase the risk of seizures [27]. Other drug-drug interactions related to the P-450 system are unlikely.

Adverse effects

Overall, linezolid has shown little toxicity and few adverse effects in phase III clinical trials [27], with no evidence of significant adverse effects on hepatic function, renal function, or hematologic variables, although the incidence of reversible thrombocytopenia was slightly higher in patients who received linezolid, compared with controls [27]. All of these trials were relatively short and used standard dosages that did not exceed 1200 mg/day. All of the oxazolidinones studied to date have shown the potential for reversible myelosuppression in animals. Dose- and time-dependent myelosuppression occurred in dogs and rats receiving prolonged high-dose linezolid in preclinical trials [27]. Except for a few cases of reversible thrombocytopenia, no significant myelosuppression occurred in phase III trials, but reversible myelosuppression with red cell hypoplasia has been reported [37]. Coupled with the data from preclinical and clinical trials, the FDA issued a report that myelosuppression, including anemia, leukopenia, pancytopenia, and thrombocytopenia, has been documented in patients receiving linezolid. As such, weekly complete blood counts are now warranted for patients who receive linezolid and especially for those patients receiving the drug for more than 2 weeks, those with pre-existing myelosuppression, those receiving concomitant drugs that produce bone marrow suppression, and those with chronic infection who have received previous or concomitant antibiotic therapy. Aplastic anemia has not occurred in patients receiving linezolid, and all cases of myelosuppression documented thus far have been reversible after discontinuation of therapy.

Caution is necessary regarding the use of linezolid in patients with uncontrolled hypertension, pheochromocytoma, carcinoid syndrome, or untreated hyperthyroidism. Patients should avoid foods that are high in tyramine content, including those foods that are changed by aging, fermentation, pickling, or smoking (eg, cheeses, fermented or air-dried meats, sauerkraut, soy sauce, beers, and red wines). The tyramine content of any protein-rich food increases with storage or improper refrigeration. Patients should also avoid alcohol, which may contain tyramine.

In summary, linezolid is a new antibiotic with a broad spectrum of activity against virtually all important gram-positive bacterial pathogens and a unique mechanism of action, with no cross-resistance with other classes of antimicrobial agents. It has been effective in clinical trials for the treatment of infection of skin and skin structures, respiratory tract infections, and systemic infections (including bacteremia) caused by vancomycin-resistant enterococci. Its efficacy against both vancomycin-resistant *E faecalis* and *E faecium* makes it a particularly attractive treatment for infections with vancomycin-resistant enterococci. The available data on animal osteomyelitis are conflicting. Despite its efficacy, linezolid is expensive ($53 for one 600-mg tablet or 30 mL of oral suspension and $72 for one 600-mg intravenous vial) [38]. The cost for a week of therapy with oral linezolid would be $371 and $512 for IV linezolid. Nonetheless, linezolid is effective against several types of bacteria that are resistant to β-lactam, vancomycin, and a host of other agents.

Quinupristin-Dalfopristin (Synercid)

Historical perspective

Synercid, a semisynthetic pristinamycin combination of quinupristin and dalfopristin, is a streptogramin, a family of compounds including pristinamycin, oestreomycin, mikamycin, and virginiamycin isolated from *Streptomyces pristinaespiralis.* Streptogramins are categorized as either group A or B, based on molecular structure. Dalfopristin, a group-A streptogramin and quinupristin, a group-B streptogramin, are water-soluble streptogramins combined in a commercially available injectable form, in a fixed 30:70 weight-to-weight ratio [39].

Mechanism of action

Individually, quinupristin and dalfopristin have only modest in vitro bacteriostatic activity, but the combination produces in vitro bactericidal activity 8 to 16 times higher than the component activity of each against many gram-positive organisms [39]. Quinupristin-dalfopristin acts synergistically: quinupristin blocks the binding of aminoacyl-tRNA complexes to the ribosome, and dalfopristin inhibits the peptide bond formation and distorts the ribosome, promoting further binding of quinupristin [40].

Indications

Quinupristin-dalfopristin is approved in the United States and the United Kingdom for the treatment of serious infections caused by vancomycin-resistant *E* (VR*E*) *faecium* associated with bacteremia and for complicated infections of skin and skin structures caused by group-A streptococci or methicillin-susceptible *Staphylococcus aureus* [41]. Quinupristin-dalfopristin may be an effective treatment for serious infections caused by *Staphylococcus* species, including those that are methicillin-resistant strains. Quinupristin-dalfopristin is usually ineffective against vancomycin-resistant VR*E faecalis* infection, which comprises 80% to 90% of clinical isolates of enterococci, a species with an efflux pump that confers intrinsic resistance [42].

Clinical data

The efficacy and safety of quinupristin-dalfopristin in complicated infections of skin and skin structures were evaluated in two open-label, multicenter studies in the United States and elsewhere [43,44]. In the US study [43], patients received either quinupristin-dalfopristin (7.5 mg/kg every 12 hours [n = 229]) or standard therapy (n = 221) consisting of either vancomycin (1 g every 12 hours [n = 78]) or oxacillin (2 g every 6 hours [n = 134]) or vancomycin and oxacillin (n = 9). In the global trial [44], quinupristin-dalfopristin was compared with cefazolin (1 g every 8 hours [n = 170]) or vancomycin (1 g every 12 hours [the dose was adjusted for weight or abnormal renal function] [n = 44]) or vancomycin and cefazolin (n = 8). The use of aztreonam was permitted for treating co-infection of gram-negative pathogens. In both studies, patients received treatment for 72 hours.

In the US trial, the clinical success rates were 64.7% (88 of 136) for quinupristin-dalfopristin and 68.3% (82 of 120) for vancomycin and/or oxacillin. In the global study, the clinical success rate was 71.2% (109 of 153) for the quinupristin-dalfopristin group compared and 72.5% (111 of 153) for the vancomycin and/or cefazolin group [45]. Bacteriologic success rates were lower for quinupristin-dalfopristin, perhaps because of the more frequent presence of polymicrobial infection in this group and presumed bacteriologic failure when treatment was altered.

Two hundred ninety-eight patients with nosocomial pneumonia in 74 centers in five countries, including a subgroup of 171 (87 quinupristin-dalfopristin-treated and 84 vancomycin-treated patients), were available for evaluation. One hundred fifty patients received quinupristin-dalfopristin, 7.5 mg/kg of every 8 hours, and 148 patients received vancomycin, 1 g every 12 h. Aztreonam, 2 g every 8 hours, could be administered in both groups for the coverage of gram-negative organisms, and tobramycin was added for coverage against *P aeruginosa*. The primary endpoint was the clinical response observed between the 7th and the 13th day after the end of treatment. Therapy was successful (cure or improvement) in 49 patients (56.3%) receiving quinupristin-dalfopristin and in 49 (58.3%) patients receiving vancomycin [45].

Pharmacokinetics

Quinupristin is converted to two active metabolites, and dalfopristin is converted to one. Both agents are primarily excreted in the bile and feces, with approximately 15% to 20% excreted in the urine. As such, the dosage of the drug does not need adjustment in the setting of renal impairment, and the drug is not removed by hemodialysis or peritoneal dialysis. Quinupristin-dalfopristin has a short half-life (1 to 2 hours), but the prolonged postantibiotic effect and additional growth inhibition at sub-minimum inhibitory concentration levels suggest that dosing intervals of 8 or 12 hours will suffice [46].

Dosing

For VR*E faecium* infections, the dosage of quinupristin-dalfopristin should be 7.5 mg/kg every 8 hours [46]. For complicated infections of skin and skin structures, the dosage should be 7.5 mg/kg every 12 hours [46]. Dose adjustment in renal failure, hemodialysis, or peritoneal dialysis is not required. With hepatic impairment, pharmacokinetic data warrant dosage adjustment, although specific recommendations are not available. In the elderly, no adjustment is required.

Drug interactions

Quinupristin-dalfopristin, an inhibitor of the cytochrome P-450 3A4 enzymatic pathway, may produce elevated levels of substrate drugs such as cyclosporine, nifedipine, midazolam, and terfenidine [47], hence, caution is necessary with these drugs. Concurrent therapy with astemizole and cisapride (which may prolong the Q-Tc interval and lead to arrhythmias) should be avoided. Other medications metabolized by cytochrome P-450 3A4, including protease inhibitors, non-nucleoside reverse transcriptase inhibitors, benzodiazepines, calcium channel blockers, some β-hydroxy-β-methylglutaryl-CoA reductase inhibitors, immunosuppressive agents, corticosteroids, carbamazepine, quinidine, lidocaine, and disopyramide, may lead to increased plasma concentrations during concurrent dosing [46].

Adverse effects

Quinupristin-dalfopristin commonly causes phlebitis (75% of patients) when administered through a peripheral vein. As such, it should be administered through a peripherally inserted central catheter or a central venous catheter. Five to six percent of patients develop elevated total and conjugated bilirubin [47], and many patients (5%–50%) may develop arthralgias and myalgias [48]. Nausea was a common side effect in one study [49].

In summary, quinupristin-dalfopristin is the first streptogramin available in parenteral form that possesses activity against multiresistant gram-positive pathogens, including methicillin-resistant *Staphylococcus aureus* (MRSA) and VR*E faecium*. Its advantages include potency, bactericidal capability, long postantibiotic effect, and infrequent resistance. Disadvantages include significant drug interactions, intravenous formulation, phlebitis when the drug is administered peripherally, and occasional myalgias and arthralgias.

Third-generation fluoroquinolones: gatifloxacin (Tequin) and moxifloxacin (Avelox)

Historical perspective

Quinolones were first introduced in 1962. Several, for example, ciprofloxacin, remain highly effective against gram-negative pathogens, but others have quickly lost activity against gram-positive organisms, including *Streptococcus pneumoniae* and *Staphylococcus aureus*, primarily through resistance. Moxifloxacin and gatifloxacin, which are fourth-generation fluoroquinolones, recently became available for the treatment of uncomplicated infections of skin and skin structures. These agents are available in parenteral and oral forms and offer improved coverage against gram-positive pathogens [1].

Mechanism of action

The third-generation fluoroquinolones bind to bacterial topoisomerase II (DNA gyrase) and IV, which impedes DNA replication, repair, and transcription, thereby resulting in bacterial death. The ability to target both enzymes helps to prevent or delay resistance [50].

Indications

Both drugs inhibit gram-positive bacteria, most notably penicillin-susceptible and -resistant strains of *Staphylococcus pneumoniae* [50]. Compared with ciprofloxacin, moxifloxacin and gatifloxacin have enhanced activity against *Staphylococcus aureus* but less activity against methicillin-resistant strains than against methicillin-susceptible strains. Activity against methicillin-resistant strains is poor because inhibitory concentrations often exceed achievable serum concentrations [50]. The activity against gram-negative organisms is preserved, although it is less than the activity of ciprofloxacin against *P aeruginosa* [50]. In addition to respiratory tract infections, gatifloxacin is approved for skin infections, cystitis, pyelonephritis, complicated urinary tract infections, and gonorrhea. For diabetic foot infections, fluoroquinolone monotherapy should be avoided [50].

Clinical data

A multicenter study [51] showed that gatifloxacin, 400 mg daily, was as safe and efficacious, both clinically and microbiologically, as levofloxacin, 500 mg daily for 7 to 10 days, as a treatment for uncomplicated infections of skin and skin structures [51]. Cure rates were 91% for gatifloxacin and 84% for levofloxacin, for either 7 or 10 days of treatment. For patients with *Staphylococcus aureus* infection, the cure rates were 96% and 87%, respectively, for each group [51].

Moxifloxacin, 400 mg once daily, or cephalexin, 500 mg three times daily for 7 days, resulted in a clinical resolution in 90% of patients during a double-blind, randomized trial [52] in 401 patients with uncomplicated infections of skin and skin structures. Similar results were obtained in two other randomized, double blind trials published as abstracts [52].

Pharmacokinetics

Fluoroquinolones provide concentration-dependent killing, and both moxifloxacin and gatifloxacin penetrate tissues well. Protein binding is 20% for gatifloxacin and 50% for moxifloxacin. Gatifloxacin is excreted primarily in the urine (70% as unchanged drug). Approximately 45% of a dose of moxifloxacin is excreted in feces (25%) and in urine (20%) as unchanged drug [53], negating its use for urinary tract infections.

Dosing

The dose for both oral and intravenous preparations of gatifloxacin and moxifloxacin is 400 mg daily, with no dosage adjustment for age. Patients with a creatinine clearance of less than 40 mL/minute or those undergoing hemodialysis or peritoneal dialysis should receive 400 mg initially followed by 200 mg every 24 hours, and always after hemodial-

ysis. No dosage adjustment is required in mild to moderate hepatic disease [53].

Drug interactions

Reports of possible drug-drug interactions between fluoroquinolones and glyburide suggest the potential for a drug class effect [54]. Package inserts for all marketed fluoroquinolones mention such potential interactions. Gatifloxacin and moxifloxacin may enhance the hypoprothrombinemic effect of warfarin, and the manufacturer recommends monitoring of the international normalized ratio during concurrent therapy [55]. Caution is warranted for patients who receive newer fluoroquinolones concomitantly with drugs that prolong the Q-T interval (including class Ia and class III antiarrhythmics, erythromycin, cisapride, antipsychotics, cyclic antidepressants, and the azole antifungal agents).

Adverse effects

The most common side effects include gastrointestinal distress (eg, nausea, vomiting, diarrhea, and abdominal pain) [50]. Central nervous system effects include headache, dizziness, occasional confusion, agitation, insomnia, depression, somnolence, vertigo, light-headedness, and tremors [50]. Compared with other fluoroquinolones, gatifloxacin and moxifloxacin have less potential to cause seizures and less demonstrated phototoxicity [50]. Arthritis or tendonitis did not manifest in volunteers given gatifloxacin to evaluate safety and pharmacokinetics [56]. Cardiac toxicity, with rate-corrected electrocardiographic Q-Tc interval prolongation and the possible development of fatal ventricular arrhythmias such as torsades de pointes, is uncommon [50]. There have been only three reports of torsades de pointes in association with gatifloxacin and one with moxifloxacin [57]. Symptomatic hyper- and hypoglycemia have occurred with gatifloxacin, usually in diabetic patients. Prescribing information for gatifloxacin includes precautions against possible disturbances of glucose homeostasis [55]. Colitis caused by *Clostridium difficile* may occur with the use of gatifloxacin, given its increased anaerobic spectrum of activity [58].

In summary, the new fluoroquinolones gatifloxacin and moxifloxacin exhibit better in vitro activity against gram-positive organisms than levofloxacin or ciprofloxacin. They are well tolerated and provide good bioavailabilty, and they can be administered once daily. Nonetheless, the potential for emerging resistance is real, especially with upper respiratory tract infections in which a bacterial cause is unclear [50]. Scheld [59] recommends a focused therapeutic approach to reduce the development of antimicrobial resistance and maintain class efficacy.

Antibiotics in development: dalbavancin and oritavancin

Two glycopeptide antibiotics may soon be available, dalbavancin, a novel semisynthetic glycopeptide with a half-life of 9 to 12 days, and oritavancin, another semisynthetic with a chemical structure that enhances better anchoring to bacterial cytoplasmic membranes. Both agents have the same mechanism of action, that is, the inhibition of cell-wall peptidoglycan cross-linking.

In vitro and in vivo studies [60] of antibacterial activity showed that dalbavancin had excellent activity against all tested gram-positive bacteria, with high activity against *Staphylococcus aureus*, coagulase-negative staphylococci (including *Staphylococcus haemolyticus*), and streptococci. Activity against staphylococci was significantly better than that of oritavancin, teicoplanin, or vancomycin and even against strains that were methicillin-resistant or less susceptible to teicoplanin. The activity was comparable to teicoplanin and better than vancomycin against *Streptococcus pneumoniae*. The activity against Van-S strains of enterococci was the same for dalbavancin, oritavancin, and teicoplanin but better than vancomycin itself. Dalbavancin maintained the activity against Van-B isolates, suggesting efficacy for infections caused by multiresistant gram-positive bacteria, particularly staphylococci and streptococci. In two animal studies investigating distribution and excretion, dalbavancin showed good cutaneous penetration. The drug has dual routes of elimination, with approximately 40% of intact drug excreted in urine. The drug did not accumulate in any one tissue, compartment, or organ [61].

A randomized, controlled, open-label phase II proof-of-concept trial [62] compared once-weekly dalbavancin therapy with standard treatment regimens of skin and soft tissue infections. The trial was conducted at 10 centers in the United States among men and nonpregnant women 18 years of age or older who had a skin and soft tissue infections that were suspected or known to be caused by gram-positive bacteria. Results demonstrated clinical success rates of 94.1% in patients treated with dalbavancin (two doses), 61.5% among patients treated with one dose, and 76.2% in patients treated with a standard regimen. All treatment regimens were well tolerated, and drug-related adverse reactions were similar in all groups. Phase III clinical trials to evaluate the safety and efficacy of dalbavancin, relative to vancomycin, for the treatment of skin and skin structure infections caused by suspected or diagnosed MRSA are in progress.

In summary, dalbavancin is a new glycopeptide specifically designed as an alternative to vancomycin for treating hospitalized patients with gram-positive infections. The drug is effective against MRSA, and its potency, tissue penetration, and long half-life may allow more flexibility and convenience in dosing once weekly compared with vancomycin (eg, a 500 to 1000 mg once-weekly regimen). Nonetheless, the activity of the drug against resistant pathogens such as MRSA may lead to reserving it for last-line therapy, despite its improved dosage regimen.

Oritavancin can anchor to the cytoplasmic membrane, providing better binding against vancomycin-susceptible and -resistant *Enterococcus* species. It is most active against VRE [63] (both *E faecalis* and *E faecium*) and even enterococci with the Van-A-, Van-B-, or Van-C-resistance determinants. The drug is active against oxacillin-susceptible *Staphylococcus aureus*, oxacillin-resistant *Staphylococcus aureus*, oxacillin-susceptible *Staphylococcus epidermis*, oxacillin-resistant *Staphylococcus aureus*, *Streptococcus* serogroups A, B, C, and G, and *Streptococcus pneumoniae* [64].

In rabbit studies [65], oritavancin was effective in the treatment of endocarditis caused by MRSA. Its long half-life ($\geq$ 10 days) offers a shorter duration of treatment [66]. A study [67] comparing a regimen of intravenous oritavancin (either 1.5 or 3.0 mg/kg once daily) followed by placebo with a regimen of intravenous vancomycin (15 mg/kg once daily) followed by oral cephalexin in 517 patients with complicated skin and soft tissue infections was statistically efficacious and equivalent in the two groups. Results showed a 76% clinical success rate in the oritavancin group and 80% in the vancomycin-cephalexin group. Patients in the oritavancin group required 5.7 days of treatment for dosages of 1.5 mg/kg/day and 5.3 days of treatment for dosages of 3.0 mg/kg/day, compared with 11.5 days for patients in the vancomycin-cephalexin group.

The antibiotics described in this article represent a powerful and efficacious way of treating skin and skin structure infections. Their benefits must be balanced against their side effects, interactions, and the potential for the development of resistance. Their prolonged effectiveness may well rest on prudent and judicious use by clinicians.

References

[1] Schweiger E, Weinberg MJ. Novel antibacterial agents for skin and skin structure infections. J Am Acad Dermatol 2004;50(3):331–40.

[2] Tally FP, DeBruin MF. Development of daptomycin for Gram-positive infections. J Antimicrob Chemother 2000;46:523–6.

[3] Tally FP, Zeckel M, Wasilewski MM, et al. Daptomycin: a novel agent for Gram-positive infections. Expert Opin Investig Drugs 1999;8:1223–38.

[4] Canepari P, Boaretti M, del Mar Lleó M, et al. Lipoteichoic acid as a new target for activity of antibiotics: mode of action of daptomycin (LY 146032). Antimicrob Agents Chemother 1990;34:1220–6.

[5] Boaretti M, Canepari P, Lleó MM, et al. The activity of daptomycin on Enterococcus faecium protoplasts: indirect evidence supporting a novel mode of action on lipoteichoic acid synthesis. J Antimicrob Chemother 1993;31:227–35.

[6] Alborn WE, Allen NE, Preston DA. Daptomycin disrupts membrane potential in growing Staphylococcus aureus. Antimicrob Agents Chemother 1991;35:2282–7.

[7] Wale LJ, Shelton AP, Greenwood D. Scanning electronmicroscopy of Staphylococcus aureus and Enterococcus faecalis exposed to daptomycin. J Med Microbiol 1989;30(1):45–9.

[8] US Food and Drug Administration. Drug approvals list [cited 29 October 2003]. Available at: http://www.fda.gov/cder/foi/label/2003/21572_cubicin_lbl.pdf. (2003). Accessed April 10, 2004.

[9] Kotra LP. Daptomycin. Curr Opin Investig Drugs 2000;2:185–205.

[10] Carpenter CF, Chambers HF. Daptomycin for grampositive infections. Clin Infect Dis 2004;38:994–1000.

[11] Leggett J, Totsuka K, Ebert S, et al. Pharmacodynamic and pharmacokinetic parameters (PKPs) affecting activity of LY146032 against Staphylococcus aureus [abstract 154]. In: Program and Abstracts of the Twenty-Seventh Interscience Conference on Antimicrobial Agents and Chemotherapy. Washington, DC: American Society for Microbiology; 1987. p. 123.

[12] Safdar N, Andes DR, Craig WA. In vivo pharmacodynamic activity of daptomycin (DAP) against multiple bacterial pathogens [abstract 1769]. In: Program and Abstracts of the Thirty-Ninth Interscience Conference on Antimicrobial Agents and Chemotherapy. Washington, DC: American Society of Microbiology; 1999. p. 42.

[13] Louie A, Kaw P, Liu W, et al. The pharmacodynamics of daptomycin as determined for Staphylococcus aureus in a mouse thigh infection model [abstract 1770]. In: Program and Abstracts of the Thirty-Ninth Interscience Conference on Antimicrobial Agents and Chemotherapy. Washington, DC: American Society for Microbiology; 1999. p. 42.

[14] Lee BL, Sachdeva M, Chambers HF. Effect of protein binding of daptomycin on MIC and antibacterial activity. Antimicrob Agents Chemother 1991;35:2505–8.

[15] Oleson FB, Berman CL, Kirkpatrick JB, et al. Once-daily dosing decreases toxicity of daptomycin. Toxicol Sci 1999;48(Suppl 1):S322.

[16] Brickner SJ. Oxazolidinone antibacterial agents. Curr Pharm Des 1996;2:175–94.

[17] Moellering Jr RC. A novel antimicrobial agent joins the battle against resistant bacteria [editorial]. Ann Intern Med 1999;130:155–7.

[18] Ford C, Hamel J, Stapert D, et al. Oxazolidinones: a new class of antimicrobials. Infect Med 1999;16:435–45.

[19] Daly JS, Eliopoulos GM, Willey S, et al. Mechanism of action and in vitro and in vivo activities of S-6123, a new oxazolidinone compound. Antimicrob Agents Chemother 1988;32:1341–6.

[20] Lin AH, Murray RW, Vidmar TJ, et al. The oxazolidinone eperezolid binds to the 50S ribosomal subunit and competes with binding of chloramphenicoland lincomycin. Antimicrob Agents Chemother 1997;41:2127–31.

[21] Swaney SM, Aoki H, Ganoza MC, et al. The oxazolidinone linezolid inhibits initiation of protein synthesis in bacteria. Antimicrob Agents Chemother 1998;42:3251–5.

[22] Diekema DI, Jones RN. Oxazolidinones: a review. Drugs 2000;59:7–16.

[23] Zurenko GE, Yagi BH, Schaadt RD, et al. In vitro activities of U-100592 and U-100766, novel oxazolidinone antibacterial agents. Antimicrob Agents Chemother 1996;40:839–45.

[24] Wallace Jr RJ, Brown-Elliott BA, Ward SC, et al. Activities of linezolid against rapidly growing mycobacteria. Antimicrob Agents Chemother 2001;45:764–7.

[25] Peters J, Kondo KL, Lee RK, et al. In-vitro activity of oxazolidinones against Mycobacterium avium complex. J Antimicrob Chemother 1995;35:675–9.

[26] Brown BA, Ward SC, Crist CJ, et al. In vitro activity of linezolid against multiple species of Nocardia: a new drug of choice for a difficult disease? [abstract U-57]. In: Program and Abstracts of the 100th General Meeting of the American Society for Microbiology. Washington, DC: American Society for Microbiology; 2000.

[27] Zyvox [package insert]. Kalamazoo, MI: Pharmacia & Upjohn; 2000.

[28] Moellering Jr RC. Linezolid: the first oxazolidinone antimicrobial. Ann Intern Med 2003;138:135–42.

[29] Duvall SE, Bruss JB, McConnell-Martin MA, et al. Comparison of oral linezolid to oral clarithromycin in the treatment of uncomplicated skin infections: results from a multinational phase III trial [abstract 80.005]. In: Program and Abstracts of the 9th International Congress on Infectious Diseases. Boston: International Society of Infectious Diseases; 2000.

[30] Plouffe JF. Emerging therapies for gram-positive bacterial infections. Clin Infect Dis 2000;31(Suppl 4):S144–9.

[31] Bruss JB, Duvall SE, McConnell-Martin MA, et al. Comparison of linezolid to oxacillin followed by oral dicloxacillin in the treatment of complicated skin in-

fections: results from a multinational phase III trial [abstract]. In: Program and Abstracts of the 9th International Congress on Infectious Diseases. Boston: International Society of Infectious Diseases; 2000.

[32] Stevens DL, Smith LG, Bruss JB, et al. Randomized comparison of linezolid (PNU-100766) versus oxacillin/dicloxacillin for the treatment of complicated skin and soft tissue infections. Antimicrob Agents Chemother 2000;44:3408–13.

[33] Cammarata SK, San Pedro GS, Timm JA, et al. Comparison of Linezolid versus ceftriaxone/cefpodoxime in the treatment of hospitalized patients with community-acquired pneumonia [abstract]. Presented at the European Congress of Clinical Microbiology and Infectious Diseases. Stockholm, Sweden, May 28–31, 2000.

[34] Brier ME, Stalker DJ, Aronoff GR, et al. Pharmacokinetics of linezolid in subjects with varying degrees of renal function and on dialysis [abstract A-54]. In: Program and Abstracts of the 38th Interscience Conference on Antimicrobial Agents and Chemotherapy. Washington, DC: American Society for Microbiology; 1998.

[35] Rao N, Ziran BH, Wagener MM, et al. Similar hematologic effects of long-term linezolid and vancomycin therapy in a prospective observational study of patients with orthopedic infections. Clin Infect Dis 2004;38:1058–64.

[36] Hendershot PE, Antal EJ, Welshman IR, et al. Linezolid: pharmacokinetic and pharmacodynamic evaluation of coadministration with pseudoephedrine HCl phenylpropanolamine HCl, and dextromethorphan HBr. J Clin Pharmacol 2001;41:563–72.

[37] Green SL, Maddox JC, Huttenbach ED. Linezolid and reversible myelosuppression [letter]. JAMA 2001; 285:1291.

[38] Linezolid (Zyvox). Med Lett Drugs Ther 2000;42: 45–6.

[39] Allington DR, Rivey MP. Quinupristin/dalfopristin: a therapeutic review. Clin Ther 2001;23:24–44.

[40] David M. Livermore Quinupristin/dalfopristin and linezolid: where, when, which and whether to use? J Antimicrob Chemother 2000;46:347–50.

[41] Batts DH, Lavin BS, Eliopoulos GM. Quinupristin/dalfopristin and linezolid: spectrum of activity and potential roles in therapy: a status report. Curr Clin Top Infect Dis 2001;21:227–51.

[42] Singh KV, Weinstock GM, Murray BE. An *Enterococcus faecalis* ABC homologue (Lsa) is required for the resistance of this species to clindamycin and quinupristin-dalfopristin. Antimicrob Agents Chemother 2002;46:1845–50.

[43] Nichols RL, Graham DR, Barriere SL, et al, for the Synercid Skin and Skin Structure Infection Group. Treatment of hospitalized patients with complicated gram-positive skin and skin structure infections: two randomized, multicentre studies of quinupristin/dalfopristin versus cefazolin, oxacillin or vancomycin. J Antimicrob Chemother 1999;44:263–73.

[44] Beal J, for the Global Synercid SSSI Study Group. Randomized, comparative, multicenter, open study of quinupristin/dalfopristin (Q/D, RP 59500, Synercid) versus standard therapy (cefazolin or vancomycin) in the treatment of complicated Gram-positive skin and skin structure infections (C-SSSI) [abstract 2318]. Programme and Abstracts of the Twentieth International Congress of Chemotherapy. Sydney, Australia: International Society of Chemotherapy; 1997.

[45] Fagon J-Y, Patrick H, Haas DW, et al, for the Nosocomial Pneumonia Group. Treatment of gram-positive nosocomial pneumonia. prospective randomized comparison of quinupristin/dalfopristin versus vancomycin. Am J Respir Crit Care Med 2000;161: 753–62.

[46] Nadler H, Dowzicky MJ, Feger C, et al. Quinupristin/dalfopristin: a novel selective-spectrum antibiotic for the treatment of multi-resistant and other gram-positive pathogens. Clinical Microbiology Newsletter July 1, 1999;21:103–12.

[47] Rubinstein E, Prokocimer P, Talbot GH. Safety and tolerability of quinupristin/dalfopristin: administration guidelines. J Antimicrob Chemother 1999;44:37–46.

[48] Olsen KM, Rebuck JA, Rupp ME. Arthralgias and myalgias related to quinupristin-dalfopristin administration. Clin Infect Dis 2001;32:83–6.

[49] Rehm SJ, Graham DR, Srinath L, et al. Successful administration of quinupristin/dalfopristin in the outpatient setting. J Antimicrob Chemother 2001;47: 639–45.

[50] Saravolatz DL, Leggett J. Gatifloxacin, gemifloxacin, and moxifloxacin: the role of 3 newer fluoroquinolones. Clin Infect Dis 2003;37:1210–5.

[51] Tarshis GA, Miskin BM, Jones TM, et al. Once-daily oral gatifloxacin versus oral levofloxacin in treatment of uncomplicated skin and soft tissue infections: double-blind, multicenter, randomized study. Antimicrob Agents Chemother 2001;45:2358–62.

[52] Muijsers R, Jarvis B. Moxifloxacin in uncomplicated skin and skin structure infections. Drugs 2002;62: 967–73.

[53] Gatifloxacin and moxifloxacin: two new fluoroquinolones. Med Lett 2000;42:15–7.

[54] Roberge RJ, Kaplan R, Frank R, et al. Glyburide-ciprofloxacin interaction with resistant hypoglycemia. Ann Emerg Med 2000;36:160–3.

[55] Tequin (gatifloxacin) [package insert]. Princeton, NJ: Bristol-Myers Squibb; 2002.

[56] Grasela DM. Clinical pharmacology of gatifloxacin, a new fluoroquinolone. Clin Infect Dis 2000;31(Suppl 2): S51–8.

[57] Tristani-Firouzi M, Chen J, Mitcheson JS, et al. Molecular biology of K+ channels and their role in cardiac arrhythmias. Am J Med 2001;110:50–9.

[58] Gaynes R, Rimland D, Killum E, et al. Outbreak of *Clostridium difficile* infections in a long-term nursing facility: association with gatifloxacin use. Clin Infect Dis 2004;38:640–5.

[59] Scheld WM. Maintaining fluoroquinolone class effi-

cacy: review of influencing factors. Emerg Infect Dis 2003;9:1–9.

[60] Candiani G, Abbondi M, Borgonovi M, et al. In-vitro and in-vivo antibacterial activity of BI 397, a new semi-synthetic glycopeptide antibiotic. J Antimicrob Chemother 1999;44:179–92.

[61] Stogniew M, Pu F, Dowell J. Attributes of dalbavancin: well distributed, weekly dosing, and completely eliminated. Clin Microbiol Infect 2003;9(Suppl 1):S291.

[62] Seltzer E, Dorr MB, Goldstein BP, et al. Once-weekly dalbavancin versus standard-of-care antimicrobial regimens for treatment of skin and soft-tissue infections. Clin Infect Dis 2003;37:1298–303.

[63] Allen NE, Nicas TI. Mechanism of action of oritavancin and related glycopeptide antibiotics. FEMS Microbiol Rev 2003;26:511–32.

[64] Jones RN, Barrett MS, Erwin ME. In vitro activity and

spectrum of LY333328, a novel glycopeptide derivative. Antimicrob Agents Chemother 1997;41:488–93.

[65] Kaatz GW, Seo SM, Aeschlimann JR, et al. Efficacy of LY333328 against experimental methicillin-resistant *Staphylococcus aureus* endocarditis. Antimicrob Agents Chemother 1998;42:981–3.

[66] Woodford N. Novel agents for the treatment of resistant gram-positive infections. Expert Opin Investig Drugs 2003;12:117–37.

[67] Wasilewski M, Disch D, McGill J, et al. Equivalence of shorter course therapy with oritavancin compared to vancomycin-cephalexin in complicated skin/skin structure infections. Presented at the 41st Interscience Conference on Antimicrobial Agents and Chemotherapy. Chicago, Illinois, December 16–19, 2001 [Abstract no. UL-18].

ELSEVIER
SAUNDERS

Dermatol Clin 23 (2005) 313 – 322

DERMATOLOGIC
CLINICS

Advances in Antiviral Therapy

Jashin J. Wu, MD[a], Katie R. Pang, MD[b], David B. Huang, MD, MPH[c,d,e],
Stephen K. Tyring, MD, PhD, MBA[f,g,*]

[a]Department of Dermatology, University of California at Irvine, C340, Medical Science I, Irvine, CA 92697-2400, USA
[b]Department of Dermatology, Wayne State University School of Medicine, 5E University Health Center,
4201 St. Antoine, Detroit, MI 48201, USA
[c]Division of Infectious Diseases, Department of Medicine, Baylor College of Medicine, 1 Baylor Plaza,
BCM286, N1319, Houston, TX 77030, USA
[d]University of Texas at Houston School of Public Health, University of Texas Health Science Center at Houston,
1200 Herman Pressler Box #693, Houston, TX 77030, USA
[e]Division of Infectious Diseases, Department of Medicine, University of Texas Health Science Center at Houston,
6431 Fannin Street, Houston, TX 77030, USA
[f]Department of Dermatology, University of Texas Health Science Center at Houston, 6655 Travis, Suite 820,
Houston, TX 77030, USA
[g]Center for Clinical Studies, 2060 Space Park Drive, Suite 200, Houston, TX 77058, USA

Infections caused by herpes simplex virus 1 (HSV-1), HSV-2, varicella zoster virus (VZV), Epstein-Barr virus (EBV), cytomegalovirus (CMV), human papillomaviruses (HPVs), and molluscum contagiosum virus (MCV) are common, and their incidence continues to grow despite a wide range of available and experimental therapies. There are multiple vaccines available for certain viral diseases and others in development for HSV-2 and HPV. This article discusses the pathogenesis, clinical manifestations, and available and experimental therapies for viral infections of the skin.

Herpesviruses

Herpes simplex virus 1

HSV-1 is the typical cause of herpes labialis and the cause of 30% of cases of first-episode genital herpes [1]. Approximately 90% of people aged be-

tween 20 and 40 years have antibodies to HSV-1 [1]. The primary infection usually occurs early in life, with latency of the virus established in ganglia. Reactivation can occur from many different "triggers," including immunosuppression, psychologic stress, physical trauma, or sun exposure. Prodromal symptoms, such as burning, itching, or tingling, may occur first, and lesions appear as erythematous vesicles that develop into ulcerations. The transmission of HSV-1 occurs with viral shedding during asymptomatic and symptomatic periods, usually through direct contact with infected secretions such as saliva.

Herpes simplex virus 2

HSV-2 is one of the most common sexually transmitted diseases in the world. It causes 70% of cases of primary genital herpes and more than 95% of recurrent genital herpes [1]. In the United States, the incidence of genital herpes is 500,000 to 1,000,000 per year, with a prevalence of 40 to 60 million affected individuals [1]. Similar to HSV-1, HSV-2 produces primary, latent, and recurrent infections and is transmitted during asymptomatic and symptomatic phases, typically through sexual con-

* Corresponding author. Center for Clinical Studies, 2060 Space Park Drive, Suite 200, Houston, TX 77058.

E-mail address: styring@ccstexas.com (S.K. Tyring).

tact. HSV-2 can also cause neonatal herpes when the virus is transmitted from an infected mother to the neonate, with the highest risk occurring when the mother has primary genital herpes during delivery. In addition to cutaneous lesions, the infected neonate may develop multiorgan involvement, and the infection carries a high mortality rate.

Up to 90% of patients infected with HSV-2 become infected because of asymptomatic, subclinical viral shedding [2]. In immunocompromised patients, recurrent episodes of genital herpes are more painful, have a longer duration of viral shedding, take longer to heal, and are more likely to occur in multiple sites or disseminate.

Herpes zoster

Herpes zoster or shingles is caused by the reactivation of varicella zoster virus (VZV), which resides in a latent state in the sensory ganglia following primary VZV infection (chickenpox). It has the highest incidence of all neurologic diseases, occurring annually in more than 1,000,000 people each year in the United States and during the lifetime in 20% of the population [3].

The appearance of the characteristic dermatomal rash is accompanied by severe pain. The rash usually heals within 2 to 4 weeks, and the pain associated with herpes zoster is its most distressing symptom. Pain that persists beyond cutaneous healing is termed postherpetic neuralgia, a chronic neuropathic pain syndrome that can last for months or even years.

Epstein-Barr virus

More than 90% of adults in the world have been infected with EBV and carry the virus as a lifelong persistent infection [4]. EBV causes various diseases, including infectious mononucleosis, post-transplant lymphoproliferative disease, and chronic active EBV infection, and it has been linked to many cancers, such as Burkitt's lymphoma, nasopharyngeal carcinoma, Hodgkin's disease, and gastric carcinoma.

Cytomegalovirus

CMV infection is common among the patients who have undergone bone marrow transplant, solid organ transplant, or hematopoietic stem cell transplant, and in those who are immunocompromised. CMV is one of the most common members of the herpesviruses. Seroprevalence studies indicate that infection occurs in 60% to 70% of people living in US urban cities and in almost 100% of persons living

in some areas of Africa [5]. It is one of the most important viral opportunistic infections in patients who have AIDS. Before the era of highly active antiretroviral therapy (HAART), the prevalence of CMV disease during the course of HIV infection was estimated to be between 20% and 44% [6]. The most common clinical manifestations of CMV infection include retinitis, esophagitis, pneumonitis, adrenalitis, colitis, hepatitis, and central nervous system (CNS) involvement (transverse myelitis, polyradiculopathy, and ventriculitis).

Available antiviral agents

Nucleoside antiviral agents

Viral replication depends primarily on the machinery of the host cell. The nucleoside antiviral drugs inhibit viral replication at the cellular level, such as the assembly of progeny virions or the inhibition of virus directed at the macromolecular synthesis at the viral nucleic acid synthesis level. Most antiviral drugs do not have activity against and do not eradicate nonreplicating or latent viruses. Because viral replication depends on the host cell function, antiviral therapy may have associated host toxicity.

Acyclovir

The synthetic guanosine analog acyclovir is the most extensively used antiviral drug worldwide. It requires the herpesvirus thymidine kinase to phosphorylate the drug for activation, after which bi- and triphosphorylation irreversibly hinders viral DNA synthesis. The most severe adverse event is when intravenous (IV) administration causes reversible crystalline nephropathy.

Although not specifically FDA-approved for this indication, oral acyclovir 400 mg five times daily for 5 days can be used for the treatment of herpes labialis. This antiviral agent has clinical benefit, reducing duration of pain by 36% and time to loss of crust by 27% [7]. The recommended dosage of acyclovir is 200 mg, five times a day for 10 days for first-episode genital herpes, and 200 mg, five times a day for 5 days for recurrent genital herpes. For enhanced compliance and convenience, acyclovir can be given in 400-mg doses, three times a day for 5 days or 10 days for recurrent genital herpes. The suppressive therapy is 400 mg twice a day, which can reduce recurrences by 80% to 90% and reduce asymptomatic viral shedding of HSV-2 by 95% [8].

Acyclovir is given at dosages of 800 mg, five times a day for 7 to 10 days for acute herpes zoster, which accelerates zoster rash healing and reduces pain. IV acyclovir is sometimes used for immunocompromised patients who have herpes zoster at a dosage of 5 to 10 mg/kg every 8 hours for 7 days.

Valacyclovir

Valacyclovir is a prodrug of acyclovir (the L-valyl ester of acyclovir), and it seems to have a similar safety profile to acyclovir. No crystalline nephropathy has been reported, however.

It is very effective against HSV-1 and HSV-2 in immunocompetent patients for treatment of the following conditions: an initial episode of genital herpes (1 g twice daily for 10 d), episodic therapy for recurrent herpes labialis (2 g, 2×/d for 1 d) and recurrent genital herpes (1 g or 500 mg, 2×/d for 3–5 d), and suppression of recurrent genital herpes (1 g or 500 mg 1×/d). For immunocompromised patients, valacyclovir is effective for episodic therapy (1 g, 2×/d for ≥5 d) and suppression of recurrent genital herpes (500 mg, 2×/d, or 1 g, 1×/d) [9]. Daily suppressive therapy with 500 mg of valacyclovir decreases the risk of transmission of genital herpes by 53% in heterosexual, HSV-2–discordant couples by reducing asymptomatic viral shedding [10].

Valacyclovir at a dosage of 1 g, 3 times daily for 7 days is as effective as acyclovir in reducing time to crusting, time to 50% healing, and the appearance of new zoster lesions [11]. Further, the median duration of pain after healing is reduced from 60 days with acyclovir to 40 days with valacyclovir. Valacyclovir and famciclovir have similar efficacy in the reduction of postherpetic neuralgia [12]. Valacyclovir is more convenient, more effective, and is as safe as acyclovir and less expensive than famciclovir.

In the absence of induction therapy, high-risk EBV-seronegative recipients who receive prophylactic valacyclovir are significantly less likely to develop post-transplant lymphoproliferative disease after lung transplantation [9]. Valacyclovir also reduces the incidence or delays the onset of CMV infection in transplant recipients [9].

Famciclovir

Famciclovir is an acyclic guanosine analog that is metabolized into penciclovir, the active metabolite. It requires phosphorylation by herpesvirus thymidine kinase and cellular kinases and, once activated, inhibits DNA polymerase. When compared with acyclo-

vir, however, famciclovir has a higher bioavailability and achieves higher concentrations in HSV-infected cells. Because famciclovir is more stable, it has longer antiviral activity, allowing for less frequent dosing. Adverse effects are rare and are no different than with acyclovir. Concomitant use of famciclovir with medications that are eliminated by active renal tubular secretion, such as probenecid, can lead to elevated serum concentrations of penciclovir.

Famciclovir is effective against HSV-1, HSV-2, and VZV. It is used in the treatment of the following conditions: initial episodes of genital herpes (250 mg, 3×/d for 10 d), episodic treatment of recurrent genital herpes (125 mg, 2×/d for 5 d), suppression of recurrent genital herpes (250 mg, 2×/d), and for shingles (500 mg every 8 h for 7 d). For immunocompromised patients, famciclovir is efficacious for episodic treatment of recurrent genital herpes (500 mg, 2×/d for 7 d).

Compared with acyclovir, famciclovir is as effective, safe, and well-tolerated in the treatment of HSV infections in HIV-positive patients [13]. Famciclovir is also at least as effective as acyclovir for ophthalmic zoster [14] and for shingles and acute zoster pain in immunocompromised patients [15]. Compared with valacyclovir, famciclovir is as effective, safe, and convenient in the treatment of zoster [12].

Penciclovir

Another acyclic guanosine analog that has activity against HSV-1, HSV-2, and VZV is penciclovir, the metabolite of famciclovir. Because it has low oral bioavailability, it is an FDA-approved topical treatment for herpes labialis. Similar to acyclovir, penciclovir is phosphorylated by viral thymidine kinase and cellular kinases before it can inhibit viral DNA polymerase. Topical penciclovir 1% is approved for episodic therapy of herpes labialis and is applied every 2 hours during waking hours for 4 days. It has been found to speed healing and decrease pain by about 1 day [16].

Ganciclovir/valganciclovir

Ganciclovir is a deoxyguanosine analog that hinders viral DNA synthesis. Viral enzymes phosphorylate intracellular ganciclovir, which then concentrates within CMV-infected cells by being a competitive inhibitor of deoxyguanosine triphosphate incorporation into viral DNA.

Ganciclovir is approved for treatment and chronic suppression of CMV retinitis in AIDS patients and prevention of CMV disease in transplant recipients. Ganciclovir is also effective for CMV syndromes, including CMV pneumonia, CMV colitis, and gastrointestinal infections in patients with AIDS and transplant recipients. Oral valganciclovir is convenient to use and may replace IV ganciclovir for initial and maintenance treatment [17].

Ganciclovir toxicities include metabolic abnormalities, myelosuppression, and central nervous system abnormalities.

Cidofovir

Cidofovir is an acyclic phosphonate nucleotide analog of deoxycytidine monophosphate and inhibits viral DNA synthesis. The active diphosphate form of cidofovir is a competitive inhibitor and acts as an alternative substrate for HSV and CMV DNA polymerase. Cidofovir does not depend on herpes thymidine kinase enzymatic activity, so it is active against acyclovir-resistant HSV strains and ganciclovir-resistant CMV strains.

Cidofovir is FDA-approved for the therapy for CMV retinitis in AIDS patients. It is administered at 5 mg/kg once a week for 2 weeks followed by every-other-week dosing. This treatment has not been proved for non-HIV infected persons and patients who have other CMV syndromes, however.

The major toxicity with cidofovir is nephrotoxicity, typically from proximal tubular dysfunction. Other reported side effects include neutropenia, fever, diarrhea, nausea, vomiting, asthenia, headache, rash, anterior uveitis, and ocular hypotony.

Recent studies have shown that topical cidofovir (1% gel or cream) is effective in the treatment of recalcitrant and otherwise unmanageable viral cutaneous lesions induced by herpesviruses, HPVs, and MCV. Cidofovir in IV form can be extemporaneously compounded for topical use, which costs approximately $50 to $75 per gram when compounded in a cream base containing a 3% concentration. There are no studies to investigate the bioavailability of topical or intralesional cidofovir in humans [18].

Various case reports have shown success in using topical cidofovir for acyclovir-resistant HSV-2 infections [19,20]. A randomized, double-blind, multicenter trial evaluated the safety and efficacy of cidofovir gel in 30 AIDS patients for acyclovir-resistant HSV infections [21]. None of the 10 patients in the placebo group showed complete healing or more than 50% improvement in the infection, whereas 50% in the cidofovir group did experience improvement [21]. Further, one third of cidofovir-treated subjects experienced complete healing versus none of the placebo-treated subjects. Application site reactions were comparable in both groups.

Fomivirsen

Fomivirsen is a 21-nucelotide phosphorothioate oligonuceotide that has a novel mechanism of action by inhibition of human CMV replication through an antisense mechanism. It has activity against cidofovir- and ganciclovir-resistant strains of CMV.

Fomivirsen is indicated for use in HIV patients with CMV retinitis who are not responsive to or are unable to take cidofovir and ganciclovir. Fomivirsen is given by intravitreal injection at dosages of 330 μg every 2 weeks.

Adverse events of fomivirsen include iritis, vitritis, and increased intraocular pressure. The vitritis and iritis occur in 25% of fomivirsen recipients and can be treated with topical corticosteroids [22].

Foscarnet

Foscarnet is an organic pyrophosphatase analog that directly inhibits herpesvirus DNA polymerase by reversibly blocking the pyrophosphate binding site of the viral polymerase. Foscarnet is active against HSV, VZV, EBV, CMV, and human herpes virus 8 (HHV-8). Foscarnet also has activity against acyclovir-resistant HSV and VZV strains, ganciclovir-resistant CMV strains, and HIV by directly inhibiting the HIV reverse transcriptase.

Foscarnet is approved for therapy for CMV retinitis in AIDS patients and in acyclovir-resistant HSV mucocutaneous infections. It also has been used successfully in ganciclovir-resistant CMV retinitis and gastrointestinal and pulmonary infections in AIDS patients. For acyclovir-resistant mucocutaneous HSV infections, 40 mg/kg every 8 hours is administered for 14 to 21 days.

Box 1. Available antiviral therapies for herpesvirus infections

Acyclovir
Valacyclovir
Famciclovir
Penciclovir
Ganciclovir/valganciclovir
Cidofovir
Fomivirsen
Foscarnet

Foscarnet toxicity includes mainly nephrotoxicity, metabolic and hematologic abnormalities, and CNS side effects. Patients may develop isolated or combined hypomagnesemia (15%–44%), hypocalcemia (15%–35%), hypokalemia (10%–16%), and hypophosphatemia [23]. CNS side effects include headache (25%), seizures (up to 10%), irritability, tremor, and hallucinations [24]. Other reported side effects include fever, rash, painful genital ulcerations, diarrhea, nausea, and vomiting. Box 1 lists the available antiviral therapies for herpesvirus infections.

Experimental therapy for herpesvirus infections

Helicase–primase inhibitors

A new type of drug, helicase–primase inhibitors, recently has been shown to be effective in antiviral-resistant HSVs. The helicase–primase inhibitors comprise two new classes of drugs: amino-thiazolyl-phenyl–containing drugs [25] and thiazole urea derivatives [26]. These drugs inhibit the helicase–primase complex, which is essential for the HSV DNA replication process.

Both newly described drug classes are active orally and show significant effectiveness in HSV-1 and HSV-2 in the guinea pig, mouse, and rat model. They also show great efficacy when given several hours or even days after the cutaneous lesions appear. Compared with acyclovir and valacyclovir, the helicase–primase inhibitors were superior in the same experiments [25,26]. Both classes were safe and well tolerated in the animal models. They did not show evidence of anti-VZV or anti-CMV activity, however.

Human papillomaviruses

There are more than 100 genotypes of HPV, which are DNA tumor viruses that infect the epithelial cells of skin and mucosa and cause warts or benign papillomas. There are some types of HPV that are considered "high risk," including types 16 and 18, because they are the primary causal agents for cervical cancer, anogenital cancers, and upper aerodigestive tract and skin cancers.

Among sexually active women, infection with HPV is common, with an incidence of 15% to 40% [27]. More than 25 types of HPV can infect the oral and anogenital mucosa. The International Association for Research in Cancer conducted an international study that showed that the most common high-risk HPV types that infect the cervix are HPV-16 (53%), HPV-18 (15%), HPV-45 (9%), HPV-31 (6%), and HPV-33 (3%) [28].

Box 2. Available therapies for human papillomavirus infections

Most commonly used therapies

> Cryotherapy
> Trichloroacetic acid
> Podofilox
> Surgical removal
> Laser surgery
> Imiquimod
> Interferon
> Topical cidofovir

Less commonly used therapies

> Electrosurgery
> 5-Fluorouracil
> Retinoids
> Bleomycin (intralesional and systemic)
> Salicylic acid

There is no curative therapy for HPV infections. The 2002 Centers for Disease Control and Prevention (CDC) recommendations for HPV treatment include the following: treatment with cryotherapy, trichloroacetic acid, or podofilox; surgical removal; or laser surgery (Box 2) [29]. The CDC also recommends imiquimod or interferon, which modulates the host's immune response against infected cells [29]. Other less commonly used therapies include electrosurgery, 5-fluorouracil, retinoids, bleomycin (intralesional and systemic), and salicylic acid [30]. Recurrence rates of anogenital warts are unacceptably high following surgical or cytodestruction therapy but are very low following successful therapy with imiquimod [31].

Immunomodulators

In the 1980s, the first immune response modifier (IRM) was discovered, and the chemical family was named the imidazoquinolines. The IRMs induce the endogenous production of cytokines, including interferon α (IFN-α), interleukin 12, and tumor necrosis factor α, primarily from monocytes/macrophages. They also indirectly induce IFN-γ, a Th1-type cytokine that induces cell-mediated immunity and antigen presentation.

Imiquimod was the first commercially available imidazoquinoline approved for the therapy of anogenital warts and was subsequently approved for superficial basal cell carcinoma and actinic keratosis. Some case reports show improvement in recurrent genital herpes with imiquimod, but a phase 2 trial showed that it did not have any significant short-term benefits when compared with placebo [32].

Imiquimod is typically applied in three doses per week for HPV infections. Multiple clinical trials have shown the safety and efficacy of imiquimod for HPV infections [31,33,34]. Up to half of patients may have local adverse effects, such as mild to moderate erythema, edema, erosion, and excoriation [33,34]. These effects are mild and only 1% to 2% of patients cannot tolerate therapy and discontinue [35]. Systemic symptoms, such as diarrhea, headache, fatigue, fever, malaise, and myalgias, were no different than those with placebo. Increasing the frequency of application beyond 3 times weekly does not improve success rates but instead increases side effects [36].

The most recently studied IRM, resiquimod (R-848, S-28463, 4-amino-2-ethoxymethyl-α,α-dimethyl-1H-imidazo[4,5-c]quinolin-1-ethanol), is a more potent analog of imiquimod. In a phase 2 clinical study, resiquimod improved median time to first recurrence and reduced recurrences of genital herpes, even after the end of therapy [37]. The median time to first recurrence in the resiquimod-treated group was 169 days, compared with 57 days for the placebo-treated group ($P = 0.0058$).

Topical cidofovir

Topical cidofovir also has shown efficacy in the treatment of anogenital warts and verruca vulgaris. In the first double-blind, placebo-controlled study using topical cidofovir for the treatment of genital HPV infections in 30 immunocompetent patients, 9 of 19 cidofovir-treated patients (47%) had a complete response, compared with none of the patients in the placebo-treated group ($P = 0.006$) [38]. None of the cidofovir-treated patients had disease progression versus 5 of 11 patients (45%) in the placebo-treated group. Adverse events were comparable in both treatment groups.

A randomized, placebo-controlled, single-blind, crossover pilot study examined external anogenital warts in HIV-infected patients [39]. Patients received either 1% cidofovir cream or placebo applied once daily, 5 days a week for 2 weeks, followed by 2 weeks of observation. Seven cidofovir treatments resulted in a reduction of more than 50% in the total wart area, compared with no reductions in patients treated with placebo ($P = 0.02$).

Molluscum contagiosum

Molluscum contagiosum (MC), which is caused by the MCV of the DNA poxvirus group, is a benign skin infection that affects children and young adults worldwide. In addition, MC commonly affects immunocompromised patients, and the prevalence of MC infection among HIV-infected patients ranges from 5% to 18% [30]. MC has not been reported to progress to malignancy, and most lesions regress spontaneously within 9 to 12 months, because the infection is limited to the epidermis [40].

The prevalence of this skin infection in the general population is unknown because it has not been cultured. In the United States, it is believed that the incidence of genital MC is low compared with other sexually transmitted diseases (STDs; 1 case per 42–60 cases of gonorrhea) [41], and the age distribution of patients with genital MC is similar to that of other STDs [40]. Outbreaks of MC are also possible between family members and from sauna baths, swimming pools, and school.

In sexually active young adults, MC lesions present as small, smooth, umbilicated papules on the inner thighs, genital, and pubic areas. MC is treated with similar therapies available for warts to control transmission and for cosmetic reasons. Cold steel surgery, electrosurgery, cryotherapy, cantharidin, and imiquimod are all effective therapies (Box 3) [30]. Less commonly used therapies are podofilox, lasers, trichloroacetic acid, and retinoids [30].

Box 3. Available therapies for molluscum contagiosum

Most commonly used therapies

>   Cold steel surgery
>   Electrosurgery
>   Cryotherapy
>   Cantharidin
>   Imiquimod
>   Topical cidofovir

Less commonly used therapies

>   Podofilox
>   Lasers
>   Trichloroacetic acid
>   Retinoids
>   HAART (if patient is HIV-positive)

Topical cidofovir also has been used successfully in HIV-positive patients infected with MCV [42–44]. A pilot study reported on 14 patients with AIDS, 10 with extensive HPV lesions and 4 with MC, who underwent treatment with topical cidofovir [45]. One patient dropped out, and the remaining 13 patients cleared their HPV or MC infections over varying periods of time. All the patients experienced adverse events, of which inflammation, erosion, and a burning sensation were the most common [45].

HAART in HIV-positive patients has been reported to resolve resistant MC [46–48]. In a retrospective study of 456 HIV-positive patients, the prevalence of MC was 18% before HAART was initiated compared with 5% during HAART [48].

Experimental vaccines

Many vaccines are available to prevent viruses with cutaneous manifestations, such as smallpox, hepatitis A and B, varicella zoster, measles, mumps, and rubella [49]. The following section discusses some of the vaccines in development for HSV and HPV.

Herpes simplex virus

Two different recombinant subunit vaccines have been investigated in phase 3 trials. One candidate, developed by Chiron (Emeryville, California), contains HSV-2 surface glycoproteins B and D and the adjuvant MF59. The development of this vaccine was stopped prematurely because results showed overall lack of efficacy for both preventive and therapeutic use [50]. A second recombinant vaccine was developed by SmithKlineBeecham and consists of glycoprotein D and the adjuvant monophosphoryl lipid A immunostimulant, or MPL. Clinical trials indicate that this vaccine has a clinical efficacy of 73% in protecting women who are serologically negative for both HSV-1 and HSV-2 from acquiring HSV-2 disease [51]. Currently, it is being further studied in a phase 3, double-blinded, randomized, controlled trial sponsored by GlaxoSmithKline Biologicals (Brentford, Middlesex, United Kingdom) and the National Institutes of Health. As of November 2004, more than 2600 women who are seronegative for HSV-1 and HSV-2 have been enrolled, but no cases of genital herpes have been reported. The enrollment goal is 7550 women.

DNA vaccines are also in development for HSV. Animal studies involving inoculations of plasmid DNA carrying the desired viral genes have shown promising results for the prevention of infection. The vaccines express one or two viral antigens, but they can induce cell-mediated immunity without the need for potent adjuvant agents. One such candidate that encodes glycoprotein D2 is currently in phase 1 clinical trials, and several others are in preclinical development.

The disabled infectious single cycle, or DISC, vaccine lacks the glycoprotein H gene required for virus entry into cells. After a single replication cycle, the virus cannot spread to surrounding cells and remains noninfectious. Studies in guinea pigs showed encouraging results for both preventive and therapeutic purposes [52,53]. Phase 1 studies show the candidate vaccine to be safe and well tolerated, but phase 2 trials show that the vaccine failed as therapy.

A randomized double-blind trial evaluated the safety and efficacy of a novel recombinant virus, ICP10deltaPK, for reduction of recurrent HSV-2 outbreaks [54]. Patients with a minimum of five documented herpetic recurrences in the previous year were injected 7, 17, and 28 days after lesion occurrence. Recurrences were prevented in 37.5% of the vaccine-treated patients, but 100% of the placebo-treated patients had at least one recurrence ($P = 0.068$). Vaccinated patients had fewer recurrences (1.58) compared with placebo-treated patients (3.13; $P = 0.028$) [54].

Human papillomavirus

Although more than 30 types of HPV are sexually transmitted, the major types associated with malignancy (types 16, 18, 31, 33, 45, 52, and 58) and condylomata (types 6 and 11) are fewer in number, allowing for more focused strategies for vaccination against these specific types.

Viruslike particles (VLPs) are produced by recombinant DNA technology and are designed to self-assemble into conformations that resemble HPV. These vaccines contain no viral DNA, thus carry no risk of infection or oncogenic exposure. VLPs have been designed for all of the major HPV subtypes, and clinical trials are currently ongoing for HPV-11 L1 VLP [55], HPV-6 L1 VLP [56], and HPV-16 L1 VLP [57]. A double-blind, placebo-controlled trial showed that HPV-16–negative individuals who received the HPV-16 vaccine had a significantly reduced incidence of HPV-16 infections and related cervical intraepithelial neoplasia at a median follow-up period of 17 months [58]. The incidence of persistent HPV-16 infection was 0 per 100 woman-years in women at risk in the vaccine group and 3.8 per 100 woman-years in women at risk in the placebo group (100% efficacy; 95% confidence interval, 90–100; $P<0.001$) [58]. All nine cases of HPV-16–related cervical intraepithelial neoplasia developed in the placebo recipients [58].

Fusion protein vaccines are currently under evaluation for the immunotherapy of genital warts and cervical cancer. For the treatment of genital warts, TA-GW is a recombinant fusion protein vaccine consisting of HPV-6 L2 and E7 proteins. A phase 2a clinical trial showed the vaccine to be immunogenic, with encouraging clinical responses [59]. TA-HPV is a live, recombinant vaccinia virus that has been engineered to express the E6 and E7 protein genes for HPV 16 and 18 as a treatment for cervical cancer [60]. Viral vector vaccines have the potential to produce immunity similar to that induced by live attenuated vaccines. A phase 1/2 clinical trial of TA-HPV [61] has shown promising results, and further studies are underway. A third protein vaccine, TA-CIN, is in preclinical development for the treatment of cervical dysplasia [60].

Peptide-based vaccines have been shown to protect against HPV-induced tumors in mice, although the T-cell repertoires in mice and humans differ. One early-stage human clinical trial involving HLA-A*0201 binding HPV16-E7 peptides is ongoing to assess the possible therapeutic implications of these vaccines. Other investigational approaches to HPV immunization include bacterial vectors [62], dendritic cells pulsed with HPV epitopes [63], and DNA vaccines [64].

Summary

Current therapies for viral infections of the skin can reduce or suppress symptoms, but there is no known cure and no available method to reduce the frequency of outbreaks after antiviral drug cessation. Despite the encouraging potential of the helicase–primase inhibitors, neither they nor current treatments can destroy the herpesvirus in the latent state. IRMs (eg, imiquimod) can eradicate HPV-associated lesions and markedly reduce recurrences. One HSV-2 prophylactic vaccine has shown promising results in preventing HSV-2 infection in women who are seronegative for HSV-1 and -2, but further trials are underway. Other prophylactic and therapeutic vaccinations are currently being investigated, and, if successful, they may help end the epidemic of these viral infections.

References

[1] Yeung-Yue KA, Brentjens MH, Lee PC, Tyring SK. Herpes simplex viruses 1 and 2. Dermatol Clin 2002; 20:249–66.

[2] Brown TJ, Yen-Moore A, Tyring SK. An overview of sexually transmitted diseases, part I. J Am Acad Dermatol 1999;41:511–29.

[3] Donohue JG, Choo PW, Manson JE, Platt R. The incidence of herpes zoster. Arch Intern Med 1995;155: 1605–9.

[4] Henle G, Henle W, Clifford P, et al. Antibodies to Epstein-Barr virus in Burkitt's lymphoma and control groups. J Natl Cancer Inst 1969;43:1147–57.

[5] Zhang LJ, Hanff P, Rutherford C, Churchill WH, Crumpacker CS. Detection of human cytomegalovirus DNA, RNA, and antibody in normal donor blood. J Infect Dis 1995;171:1002–6.

[6] Masur H, Whitcup SM, Cartwright C. Advances in the management of AIDS-related cytomegalovirus retinitis. Ann Intern Med 1996;125:126–36.

[7] Spruance SL, Stewart JC, Rowe NH, McKeough MB, Wenerstrom G, Freeman DJ. Treatment of recurrent herpes simplex labialis with oral acyclovir. J Infect Dis 1990;161:185–90.

[8] Evans TY, Tyring SK. Advances in antiviral therapy in dermatology. Dermatol Clin 1998;16:409–19.

[9] Wu JJ, Brentjens MH, Torres G, Yeung-Yue K, Lee P, Tyring SK. Valacyclovir in the treatment of herpes simplex, herpes zoster, and other viral infections. J Cutan Med Surg 2003;7:372–81.

[10] Corey L, Wald A, Patel R, et al. Once-daily valacyclovir to reduce the risk of transmission of genital herpes. N Engl J Med 2004;350:11–20.

[11] Beutner KR, Friedman DJ, Forszpaniak C, Andersen PL, Wood MJ. Valaciclovir compared with acyclovir for improved therapy for herpes zoster in immunocompetent adults. Antimicrob Agents Chemother 1995;39:1546–53.

[12] Tyring SK, Beutner KR, Tucker BA, Anderson WC, Crooks RJ. Antiviral therapy for herpes zoster: randomized, controlled clinical trial of valacyclovir and famciclovir therapy in immunocompetent patients 50 years and older. Arch Fam Med 2000;9:863–9.

[13] Romanowski B, Aoki FY, Martel AY, Lavender EA, Parsons JE, Saltzman RL. Efficacy and safety of famciclovir for treating mucocutaneous herpes simplex infection in HIV-infected individuals. Collaborative Famciclovir HIV Study Group. AIDS 2000;14: 1211–7.

[14] Tyring S, Engst R, Corriveau C, et al. Famciclovir for ophthalmic zoster: a randomised aciclovir controlled study. Br J Ophthalmol 2001;85:576–81.

[15] Tyring S, Belanger R, Bezwoda W, Ljungman P, Boon R, Saltzman RL. A randomized, double-blind trial of famciclovir versus acyclovir for the treatment of localized dermatomal herpes zoster in immunocompromised patients. Cancer Invest 2001;19:13–22.

[16] Spruance SL, Rea TL, Thoming C, Tucker R, Saltzman

R, Boon R. Penciclovir cream for the treatment of herpes simplex labialis. A randomized, multicenter, double-blind, placebo-controlled trial. Topical Penciclovir Collaborative Study Group. JAMA 1997;277:1374–9.

[17] Valganciclovir: new preparation. CMV retinitis: a simpler, oral treatment. Prescribe Int 2003;12:133–5.

[18] Toro JR, Sanchez S, Turiansky G, Blauvelt A. Topical cidofovir for the treatment of dermatologic conditions: verruca, condyloma, intraepithelial neoplasia, herpes simplex and its potential use in smallpox. Dermatol Clin 2003;21:301–9.

[19] Snoeck R, Andrei G, Gerard M, et al. Successful treatment of progressive mucocutaneous infection due to acyclovir- and foscarnet-resistant herpes simplex virus with (S)-1-(3-hydroxy-2-phosphonylmethoxy-propyl)cytosine (HPMPC). Clin Infect Dis 1994;18:570–8.

[20] Lateef F, Don PC, Kaufmann M, White SM, Weinberg JM. Treatment of acyclovir-resistant, foscarnet-unresponsive HSV infection with topical cidofovir in a child with AIDS. Arch Dermatol 1998;134:1169–70.

[21] Lalezari J, Schacker T, Feinberg J, et al. A randomized, double-blind, placebo-controlled trial of cidofovir gel for the treatment of acyclovir-unresponsive mucocutaneous herpes simplex virus infection in patients with AIDS. J Infect Dis 1997;176:892–8.

[22] Vitravene Study Group. Safety of intravitreous fomivirsen for treatment of cytomegalovirus retinitis in patients with AIDS. Am J Ophthalmol 2002;133:484–98.

[23] Jayaweera DT. Minimising the dosage-limiting toxicities of foscarnet induction therapy. Drug Saf 1997;16:258–66.

[24] Jacobson MA, Gambertoglio JG, Aweeka FT, Causey DM, Portale AA. Foscarnet-induced hypocalcemia and effects of foscarnet on calcium metabolism. J Clin Endocrinol Metab 1991;72:1130–5.

[25] Crute JJ, Grygon CA, Hargrave KD, et al. Herpes simplex virus helicase-primase inhibitors are active in animal models of human disease. Nat Med 2002;8:386–91.

[26] Kleymann G, Fischer R, Betz UA, et al. New helicase-primase inhibitors as drug candidates for the treatment of herpes simplex disease. Nat Med 2002;8:392–8.

[27] Savio de Araujo Souza P, Lina Villa L. Genetic susceptibility to infection with human papillomavirus and development of cervical cancer in women in Brazil. Mutat Res 2003;544:375–83.

[28] Munoz N. Human papillomavirus and cancer: the epidemiological evidence. J Clin Virol 2000;19:1–5.

[29] Centers for Disease Control and Prevention. Sexually transmitted diseases treatment guidelines 2002. MMWR Morb Mortal Wkly Rep 2002;51:1–78.

[30] Ting PT, Dytoc MT. Therapy of external anogenital warts and molluscum contagiosum: a literature review. Dermatol Ther 2004;17:68–101.

[31] Carrasco D, vander Straten M, Tyring SK. Treatment of anogenital warts with imiquimod 5% cream fol-lowed by surgical excision of residual lesions. J Am Acad Dermatol 2002;47(Suppl):S212–6.

[32] Schacker TW, Conant M, Thoming C, Stanczak T, Wang Z, Smith M. Imiquimod 5-percent cream does not alter the natural history of recurrent herpes genitalis: a phase II, randomized, double-blind, placebo-controlled study. Antimicrob Agents Chemother 2002;46:3243–8.

[33] Beutner KR, Tyring SK, Trofatter Jr KF, et al. Imiquimod, a patient-applied immune-response modifier for treatment of external genital warts. Antimicrob Agents Chemother 1998;42:789–94.

[34] Beutner KR, Spruance SL, Hougham AJ, Fox TL, Owens ML, Douglas Jr JM. Treatment of genital warts with an immune-response modifier (imiquimod). J Am Acad Dermatol 1998;38:230–9.

[35] Syed TA, Ahmadpour OA, Ahmad SA, Ahmad SH. Management of female genital warts with an analog of imiquimod 2% in cream: a randomized, double-blind, placebo-controlled study. J Dermatol 1998;25:429–33.

[36] Fife KH, Ferenczy A, Douglas Jr JM, Brown DR, Smith M, Owens ML. Treatment of external genital warts in men using 5% imiquimod cream applied three times a week, once daily, twice daily, or three times a day. Sex Transm Dis 2001;28:226–31.

[37] Spruance S, Tyring S, Smith M, Meng TC. Application of a topically applied immune response modifier, resiquimod gel, to modify the recurrence rate of recurrent genital herpes: a pilot study. J Infect Dis 2001;84:196–200.

[38] Snoeck R, Bossens M, Parent D, et al. Phase II double-blind, placebo-controlled study of the safety and efficacy of cidofovir topical gel for the treatment of patients with human papillomavirus infection. Clin Infect Dis 2001;33:597–602.

[39] Matteelli A, Beltrame A, Graifemberghi S, et al. Efficacy and tolerability of topical 1% cidofovir cream for the treatment of external anogenital warts in HIV-infected persons. Sex Transm Dis 2001;28:343–6.

[40] Margolis S. Genital warts and molluscum contagiosum. Urol Clin North Am 1984;11:163–70.

[41] Brown ST, Nalley JF, Kraus SJ. Molluscum contagiosum. Sex Transm Dis 1981;8:227–34.

[42] Meadows KP, Tyring SK, Pavia AT, Rallis TM. Resolution of recalcitrant molluscum contagiosum virus lesions in human immunodeficiency virus-infected patients treated with cidofovir. Arch Dermatol 1997;133:987–90.

[43] Davies EG, Thrasher A, Lacey K, Harper J. Topical cidofovir for severe molluscum contagiosum. Lancet 1999;353:2042.

[44] Toro JR, Wood L, Turner M. Topical cidofovir: a novel treatment for recalcitrant molluseum contagiosum in HIV infected children. Arch Dermatol 2000;136:983–5.

[45] Calista D. Topical cidofovir for severe cutaneous human papillomavirus and molluscum contagiosum infections in patients with HIV/AIDS. A pilot study. J Eur Acad Dermatol Venereol 2000;14:484–8.

[46] Cattelan AM, Sasset L, Corti L, Stiffan S, Meneghetti F, Cadrobbi P. A complete remission of recalcitrant molluscum contagiosum in an AIDS patient following highly active antiretroviral therapy (HAART). J Infect 1999;38:58–60.

[47] Calista D, Boschini A, Landi G. Resolution of disseminated molluscum contagiosum with highly active antiretroviral therapy (HAART) in patients with AIDS. Eur J Dermatol 1999;9:211–3.

[48] Calista D, Morri M, Stagno A, Boschini A. Changing morbidity of cutaneous diseases in patients with HIV after the introduction of highly active antiretroviral therapy including a protease inhibitor. Am J Clin Dermatol 2002;3:59–62.

[49] Wu JJ, Huang DB, Pang KR, Tyring SK. Vaccines and immunotherapies for the prevention of infectious diseases having cutaneous manifestations. J Am Acad Dermatol 2004;50:495–528.

[50] Corey L, Langenberg AG, Ashley R, et al. Recombinant glycoprotein vaccine for the prevention of genital HSV-2 infection: two randomized controlled trials. JAMA 1999;282:331–40.

[51] Stanberry LR, Spruance SL, Cunningham AL, et al. GlaxoSmithKline Herpes Vaccine Efficacy Study Group. Glycoprotein-D-adjuvant vaccine to prevent genital herpes. N Engl J Med 2002;347:1652–61.

[52] Boursnell ME, Entwisle C, Blakely D, et al. A genetically inactivated herpes simplex virus type 2 (HSV-2) vaccine provides effective protection against primary and recurrent HSV-2 disease. J Infect Dis 1997;175:16–25.

[53] McLean CS, Challanin DN, Duncan I, Boursnell ME, Jennings R, Inglis SC. Induction of a protective immune response by mucosal vaccination with a DISC HSV-1 vaccine. Vaccine 1996;14:987–92.

[54] Casanova G, Cancela R, Alonzo L, et al. A double-blind study of the efficacy and safety of the ICP10-deltaPK vaccine against recurrent genital HSV-2 infections. Cutis 2002;70:235–9.

[55] Reichman R, Balsley J, Carlin D, et al. Evaluation of the safety and immunogenicity of a recombinant HPV-11 L1 virus like particle vaccine in healthy adult volunteers. In: Gurley M, Carter CD, Bounassif S, et al, editors. Proceedings of the 17th International Papillomavirus Conference. Charleston, SC, January 9–15, 1999.

[56] Zhang LF, Zhou J, Shao C, et al. A phase 1 trial of HPV 6 B virus like particles as immunotherapy for genital warts. International Papillomavirus Conference. Charleston, SC, January 9–15, 1999.

[57] Silva DD, Nieland J, Greenstone H, Schiller J, Kast W. Chimeric papillomavirus virus-like particles induce antigen-specific therapeutic immunity against tumours expressing the HPV-16 E7 protein. In: International Papillomavirus Conference. 17th edition. 1999.

[58] Koutsky LA, Ault KA, Wheeler CM, et al. A controlled trial of a human papillomavirus type 16 vaccine. N Engl J Med 2002;347:1645–51.

[59] Lacey CJ, Monteiro EF, Thompson HS, et al. A phase IIa study of a therapeutic vaccine for genital warts. Oxford, UK: Medical Society for the Study of Venereal Disease; 1997.

[60] The Jordan report. Accelerated development of vaccines, 2002. Bethesda, MD: National Institute of Allergy and Infectious Diseases; 2002.

[61] Borysiewicz LK, Fiander A, Nimako M, et al. A recombinant vaccinia virus encoding human papillomavirus types 16 and 18, E6 and E7 proteins as immunotherapy for cervical cancer. Lancet 1996;347:1523–7.

[62] Jensen ER, Selvakumar R, Shen H, Ahmed R, Wettstein FO, Miller JF. Recombinant Listeria monocytogenes vaccination eliminates papillomavirus-induced tumors and prevents papilloma formation from viral DNA. J Virol 1997;71:8467–74.

[63] Ossevoort MA, Feltkamp MC, van Veen KJ, Melief CJ, Kast WM. Dendritic cells as carriers for a cytotoxic T-lymphocyte epitope-based peptide vaccine in protection against a human papillomavirus type 16-induced tumor. J Immunother Emphasis Tumor Immunol 1995;18:86–94.

[64] Duggan-Keen MF, Brown MD, Stacey SN, Stern PL. Papillomavirus vaccines. Front Biosci 1998;3:1192–208.

Melanoma Treatment Update

Hensin Tsao, MD, PhD[a,b,c,*], Arthur J. Sober, MD[a,b]

[a]Department of Dermatology, Massachusetts General Hospital, 48 Blossom Street, Bartlett 622, Boston, MA 02114, USA
[b]Melanoma Center, Massachusetts General Hospital, Boston, MA, USA
[c]Wellman Center for Photomedicine, Massachusetts General Hospital, Harvard Medical School, Boston, MA, USA

In 2004, the American Cancer Society estimates 55,100 cases of cutaneous melanoma, with 7910 deaths attributable to the disease [1]. Despite successes in the surgical treatment of primary melanoma, the medical management of metastatic melanoma is still a major challenge. Within the last decade, significant shifts in management have emerged, including the following: the abandonment of large, deforming surgical margins; the introduction of selective lymphadenectomy (sentinel lymph node biopsy); and the adjuvant use of interferon treatment for nodal disease. Firm guidelines on the treatment of distant disease are still lacking because no studies have convincingly shown benefit with any systemic agent.

Adjuvant therapy for stage III disease

More accurate staging of melanoma (Table 1) through sentinel lymph node sampling allows for the identification of patients whose risk of death is high enough to potentially benefit from adjuvant therapy [2]. Attempts to reduce melanoma recurrences by various forms of adjuvant therapy date back several decades. Over the past 10 years, interferon α2b (IFN-α2b) has emerged as the standard for adjuvant therapy in stage III melanoma. Currently, IFN-α2b is approved by the US Food and Drug Administration (FDA) for the treatment of patients who have primary

melanomas larger than 4 mm or patients who have metastatic tumor involvement of the lymph nodes rendered disease-free by surgical removal.

Table 2 lists the major randomized trials of interferon in the adjuvant setting. Broadly, these trials can be separated into the following regimens:

High-dose: 20 million units (MU)/m^2 intravenously (IV) daily × 5 days/week for 4 weeks, followed by 10 MU/m^2 subcutaneously (subQ) 3 times/week for 48 weeks
Intermediate-dose: 10 MU subQ × 5 days/week for 4 weeks, followed by 10 MU subQ 3 times/week for varying durations
Low-dose: 3 MU subQ 3 times/week for varying durations

Except for high-dose IFN-α2b, no prospective trial has shown any survival benefit with the interferons.

There have been three completed randomized high-dose IFN-α2b trials to date (see Table 2): Eastern Cooperative Oncology Group (ECOG) trials 1684, 1690, and 1694. Two of three interferon trials (ECOG 1684 and ECOG 1694) suggested an overall survival benefit, whereas all three reported increases in disease-free survival times [3–5]. An updated analysis of these trials showed that, for ECOG 1684, high-dose IFN-α2b no longer retained an overall survival benefit ($P = 0.18$) at a median follow-up period of 12.6 years [6]. For ECOG 1694, however, high-dose interferon continues to demonstrate superiority to the ganglioside (ie, GM$_2$-KLH/QS21 [GMK]) vaccine in terms of overall survival at a median follow-up period of 2.1 years (hazards ratio [HR], 1.32; $P = 0.04$). The updated and pooled

* Corresponding author. Department of Dermatology, Massachusetts General Hospital, 48 Blossom Street, Bartlett 622, Boston, MA 02114.
E-mail address: htsao@partners.org (H. Tsao).

0733-8635/05/$ – see front matter © 2005 Elsevier Inc. All rights reserved.
doi:10.1016/j.det.2004.09.005

derm.theclinics.com

Table 1
2002 American Joint Commission on Cancer melanoma staging

Stage	Thickness (mm)	Ulceration	No nodes	Nodal status	Distant site
IA	≤1.0	−	0	—	—
IB	≤1.0	+, Clark IV	0	—	—
	1.01−2.0	−	0	—	—
IIA	1.01−2.0	−	0	—	—
	2.01−4.0	−	0	—	—
IIB	2.01−4.0	−	0	—	—
	>4.0	−	0	—	—
IIC	>4.0	+	0	—	—
IIIA	Any	−	1	m	—
		−	2−3	m	—
IIIB	Any	+	1	m	—
		+	2−3	m	—
		−	1	M	—
		−	2−3	M	—
IIIC	Any	+	1	M	—
		+	2−3	M	—
		+ or −	—	M/m	—
IV	Any	+ or −	Any	Any	
M1a					Skin, SQ
M1b					Lung
M1c					Other visceral

Abbreviations: m, microscopic involvement; M, macroscopic involvement; SQ, subcutaneous.
Adapted from Balch CM, Buzaid AC, Soong SJ, et al. Final version of the American Joint Committee on Cancer staging system for cutaneous melanoma. J Clin Oncol 2001;19:3635−48.

analysis of trials with observation arms (ECOG 1684 and ECOG 1690; N = 713) failed to show benefit of high-dose IFN-α2b versus observation (HR, 1.07; $P = 0.42$) [6].

High-dose interferon is associated with many side effects [7], and virtually all patients undergo dose reduction during the course of therapy. High-dose IFN-α2b should be administered by a health care professional experienced with interferon side effects. Despite the toxicity and the modest improvements in survival rates, quality-of-life studies have shown that patients at high risk for recurrence prefer IFN-α2b therapy with all of its potential toxicities [8]. Future trials in the United States will probably test experimental agents against high-dose IFN-α2b, and any drug found to have fewer side effects but similar benefits would likely replace IFN-α2b as the preferred agent.

Low-dose interferon has been investigated in patients with melanoma who are at high (ie, tumor size, ≥ 4.0 mm, and regional disease) [9,10] or intermediate (ie, tumor size, 1.0−4.0 mm) [11] risk of relapse. Because overall survival has not been altered by these regimens, low-dose approaches cannot be currently considered efficacious.

The possibility that an intermediate dose between the low- and high-dose regimens may produce some

benefit in high-risk patients is being tested in two European trials. The Scandinavian multicenter group and the European Organization for Research and Treatment of Cancer (EORTC) trial number 18,952 are still ongoing, but early results do not seem to show any appreciable survival benefit [12].

Given the weight of negative results with interferon in the adjuvant setting, not all physicians are convinced of the benefits of IFN-α2b, including the high-dose regimen. For instance, IFN-α2b has not been shown to significantly benefit patients who have microscopic nodal metastases, which includes all patients who have positive sentinel lymph node disease. Nevertheless, because IFN-α2b is an FDA-approved therapy, patients for whom its use is approved should be made aware of its potential benefits and adverse effects. Patients who are unable to tolerate interferon or who prefer less toxic treatment should be encouraged to consider entry into controlled clinical trials of adjuvant therapies, which are ongoing in the United States.

Other adjuvant therapy agents that have not shown benefit after careful study include the following: (1) chemotherapy with dacarbazine, dimethyl triazino imidazole carboxomide (DTIC); (2) immunotherapy with bacillus Calmette-Guérin, *Coryne-bacterium parvum*, or the antihelminthic agent, levamisole, which has immunomodulatory properties; and (3) the hormonal agent tamoxifen [12].

Treatment of advanced disease

There is currently no highly effective therapy for patients who have distant metastases (stage IV melanoma). Meaningful disease-free survival, however, can be achieved in selected patients who have an isolated distant metastasis if the focus can be surgically or radiotherapeutically eradicated. Markowitz et al [13] noted a 5-year overall survival rate of 25% in patients who had distant disease whose known tumor deposit or deposits were surgically eliminated. In most patients, however, additional metastases appear at other locations within months.

Chemotherapy

There has been no decline in the death rate from melanoma in the United States, and the absolute number of annual deaths from melanoma continues to increase, so development of an effective treatment for advanced disease is imperative. Not all patients present with localized disease amenable to surgical cure, however. For those who have disseminated disease, the benchmark chemotherapeutic agent is DTIC, which has a response rate of approximately 20% (mainly partial responses) [14,15]. Many other chemotherapeutic agents, singly or in combination, showed promising response rates in phase 2 trials, but in phase 3 trials, response rates were not substantially better than for DTIC alone [16].

A modest improvement was noted with the introduction of temozolamide, an oral agent that transforms into the active metabolite of DTIC [17]. This agent is unique in that it crosses the blood-brain barrier and has substantial central nervous system (CNS) penetration [18]. Because many patients who have stage IV disease have CNS involvement that is frequently lethal and because most standard chemotherapy agents do not cross the blood-brain barrier, temozolamide is an important advance. Table 3 summarizes the efficacy of other single-agent chemotherapeutic agents for patients who have advanced melanoma [16].

Combination chemotherapy

Several combination chemotherapy regimens that use DTIC also exist. The three most active combinations are shown in Table 4. The popular Dartmouth regimen (cisplatin, DTIC, carmustine [BCNU], and tamoxifen) was recently tested against DTIC alone [19] and DTIC plus IFN-α2b [20] and was found not to improve median survival times beyond 7 and 6.5 months, respectively. Although response rates between 30% to 50% have been reported in single-institution phase 2 trials with these various combination regimens, none has demonstrated significant survival benefits over DTIC alone.

Early reports of estrogen receptors in melanoma [21] sparked an interest in chemohormonal therapy with tamoxifen. Two large-scale prospective randomized trials with and without tamoxifen (ie, cisplatin/DTIC/BCNU ± tamoxifen and DTIC ± interferon ± tamoxifen) clearly showed that tamoxifen does not add benefit to these combinations [22,23].

Interleukin 2

The treatment of patients who have advanced melanoma with FDA-approved interleukin 2 (IL-2) can lead to overall response rates of approximately 15%. Early studies with IL-2 used 600,000 to 720,000 IU/kg/dose given intravenously every 8 hours (high-dose IL-2), and this regimen remains the benchmark against which other treatments are evaluated. In a recent pooled analysis of all patients treated with IL-2 in the United States (N = 270), Atkins et al [24] reported a complete response rate of 6.3% (n = 17) and a partial response rate of 9.6% (n = 26).

There are currently no good clinical predictors of IL-2 response, although patients with only cutaneous and subcutaneous metastases have a 50% response rate [25], suggesting that these disease sites may be more amenable to the antitumor effects of IL-2. Furthermore, vitiligo occurs more commonly in patients who exhibit a clinical response to IL-2 [26].

High-dose IL-2 is associated with severe toxicities, including fever, chills, hypotension, and tachycardia. Weight gain, peripheral edema, and pulmonary congestion can then result because of capillary leak syndrome. Liver function abnormalities are also common [25]. Although only the high-dose IL-2 regimen is approved by the FDA, other lower dose schedules have been used in conjunction with chemotherapy (ie, biochemotherapy) in an effort to boost efficacy while minimizing toxicity.

Biochemotherapy with interleukin 2

The efficacy of chemotherapy for curing or controlling advanced melanoma has been modest, and researchers have pursued other options. The theory of biochemotherapy (administration of an

Table 2
Randomized trials of IFN-α2 in the adjuvant therapy of melanoma

Trial[a]	Eligibility (TNM stage)	Patient accrual	Agent	Dose and schedule	Duration of treatment	Outcome analysis
High-dose IFN-α2 with IV induction phase						
ECOG1684 [3]	T4N1–3	287	IFNα 2b	20 MU/m² IV daily × 5 d/wk; 10 MU/m² SC 3×/wk	4 wk 48 wk	OS* RFS**
ECOG1690 [4]	T4N1–3	642	IFN-α2b	20 MU/m² IV daily × 5 d/wk; 10 MU/m² SC 3×/wk or 3 MU SC daily 3×/wk	4 wk 48 wk 24 mo	RFS*** OS****
ECOG1694 [5]	T4N1–3	851	IFN-α2b vs GMK vaccine	20 MU/m² IV daily × 5 d/wk; 10 MU/m² SC 3×/wk or GMK SC weekly × 4 wk, every 12 wk × 8 mo	12 mo 96 wk	RFS***** OS******
ECOG1697 (Principal investigator, Agarwala ongoing trial)	T3–4N1a	1440	IFN-α2b	20 MU/m² IV daily × 5 d/wk	4 wk	Ongoing
High-dose IFN-α2 without IV induction phase						
NCCTG 83-7052 [75]	T3–4N1-3	262	IFN-α2a	20 MU/m² IM 3×/wk	12 wk	OS**** RFS****

Low-dose IFN-α2						
WHO-16 [76]	N1–3	424	IFN-α2a	3 MU SC 3×/wk	36 mo	OS**** RFS****
Aim-High [10]	T4N1–3	674	IFN-α2a	3 MU SC 3×/wk	24 mo	RFS**** OS****
Austrian trial [11]	T3–4N0	311	IFN-α2a	3 MU SC 3 daily; 3 MU sc 3×/wk	3 wk; 12 mo	RFS******** OS^b
Intermediate-dose IFN-α2						
Scandinavian trial (Principal investigator, Aamdahl)	T4N1–3	≈500	IFN-α2b	10 MU SC × 5 days/wk; 10 MU SC 3×/wk or 10 MU SC 3×/wk	4 wk 12 mo 24 mo	Ongoing
EORTC 18952 (Principal investigator, Eggermont)	T4N1-3	1000	IFN-α2b	10 MU SC × 5 d/wk; 10 MU SC 3×/wk or 10 MU SC 3×/wk	4 wk; 12 mo 24 mo	Under analysis

Abbreviations: IM, intramuscular; NCCTG, North Central Cancer Treatment Group; NS, not significant; OS, overall survival; RFS, relapse-free survival; SC, subcutaneous; TNM, tumor-node-metastasis; WHO, World Health Organization.

[a] The control arm for all trials was observation unless otherwise noted.

[b] Too early to determine *P* value.

P = 0.047; **P* = 0.004; ***P* = 0.05; ****P* = NS; *****P* = 0.0015; ******P* = 0.009; *******P* = 0.02.

Adapted from Agarwala S, Kirkwood J. Interferons and adjuvant therapy. In: Balch C, Houghton A, Sober A, Soong S, editors. Cutaneous meladoma. St. Louis, MO: Quality Medical Publishing; 2003. p. 605–22.

Table 3
Efficacy of single-agent chemotherapy

Agent	No. of evaluable patients	Complete and partial response (%)
Carboplatin	43	16
Carmustine	122	18
Cisplatin	188	23
Dacarbazine	1936	20
Docetaxel	83	15
Fotemustine	153	24
Lomustine	270	13
Paclitaxel	53	13
Temozolomide	200	17
Vinblastine	62	13
Vindesine	273	14

Adapted from Atkins MB, Buzaid AC, Houghton Jr AN. Chemotheraphy and biochemistry. In: Balch C, Houghton A, Sober A, Soong S, editors. Cutaneous melanoma. St. Louis, MO: Quality medical Publishing; 2003. p. 589–604.

immunologically active agent plus a chemotherapeutic agent) is based on the observation that each agent has demonstrable independent clinical activity. Protocols have included IL-2 plus a chemotherapeutic agent and interferon with a chemotherapeutic agent. Initial response rates of approximately 50% were reported in some of the earlier studies [27–29].

In 1991, Falkson et al [27] reported 12 complete responses and 4 partial responses in a single-institution trial in 30 patients receiving DTIC and interferon. Three subsequent, larger prospective trials have not confirmed a benefit from adding interferon to DTIC [29–31].

With inpatient regimens of IL-2 with or without IFN-α2b plus cisplatin, composite response rates of approximately 50% were observed [28,29,32–34]. Complete response rates of only 10% to 20% with a

1-year median survival time were noted, although 10% of patients had durable disease-free responses of at least 2 years. More recent reports show lower response rates with biochemotherapy protocols [35]. Results from phase 3 trials are disappointing compared with phase 2 trials, although they are still superior to single-agent therapy results [36–39]. One large-scale phase 3 study with cisplatin, vinblastine, and DTIC with or without IL-2/IFN-α2b is currently being tested in a United States intergroup trial [40]. This investigation is the largest biochemotherapy trial to date and initial reports should be available shortly. If results are positive, other approaches, such as outpatient IL-2 regimens, temozolomide substitution for DTIC, and maintenance regimens with IL-2 and granulocyte-macrophage colony–stimulating factor, may be worth exploring.

Vaccines

An immune response to melanocytes has long been inferred through phenomena such as vitiligo and halo nevi. With the success of vaccines levied against infectious agents, the challenge emerged to develop similar strategies for cancer, particularly one that has a priori evidence of immunoreactivity, such as melanoma. The advantages and disadvantages of various types of vaccines are shown in Table 5. More recent interests in vaccines for melanoma have been fueled by the isolation of tumor-specific antigens in melanoma (Table 6) [41]. Although the science behind vaccine development is advancing rapidly, the current article limits the discussion to the uses of vaccines in the clinical setting.

Many vaccination strategies exist. Vaccine components fall into two major categories: multivalent

Table 4
Selected combination chemotherapy regimens for advanced melanoma

Regimen	Combination
Dartmouth	Cisplatin, 25 mg/m² IV, on days 1 to 3 every 3 to 4 wk
	DTIC, 220 mg/m² IV, on days 1 to 3 every 3 to 4 wk
	BCNU, 150 mg/m² IV, on day 1 every 6 to 8 wk
	Tamoxifen, 10 mg/m² by mouth, twice a day continuously
CVD (modified)	Cisplatin, 20 mg/m² IV, on days 1 to 4
	Vinblastine, 2 mg/m² IV, on days 1 to 4
	DTIC, 800 mg/m² IV, on days 1; repeat every 3 wk
BHD	BCNU, 150 mg/m² IV, on day 1 every 8 wk
	Hydroxyurea, 1500 mg/m² by mouth, on days 1 to 5 every 4 wk
	DTIC, 150 mg/m² IV, on days 1 to 5 every 4 wk

Abbreviations: BHD, BCNU, hydroxyurea, DTIC; CVD, cisplatin, vinblastine, DTIC.
Adapted from Atkins MB, Buzaid AC, Houghton Jr AN. Chemotherapy and biochemotherapy. In: Balch C, Houghton A, Sober A, Soong S, editors. Cutaneous Melanoma. St. Louis, MO: Quality Medical Publishing; 2003. p. 589–604.

Table 5
Types of vaccines

Type of vaccine	Relative advantage(s)	Relative disadvantage(s)
Allogeneic cellular	Simple to prepare, presents broad spectrum of potential antigens, currently in phase 3 clinical trials	Presents irrelevant "allo" antigens, difficult to precisely characterize components, requires adjuvant
Autologous cellular	Presents patient-specific unique antigens, presents numerous antigens	Requires laborious individual vaccine production, requires adjuvant
Autologous heat-shock protein	Presents patient-specific unique antigens, presents numerous antigens	Requires laborious individual vaccine production, unproven immunogenicity
Purified protein or carbohydrate	Well-defined components, safety and immunogenicity established (carbohydrates) in mature clinical trials	Production can be difficult, requires adjuvant
Dendritic cells	Can be loaded with peptides, total tumor lysate or RNA, professional antigen-presenting cells	Requires laborious individual vaccine production
Peptide	Simple to prepare, safety established in early trials	Requires adjuvant, only presents single epitope, HLA-restricted
DNA	Simple to prepare, numerous epitopes presented, immunostimulatory sequences in vector	Little clinical data to date
Recombinant virus	Inherently immunogenic, presents numerous epitopes	Neutralizing immunity to vector

Adapted from Wolchok JD, Weber JS, Houghton AN, et al. Melanoma vaccines. In: Balch C, Houghton A, Sober A, Soong S, editors. Cutaneous melanoma. St. Louis, MO: Quality Medical Publishing; 2003. p. 645–56.

antigens (ie, whole tumor cells, whole-cell lysates, antigens shed from tumors) and specific tumor-derived antigens (ie, antibody-defined gangliosides and T-cell–defined peptides).

Multi(poly)valent vaccines

A polyvalent, allogeneic whole-cell vaccine prepared from three allogeneic melanoma cell lines (CancerVax) had encouraging phase 2 results [42] and is now awaiting maturation of data from several randomized controlled studies. An autologous whole-cell vaccine (Avax), derived from irradiated autologous tumor cells that have been modified by

Table 6
Potential vaccine targets on melanoma cells

Category of antigen	Example
Gangliosides	GM_2, GD_2, GD_3
Mutated protein	CDK4, β-catenin
Cancer-testis antigen	MAGE, BAGE, GAGE families, NY-ESO-1
Melanosomal differenttiation antigen	Tyrosinase, gp75, TRP-1, TRP-2, gp100

Abbreviations: CDK4, cyclin-dependent kinase-4; TRP, tyrosine-related protein.
Adapted from Wolchok JD, Weber JS, Houghton AN, et al. Melanoma vaccines. In: Balch C, Houghton A, Sober A, Soong S, editors. Cutaneous melanoma. St. Louis, MO: Quality Medical Publishing; 2003. p. 645–56.

dinitrophenyl [43], again showed some benefit in phase 2 trials [44] and is now in the phase 3 setting.

Vaccines derived from tumor lysates include the following: viral melanoma oncolysate [45]; a vaccinia melanoma cell lysate [46]; and Melacine, a mechanical lysate from two melanoma cell lines combined with monophosphoryl lipid A and the purified mycobacterial cell wall skeleton [47]. To date, none of these vaccines has shown significant survival benefits in phase 3 trials, although there is some suggestion that Melacine may improve survival for individuals who have HLA-A2 and HLA-C3 [48].

A shed tumor antigen vaccine developed by Bystryn et al [49] did prolong median time to disease progression when compared with placebo but did not improve overall survival times.

Univalent vaccines

Melanoma cells have gangliosides as one of their major constituents and thus vaccines targeting these carbohydrate moieties have been developed. Earlier studies suggested that patients who developed antibodies against a GM_2 ganglioside experienced improved survival times [50]. A modified GM_2 ganglioside vaccine (GMK) was recently tested against high-dose IFN-α2b, however, and found to be inferior to interferon [5]. Peptide antigens derived from melanoma proteins also have been directly inoculated or loaded on dendritic cells in an attempt to create peptide-specific vaccines [51,52]. Responses have been occasional and inconsistent, but pigmentation

loss in normal skin suggests that dendritic cell approaches do produce activity against melanocytes [53].
Although many of these vaccination strategies hold
promise, formal testing in phase 3 trials is lacking.

Radiation therapy

External radiotherapy (XRT) has little role in
treating primary melanoma. Lentigo maligna, the
precursor lesion to lentigo maligna melanoma, has
been successfully treated with superficial XRT reaching just below the hair follicles. XRT can also be
useful for large lesions in patients older than 60 years
[54–56]. For invasive primary melanoma, excisional
surgery is the treatment of choice. XRT has been
useful for unresectable in-transit metastases. Adjuvant XRT has been used in nodal areas of the head
and neck after resection of involved nodes and in
other nodal basins where the tumor has penetrated the
nodal capsule (extracapsular spread), although no
prospective randomized trials have shown efficacy
with this approach. XRT has been palliative for unresectable nodal metastases, with complete response
rates of more than 20%, partial response rates of 35%
to 45% [57–59], and a 1-year median survival duration [57,58].

In distant disease, XRT has been most frequently
used for brain and bone metastases. Whole-brain
XRT plus high-dose systemic steroids can relieve
neurologic symptoms and elevated intracranial pressure. Stereotactic radiosurgery was as good as
surgical resection for solitary metastases of 3 cm or
smaller in the cerebrum [60–67]. Megavoltage photon therapy achieved a 67% response rate in pain and
compression symptoms of malignant spinal cord
compression [68]. Bony metastases of melanoma
respond to XRT as did bone metastases from other
cancers [69].

Summary

Except for high-dose interferon as adjuvant
therapy in stage III disease, there has been little
success over the last 20 years in treating metastatic
melanoma. Recent advances in melanoma biology
suggest that disarming oncogenic mechanisms in
melanoma may be an attractive approach to therapy.
For instance, sustained expression of Bcl2 has been
associated with an increased resistance to apoptosis,
and recently, anti-sense–mediated reduction of Bcl2
levels was shown to chemosensitize patients to DTIC
[70]. Likewise, the identification of activating muta-

tions in the RAS signaling pathway, including the
NRAS and *BRAF* genes [71,72], opens up new
therapeutic options for both RAS [73] and RAF
inhibitors [74]. A more thorough understanding of
melanoma biology and tumor immunology will undoubtedly yield new promise for patients who have
advanced disease. For now, these patients are best
managed in ongoing clinical trials (see http://www.
nci.nih.gov/clinicaltrials/), and patients should always
be encouraged to consider participation in these trials.

References

[1] Jemal A, Tiwari RC, Murray T, et al. Cancer statistics,
    2004. CA Cancer J Clin 2004;54:8–29.
[2] Balch CM, Buzaid AC, Soong SJ, et al. Final version
    of the American Joint Committee on Cancer staging
    system for cutaneous melanoma. J Clin Oncol 2001;
    19:3635–48.
[3] Kirkwood JM, Strawderman MH, Ernstoff MC, Smith
    TJ, Borden EC, Blum RH. Interferon alfa-2b adjuvant
    therapy of high-risk resected cutaneous melanoma: the
    Eastern Cooperative Oncology Group trial EST 1684.
    J Clin Oncol 1996;14:7–17.
[4] Kirkwood JM, Ibrahim JG, Sondak VK, et al. High-
    and low-dose interferon alfa-2b in high-risk melanoma:
    first analysis of intergroup trial E1690/S9111/C9190.
    J Clin Oncol 2000;18:2444–58.
[5] Kirkwood JM, Ibrahim JG, Sosman JA, et al.
    High-dose interferon alfa-2b significantly prolongs
    relapse-free and overall survival compared with the
    GM2-KLH/QS-21 vaccine in patients with resected
    stage IIB-III melanoma: results of intergroup trial
    E1694/S9512/C509801. J Clin Oncol 2001;19:2370–80.
[6] Kirkwood JM, Manola J, Ibrahim J, Sondak V, Ernstoff
    MS, Rao U. A pooled analysis of Eastern Cooperative
    Oncology Group and intergroup trials of adjuvant
    high-dose interferon for melanoma. Clin Cancer Res
    2004;10:1670–7.
[7] Kirkwood JM, Bender C, Agarwala S, et al. Mecha-
    nisms and management of toxicities associated with
    high-dose interferon alfa-2b therapy. J Clin Oncol
    2002;20:3703–18.
[8] Kilbridge KL, Weeks JC, Sober AJ, et al. Patient
    preferences for adjuvant interferon alfa-2b treatment.
    J Clin Oncol 2001;19:812–23.
[9] Cascinelli N, Bufalino R, Morabito A, MacKie R.
    Results of adjuvant interferon study in WHO mela-
    noma programme. Lancet 1994;343:913–4.
[10] Hancock BW, Wheatley K, Harris S, et al. Adjuvant
    interferon in high-risk melanoma: the AIM HIGH
    Study—United Kingdom Coordinating Committee
    on Cancer Research Randomized Study of Adjuvant
    Low-Dose Extended-Duration Interferon Alfa-2a in
    High-Risk Resected Malignant Melanoma. J Clin
    Oncol 2004;22:53–61.
[11] Pehamberger H, Soyer HP, Steiner A, et al. Adjuvant

interferon alfa-2a treatment in resected primary stage II cutaneous melanoma. Austrian Malignant Melanoma Cooperative Group. J Clin Oncol 1998;16:1425–9.

[12] Agarwala S, Kirkwood J. Interferons and adjuvant therapy. In: Balch C, Houghton A, Sober A, Soong S, editors. Cutaneous melanoma. St. Louis, MO: Quality Medical Publishing; 2003. p. 605–22.

[13] Markowitz JS, Cosimi LA, Carey RW, et al. Prognosis after initial recurrence of cutaneous melanoma. Arch Surg 1991;126:703–7 [discussion: 707–8].

[14] Anderson CM, Buzaid AC, Legha SS. Systemic treatments for advanced cutaneous melanoma. Oncology 1995;9:1149–57.

[15] Hill GJ, Krementz ET, Hill HZ. Dimethyl triazeno imidazole carboxamide and combination therapy for melanoma: IV: late results after complete response to chemotherapy. Cancer 1984;53:1299–305.

[16] Atkins MB, Buzaid AC, Houghton Jr AN. Chemotherapy and biochemotherapy. In: Balch C, Houghton A, Sober A, Soong S, editors. Cutaneous melanoma. St. Louis, MO: Quality Medical Publishing; 2003. p. 589–604.

[17] Crosby T, Fish R, Coles B, Mason MD. Systemic treatments for metastatic cutaneous melanoma. Cochrane Database Syst Rev 2000;CD001215.

[18] Patel M, McCully C, Godwin K, et al. Plasma and cerebrospinal fluid pharmacokinetics of intravenous temozolomide in non-human primates. J Neurooncol 2003;61(3):203–7.

[19] Chapman PB, Einhorn LH, Meyers ML, et al. Phase III multicenter randomized trial of the Dartmouth regimen versus dacarbazine in patients with metastatic melanoma. J Clin Oncol 1999;17:2745–51.

[20] Middleton MR, Lorigan P, Owen J, et al. A randomized phase III study comparing dacarbazine, BCNU, cisplatin and tamoxifen with dacarbazine and interferon in advanced melanoma. Br J Cancer 2000;82:1158–62.

[21] Fisher RI, Neifeld JP, Lippman ME. Oestrogen receptors in human malignant melanoma. Lancet 1976;2:337–9.

[22] Rusthoven JJ, Quirt IC, Iscoe NA, et al. Randomized, double-blind, placebo-controlled trial comparing the response rates of carmustine, dacarbazine, and cisplatin with and without tamoxifen in patients with metastatic melanoma. National Cancer Institute of Canada Clinical Trials Group. J Clin Oncol 1996;14:2083–90.

[23] Falkson CI, Ibrahim J, Kirkwood JM, Coates AS, Atkins MB, Blum RH. Phase III trial of dacarbazine versus dacarbazine with interferon alpha-2b versus dacarbazine with tamoxifen versus dacarbazine with interferon alpha-2b and tamoxifen in patients with metastatic malignant melanoma: an Eastern Cooperative Oncology Group study. J Clin Oncol 1998;16:1743–51.

[24] Atkins MB, Kunkel L, Sznol M, Rosenberg SA. High-dose recombinant interleukin-2 therapy in patients with metastatic melanoma: long-term survival update. Cancer J Sci Am 2000;6(Suppl 1):S11–4.

[25] Schwartzentruber DJ, Rosenberg SA. Interleukins. In: Balch C, Houghton A, Sober A, Soong S, editors. Cutaneous melanoma. St. Louis, MO: Quality Medical Publishing; 2003. p. 623–43.

[26] Rosenberg SA, White DE. Vitiligo in patients with melanoma: normal tissue antigens can be targets for cancer immunotherapy. J Immunother Emphasis Tumor Immunol 1996;19:81–4.

[27] Falkson CI, Falkson G, Falkson HC. Improved results with the addition of interferon alfa-2b to dacarbazine in the treatment of patients with metastatic malignant melanoma. J Clin Oncol 1991;9:1403–8.

[28] Legha SS, Ring S, Eton O, Bedikian A, Plager C, Papadopoulos N. Development and results of biochemotherapy in metastatic melanoma: the University of Texas M.D. Anderson Cancer Center experience. Cancer J Sci Am 1997;3(Suppl 1):S9–15.

[29] Richards JM, Gale D, Mehta N, Lestingi T. Combination of chemotherapy with interleukin-2 and interferon alfa for the treatment of metastatic melanoma. J Clin Oncol 1999;17:651–7.

[30] Bajetta E, Di Leo A, Zampino MG, et al. Multicenter randomized trial of dacarbazine alone or in combination with two different doses and schedules of interferon alfa-2a in the treatment of advanced melanoma. J Clin Oncol 1994;12:806–11.

[31] Thomson DB, Adena M, McLeod GR, et al. Interferon-alpha 2a does not improve response or survival when combined with dacarbazine in metastatic malignant melanoma: results of a multi-institutional Australian randomized trial. Melanoma Res 1993;3:133–8.

[32] Demchak PA, Mier JW, Robert NJ, O'Brien K, Gould JA, Atkins MB. Interleukin-2 and high-dose cisplatin in patients with metastatic melanoma: a pilot study. J Clin Oncol 1991;9:1821–30.

[33] Atkins MB, O'Boyle KR, Sosman JA, et al. Multi-institutional phase II trial of intensive combination chemoimmunotherapy for metastatic melanoma. J Clin Oncol 1994;12:1553–60.

[34] Antoine EC, Benhammouda A, Bernard A, et al. Salpetriere Hospital experience with biochemotherapy in metastatic melanoma. Cancer J Sci Am 1997;3(Suppl 1):S16–21.

[35] Chapman PB, Panageas KS, Williams L, et al. Clinical results using biochemotherapy as a standard of care in advanced melanoma. Melanoma Res 2002;12:381–7.

[36] Eton O, Legha SS, Bedikian AY, et al. Sequential biochemotherapy versus chemotherapy for metastatic melanoma: results from a phase III randomized trial. J Clin Oncol 2002;20:2045–52.

[37] Keilholz U, Goey SH, Punt CJ, et al. Interferon alfa-2a and interleukin-2 with or without cisplatin in metastatic melanoma: a randomized trial of the European Organization for Research and Treatment of Cancer Melanoma Cooperative Group. J Clin Oncol 1997;15:2579–88.

[38] Rosenberg SA, Yang JC, Schwartzentruber DJ, et al. Prospective randomized trial of the treatment of

patients with metastatic melanoma using chemotherapy with cisplatin, dacarbazine, and tamoxifen alone or in combination with interleukin-2 and interferon alfa-2b. J Clin Oncol 1999;17:968–75.

[39] Dorval T, Negrier S, Chevreau C, et al. Randomized trial of treatment with cisplatin and interleukin-2 either alone or in combination with interferon-alpha-2a in patients with metastatic melanoma: a Federation Nationale des Centres de Lutte Contre le Cancer multicenter, parallel study. Cancer 1999;85:1060–6.

[40] Atkins MB, Lee S, Flaherty LE, Sosman JA, Sondak VK, Kirkwood JM. A prospective randomized phase III trial of concurrent biochemotherapy (BCT) with cisplatin, vinblastine, dacarbazine (CVD), IL-2 and interferon alpha-2b (IFN) versus CVD alone in patients with metastatic melanoma (E3695): an ECOG-coordinated intergroup trial. Proc Am Soc Clin Oncol 2003; 22:708 [abstract].

[41] Wolchok JD, Weber JS, Houghton AN, Livingston PO. Melanoma vaccines. In: Balch C, Houghton A, Sober S, Soong S, editors. Cutaneous melanoma. St. Louis, MO: Quality Medical Publishing; 2003. p. 645–56.

[42] Morton DL, Foshag LJ, Hoon D, et al. Prolongation of survival in metastatic melanoma after active specific immunotherapy with a new polyvalent melanoma vaccine. Ann Surg 1992;216:463–82.

[43] Berd D, Macguire HC, McCue P, Mastrangelo MJ. Treatment of metastatic melanoma with an autologous tumor-cell vaccine: clinical and immunologic results in 64 patients. J Clin Oncol 1990;8:1858–67.

[44] Berd D, Maguire Jr HC, Schuchter LM, et al. Autologous hapten-modified melanoma vaccine as postsurgical adjuvant treatment after resection of nodal metastases. J Clin Oncol 1997;15:2359–70.

[45] Wallack MK, Sivanandham M, Balch CM, et al. A phase III randomized, double-blind, multiinstitutional trial of vaccinia melanoma oncolysate-active specific immunotherapy for patients with stage II melanoma. Cancer 1995;75:34–42.

[46] Hersey P. Active immunotherapy with viral lysates of micrometastases following surgical removal of high risk melanoma. World J Surg 1992;16:251–60.

[47] Mitchell MS. Perspective on allogeneic melanoma lysates in active specific immunotherapy. Semin Oncol 1998;25:623–35.

[48] Sosman JA, Unger JM, Liu PY, et al. Adjuvant immunotherapy of resected, intermediate-thickness, node-negative melanoma with an allogeneic tumor vaccine: impact of HLA class I antigen expression on outcome. J Clin Oncol 2002;20:2067–75.

[49] Bystryn JC, Zeleniuch-Jacquotte A, Oratz R, Shapiro RL, Harris MN, Roses DF. Double-blind trial of a polyvalent, shed-antigen, melanoma vaccine. Clin Cancer Res 2001;7:1882–7.

[50] Livingston PO, Wong GY, Adluri S, et al. Improved survival in stage III melanoma patients with GM2 antibodies: a randomized trial of adjuvant vaccination with GM2 ganglioside. J Clin Oncol 1994;12:1036–44.

[51] Rosenberg SA, Zhai Y, Yang JC, et al. Immunizing patients with metastatic melanoma using recombinant adenoviruses encoding MART-1 or gp100 melanoma antigens. J Natl Cancer Inst 1998;90:1894–900.

[52] Nestle FO, Alijagic S, Gilliet M, et al. Vaccination of melanoma patients with peptide- or tumor lysate-pulsed dendritic cells. Nat Med 1998;4(3):328–32.

[53] Tsao H, Millman P, Linette GP, et al. Hypopigmentation associated with an adenovirus-mediated gp100/MART-1-transduced dendritic cell vaccine for metastatic melanoma. Arch Dermatol 2002;138:799–802.

[54] DeGroot WP. Provisional results of treatment of the melanose precancereuse circonscrite Dubreuilh by Bucky-rays. Dermatologica 1968;136:426.

[55] Arma-Szlachcic M, Ott F, Storck H. The x-ray treatment of melanotic precancerosis. Study of 88 follow-up cases [in German]. Hautarzt 1970;21:505–8.

[56] Braun-Falco O, Lukacs S, Schoefinius HH. Treatment of melanosis circumscripta precancerosa Dubreuilh Clinical and catamnestic experiences with special reference to dermato-x-ray-therapy [in German]. Hautarzt 1975;26:207–10.

[57] Burmeister BH, Smithers BM, Poulsen M, et al. Radiation therapy for nodal disease in malignant melanoma. World J Surg 1995;19:369–71.

[58] Corry J, Smith JG, Bishop M, Ainslie J. Nodal radiation therapy for metastatic melanoma. Int J Radiat Oncol Biol Phys 1999;44:1065–9.

[59] Sause WT, Cooper JS, Rush S, et al. Fraction size in external beam radiation therapy in the treatment of melanoma. Int J Radiat Oncol Biol Phys 1991;20: 429–32.

[60] Mori Y, Kondziolka D, Flickinger JC, Kirkwood JM, Agarwala S, Lunsford LD. Stereotactic radiosurgery for cerebral metastatic melanoma: factors affecting local disease control and survival. Int J Radiat Oncol Biol Phys 1998;42:581–9.

[61] Sansur CA, Chin LS, Ames JW, et al. Gamma knife radiosurgery for the treatment of brain metastases. Stereotact Funct Neurosurg 2000;74:37–51.

[62] Lavine SD, Petrovich Z, Cohen-Gadol AA, et al. Gamma knife radiosurgery for metastatic melanoma: an analysis of survival, outcome, and complications. Neurosurgery 1999;44:59–64 [discussion: 64–6].

[63] Seung SK, Sneed PK, McDermott MW, et al. Gamma knife radiosurgery for malignant melanoma brain metastases. Cancer J Sci Am 1998;4:103–9.

[64] Gieger M, Wu JK, Ling MN, Wazer D, Tsai JS, Engler MJ. Response of intracranial melanoma metastases to stereotactic radiosurgery. Radiat Oncol Investig 1997; 5:72–80.

[65] Fernandez-Vicioso E, Suh JH, Kupelian PA, Sohn JW, Barnett GH. Analysis of prognostic factors for patients with single brain metastasis treated with stereotactic radiosurgery. Radiat Oncol Investig 1997;5:31–7.

[66] Somaza S, Kondziolka D, Lunsford LD, Kirkwood JM, Flickinger JC. Stereotactic radiosurgery for cerebral metastatic melanoma. J Neurosurg 1993;79: 661–6.

[67] Buatti JM, Friedman WA, Bova FJ, Mendenhall WM.

Treatment selection factors for stereotactic radiosurgery of intracranial metastases. Int J Radiat Oncol Biol Phys 1995;32:1161–6.

[68] Kirova YM, Chen J, Rabarijaona LI, Piedbois Y, Le Bourgeois JP. Radiotherapy as palliative treatment for metastatic melanoma. Melanoma Res 1999;9:611–3.

[69] McKay MJ, Peters LJ, Ainslie J. Radiation therapy for distant metastases. In: Balch C, Houghton A, Sober A, Soong S, editors. Cutaneous melanoma. St. Louis, MO: Quality Medical Publishers; 2003. p. 573–86.

[70] Jansen B, Wacheck V, Heere-Ress E, et al. Chemosensitisation of malignant melanoma by BCL2 antisense therapy. Lancet 2000;356:1728–33.

[71] Davies H, Bignell GR, Cox C, et al. Mutations of the BRAF gene in human cancer. Nature 2002;417: 949–54.

[72] Tsao H, Goel V, Wu H, Yang G, Haluska FG. Genetic interaction between NRAS and BRAF mutations and PTEN/MMAC1 inactivation in melanoma. J Invest Dermatol 2004;122:337–41.

[73] Smalley KS, Eisen TG. Farnesyl transferase inhibitor SCH66336 is cytostatic, pro-apoptotic and enhances chemosensitivity to cisplatin in melanoma cells. Int J Cancer 2003;105:165–75.

[74] Flaherty KT, Brose M, Schuchter L, et al. Phase I/II trial of BAY 43-9006, carboplatin (C) and paclitaxel (P) demonstrates preliminary antitumor activity in the expansion cohort of patients with metastatic melanoma. ASCO Annual Meeting Proceedings 2004. J Clin Oncol 2004;22(14 Suppl):7507.

[75] Creagan ET, Dalton RJ, Ahmann DL, et al. Randomized, surgical adjuvant clinical trial of recombinant interferon alfa-2a in selected patients with malignant melanoma. J Clin Oncol 1995;13:2776–83.

[76] Cascinelli N, Belli F, MacKie RM, Santinami M, Bufalino R, Morabito A. Effect of long-term adjuvant therapy with interferon alpha-2a in patients with regional node metastases from cutaneous melanoma: a randomised trial. Lancet 2001;358:866–9.

ELSEVIER
SAUNDERS

Dermatol Clin 23 (2005) 335 – 342

DERMATOLOGIC
CLINICS

Adverse Drug Interactions and Reactions in Dermatology: Current Issues of Clinical Relevance

Gavin A.E. Wong, MBChB, MRCP(UK), Neil H. Shear, MD, FRCPC*

Division of Dermatology, Department of Medicine, Sunnybrook and Women's College Health Sciences Centre, University of Toronto, 2075 Bayview Avenue, Room M1-700, Toronto, ON M4N 3M5, Canada

Adverse drug interactions and reactions can cause significant morbidity and may be life-threatening. They are therefore important in all branches of medicine, including dermatology. This article discusses several adverse drug interactions and reactions that are relevant to current clinical dermatologic practice.

Adverse drug interactions: when good drugs don't work

Numerous mechanisms may be involved in the evolution of clinically significant drug interactions, and these have been reviewed extensively elsewhere [1–4]. Pharmacokinetic interactions may affect any stage of the "life of a drug"—namely, absorption, distribution, metabolism, and excretion. Bioavailability is the percentage of administered drug that reaches circulation. Most physicians are concerned about interactions that increase toxicity. The binding of drugs with cations, induction of cytochrome P450 (CYP) enzyme, and induction of P-glycoprotein (P-gp) are three interaction mechanisms that reduce drug bioavailability, which may lead to therapeutic failure. The following examples highlight some of these important potential interactions.

Adverse binding interactions between drugs and polyvalent cations

Some drugs interact with compounds containing polyvalent cations (eg, Ca^{2+}, Mg^{2+}, Al^{3+}, Zn^{2+}), with resultant formation of poorly absorbed chelates. These interactions are examples of simple, avoidable, and clinically significant pharmacokinetic drug interactions affecting drug absorption. They lead to reduced drug bioavailability and may result in reduced drug efficacy or therapeutic failure.

Sources of polyvalent cations include the following: antacid preparations, calcium supplements, iron supplements, zinc supplements, multivitamin-mineral supplements, sucralfate (sucrose aluminium sulfate), and dairy products. Aluminum, magnesium, and less commonly, calcium are the cations present in most antacid preparations [5]. The neutralization of gastric hydrochloric acid results in the release of free cations that can bind drugs and form nonabsorbable chelates.

Drugs used in dermatologic practice that are affected by interactions with polyvalent cations include tetracyclines, quinolone antimicrobial agents, bisphosphonates, and mycophenolate mofetil (MMF).

Tetracyclines

Tetracyclines are widely used to treat numerous dermatologic diseases [6]. Adverse interactions between tetracyclines and metallic cations, dairy products, and iron are well known [7]. Different tetracycline derivatives may have variable susceptibility to interact with these compounds. For instance, the absorption of tetracycline hydrochloride and minocycline were significantly decreased by the

Dr. Wong is supported by a Pfizer Canada, Inc., Fellowship in Clinical Pharmacology, from the Canadian Society for Clinical Pharmacology, and is a recipient of a Ben Fisher (Galderma Canada) Clinical Fellowship.

* Corresponding author.

E-mail address: neil.shear@sw.ca (N.H. Shear).

coadministration of milk and food. This undesired effect was greater for tetracycline hydrochloride, however. The coadministration of ferrous sulfate (300 mg) significantly reduced the absorption of both drugs [8]. Patients should be advised to take tetracyclines on an empty stomach to avoid interactions that reduce drug absorption.

Quinolone antimicrobial agents

Quinolones are a class of broad-spectrum antimicrobial agents increasingly used to treat cutaneous infections [9]. Quinolones are rapidly absorbed and have good oral bioavailability. Concurrently administered magnesium-aluminum antacids drastically reduce the bioavailability of ciprofloxacin (by 75%–91%), norfloxacin (by 91%), ofloxacin (by 73%), and enoxacin (by 73%). Chelation reactions are a common clinical issue and occur in 22% to 76% of patients who are prescribed quinolones [10]. The coadministration of magnesium-aluminum antacids and sucralfate has the greatest effect on quinolone bioavailability, followed by iron, calcium, and zinc [10]. Milk and dairy products with high calcium content may also reduce quinolone absorption. To reduce these adverse interactions, quinolone ingestion should be followed by a 2-hour interval before potential interactants are administered.

Bisphosphonates

Bisphosphonates are recommended for minimizing bone loss and fracture risk in patients at risk for glucocorticoid-induced osteoporosis [11]. Bisphosphonates are poorly absorbed after oral intake, with a bioavailability of approximately 0.7% for alendronate, 0.3% for pamidronate, and 3% to 7% for etidronate [12]. The coadministration of polyvalent cations and bisphosphonates results in insoluble chelate formation, further reducing drug bioavailability, and therefore should be avoided. Food intake may completely inhibit bisphosphonate absorption, and therefore, bisphosphonates ideally should be taken on an empty stomach, 2 hours before breakfast. Weekly bisphosphonate dosing may be more convenient for patients.

Mycophenolate mofetil

MMF is an immunosuppressive agent increasingly used in dermatologic practice [13]. Concomitant administration of MMF and metallic cations results in significant reduction in MMF absorption and bioavailability. Studies have shown that the bioavailability of MMF was decreased by 50% with concomitant administration of calcium polycarbophil and by 89.7% with iron ion coadministration [14,15]. An

interval of 2 to 3 hours between ingestion of potential interactants is therefore recommended [13].

Adverse interaction between herbal and conventional medicines: cytochrome P450 enzyme and P-glycoprotein induction

Herbal medicines are increasingly used by the general population. These products are perceived to be "natural" and therefore safe [16]. Most herbal products in the United States are considered dietary supplements and are marketed without approval of efficacy and safety by the US Food and Drug Administration [17]. Herbal medicines have the potential to interact adversely with conventional drugs. Therefore, physicians should specifically ask patients about ingestion of herbal supplements, because this information may not be divulged voluntarily.

Recent reviews have highlighted potential herb–drug interactions, with some attempts to evaluate the quality of the evidence and the clinical significance of these interactions [18–22]. Many of these reports are single cases and small-case series with speculative causality of the herb–drug interaction. The best evidence for mechanisms of interaction and clinical significance exists for St. John's wort (SJW), which is discussed in the following section.

Pharmacokinetic interactions with St. John's wort

SJW is an herbal product, derived from the plant *Hypericum perforatum*, available over-the-counter to treat various conditions, including depression. Long-term SJW administration (>14 d) has inductive effects on CYP isoenzymes, predominantly CYP3A4. Induction of CYP3A4 expression is caused by SJW's activation of the pregnane X receptor, a nuclear receptor that interacts with numerous xenobiotics. SJW also increases expression of P-gp, a transport protein present in cell membranes with an important role in drug efflux from tissues [23–29].

Because of its effects on CYP and P-gp, SJW potentially interacts with many drugs, including the following: amitriptyline [30], cyclosporine [31], digoxin [32], fexofenadine [33], indinavir [34], nevirapine [35], omeprazole [36], phenprocoumon [37], simvastatin [38], tacrolimus [39], theophylline [40], and warfarin [41]. In these examples, the coadministration with SJW causes reduced blood concentrations of the conventional drugs and may result in clinically significant consequences. In addition, contraceptive failures have been reported in women taking SJW concurrently with oral contraceptive pills, possibly related to increased incidence of breakthrough bleeding [23,42–44]. Many other drugs are substrates for CYP3A4 and P-gp, and therefore, despite the lack of specific studies, these drugs potentially interact with SJW.

Pharmacodynamic interactions with St. John's wort

Combining selective serotonin reuptake inhibitors (SSRIs) with SJW may lead to symptoms compatible with serotonin excess. These symptoms include confusion, agitation, tremor, restlessness, flushing, fever, gastrointestinal upset, headache, and myalgia [23]. This interaction is believed to occur because of the additive effects of SSRIs and SJW on serotonin uptake in the brain. The coadministration of SSRIs and SJW should therefore be avoided.

Adverse drug reactions

The changing meaning of sulfa allergy

The term *sulfa allergy* refers to intolerance of sulfonamide drugs; and when this term is used by patients, it usually refers to intolerance of sulfonamide antimicrobial agents. The term does not imply allergy to sulfur, sulfates, and sulfites [45]. Much confusion is associated with this term, particularly with regard to its exact meaning and implications for future drug prescribing. This section highlights some current issues and controversies in this area.

What is a sulfonamide?

Sulfonamide drugs are any compounds containing an SO_2NH_2 moiety. These include sulfonamide antimicrobial agents (eg, sulfamethoxazole) and members of other drug classes, including the following: thiazide diuretics (eg, hydrochlorothiazide), loop diuretics (eg, furosemide), sulfonylurea oral hypoglycemic agents (eg, glyburide), carbonic anhydrase inhibitors (eg, acetazolamide), and selective cylooxygenase 2 inhibitors (eg, celecoxib) [45].

How do sulfonamide antimicrobial agents and other sulfonamide drugs differ?

Sulfonamide antimicrobial agents are derived from sulfanilamide and are structurally differentiated from sulfonamide nonantimicrobial agents by the presence of (1) an aromatic amine group at the N4 position and (2) an aromatic ring at the sulfonamide-N1 position (Fig. 1).

Do patients with hypersensitivity to sulfonamide antimicrobial agents experience cross-reactions with other sulfonamide drugs?

Cross-reactivity suggests that two drugs will cause a similar reaction in a susceptible patient because of their similar mechanisms. The previous question is often asked and difficult to answer with authority. Some evidence from the literature is helpful to consider, however.

Sulfonamide antimicrobial agents can cause a wide spectrum of adverse reactions [46]. Hypersensitivity syndrome reaction describes the triad of rash, fever, and internal organ involvement. Oxidation of the aromatic amine portion of sulfamethoxazole and subsequent generation of reactive hydroxylamine and nitroso metabolites is believed to be involved in the pathogenesis of this syndrome [47]. IgE-mediated reactions to sulfamethoxazole are believed to be related to the N1 substituent and not the sulfonamide (SO_2NH_2) moiety [48]. Sulfonamide nonantimicrobial agents do not have either of the groups implicated in the pathogenesis of these two adverse reaction types and therefore would not be expected to cross-react through similar mechanisms.

It has been suggested that a previous sulfonamide allergy may not predict future adverse reactions to other sulfonamides caused by cross-reactivity but may instead simply be a marker for individuals prone to hapten allergies [49]. A recent retrospective cohort study, although not without some limitations in study design, does provide some interesting evidence for this concept [50,51]. First, in patients with prior sulfonamide antibiotic allergic reactions, there was an increased risk of subsequent allergic reaction to sulfonamide nonantibiotics. Second, this group of patients (with prior sulfonamide antibiotic allergic reactions) had an even greater risk of subsequently reacting to penicillin. Third, patients with a history of penicillin hypersensitivity had a greater risk of subsequently having an allergic reaction to sulfonamide nonantibiotic agents as compared with patients with a history of sulfonamide antibiotic hypersensitivity. This study concluded that, although prior sulfonamide antibiotic hypersensitivity does increase the risk of subsequent allergic reaction to sulfonamide nonantibiotic agents, this association may be caused by a predisposition to allergic reactions rather than to cross-reactivity with sulfonamide-based drugs.

Recent in vitro studies have shown that some drugs can interact directly with T-cell receptors to elicit immune responses, the so-called "p-i" (pharmacologic interaction with immune receptors) concept [52]. Studies of sulfamethoxazole-reactive T-cell

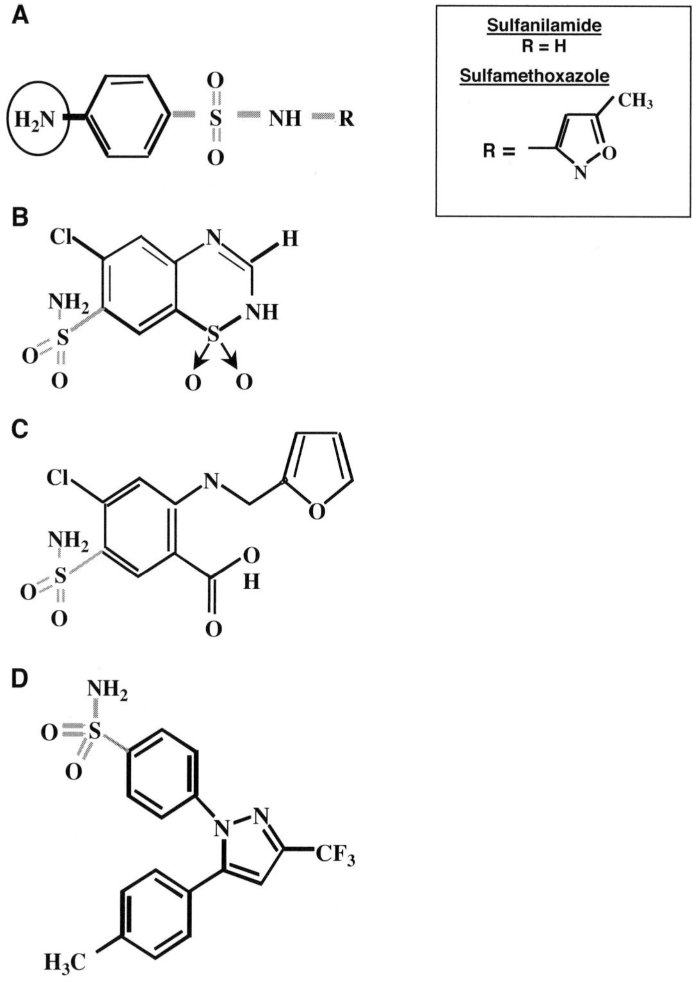

A

Sulfanilamide
R = H

Sulfamethoxazole

R =

B

C

D

Fig. 1. (*A*) Sulfonamide antimicrobial core structure. (*B*) Cholorothiazide. (*C*) Furosemide. (*D*) Celecoxib.

clones generated from sulfamethoxazole-hypersensitive patients have shown cross-reactivity with compounds containing the sulfanilamide-core structure but no cross-reactivity with celecoxib and furosemide. This finding suggests that cross-reactivity requires a similarity in the whole compound structure, such as the sulfanilamide-core structure common to sulfonamide antimicrobial agents, and not simply the SO_2NH_2 moiety common to all sulfonamide drugs [53].

A pilot study showed that in six patients with sulfonamide antimicrobial allergy confirmed by positive intradermal testing or in vitro lymphocyte toxicity assay, all six patients tolerated oral challenge with celecoxib [54]. In addition, four of these six patients continued celecoxib without problems, one patient discontinued the drug because of gastro-

intestinal side effects, and one patient was advised by her physician not to take the drug despite tolerating the oral challenge. This study was limited by its small sample size but does provide some in vivo clinical evidence that certain sulfonamide non-antibiotic agents can be tolerated in patients with confirmed sulfonamide antimicrobial allergy. A review of the literature, summarized in this study, did not reveal substantial evidence of cross-reactivity between sulfonamide antimicrobial agents and other sulfonamide drugs described in previous clinical reports [54].

What advice should be given to patients?

Based on current evidence, patients with a history of adverse reactions to sulfonamide antimicrobial agents should avoid other sulfonamide antimicrobial agents. Other sulfonamide-containing drugs are not of equivalent risk for cross-reactivity and do not need to be avoided.

Patients with a prior history of adverse reactions, both to sulfonamide antimicrobial agents and to penicillin, may be at increased risk from future adverse drug reactions caused by as yet unknown mechanisms. It is hoped that as further in vitro and clinical studies are undertaken, clinicians will be able to advise their patients about potential cross-reactivity of sulfonamide drugs more rationally based on sound scientific evidence.

New adverse reactions from new drugs: cutaneous reactions from epidermal growth factor receptor inhibitors

Epidermal growth factor receptors (EGFRs) are widely expressed in normal tissue [55]. EGFRs are transmembrane proteins with an extracellular ligand-binding domain, a lipophilic transmembrane domain, and an intracellular tyrosine kinase (TK) domain. Ligands, such as epidermal growth factor, transforming growth factor α, amphiregulin, and betacellulin, bind to EGFRs, leading to receptor dimerization, TK activation, and subsequent triggering of intracellular signaling events. Cutaneous EGFRs are expressed on basal keratinocytes, hair follicle outer root sheath, sebocytes, and eccrine ducts [56]. EGFRs and their ligand interactions are integral to epidermal homeostasis. The activation of EGFRs leads to effects on keratinocyte proliferation, differentiation, migration, and survival by way of complex signaling pathways [57].

EGFRs are overexpressed in many solid tumor types, including non–small cell lung, prostate, colorectal, breast, ovarian, and head and neck cancers. EGFR activation contributes to tumor progression with cell proliferation, angiogenesis, and apoptosis inhibition. Therefore, EGFR inhibition has emerged as a potential target mechanism for cancer chemotherapy (Table 1) [58].

Many EGFR inhibitors are in varying stages of drug development. These drugs include the orally bioavailable EGFR-TK inhibitors gefitinib (Iressa, ZD1839) and erlotinib (Tarceva, OSI-774) and intravenously administered monoclonal anti-EGFR antibodies, such as cetuximab (Erbitux, C225). Numerous other agents are in earlier stages of development [59–62]. Adverse cutaneous reactions with these agents are common and will become increasingly prevalent as clinical trials proceed. Therefore, knowledge of these agents and their potential skin side effects are relevant to practicing dermatologists.

Clinical presentation

Several reports have focused on the cutaneous consequences of EGFR inhibition [63–68]. Adverse skin reactions occur in approximately 40% to 80% of patients treated with EGFR inhibitors and are generally mild, well tolerated, reversible, and do not necessitate treatment discontinuation. There is an increased incidence of rash with increasing gefitinib dosage. The degree of skin toxicity does not seem to correlate with response to gefitinib treatment, however [69].

The most common skin problems reported are acneiform eruptions, dry skin, and pruritus. These reactions usually develop 1 to 2 weeks after initiation of therapy. Dryness affects any part of the skin surface, with fine scaling and an asteatotic, or xerotic, pattern. Some women have reported vaginal dryness and dysuria [66].

Acneiform eruptions typically present as erythematous follicular papules and pustules on the face, scalp, upper chest, and upper back (Fig. 2). Less commonly, this follicular eruption can be widespread [64]. Other hair changes, including finer hairs, curling, and brittleness, also have been described [65].

A less common cutaneous side effect described is painful paronychial inflammation and in-growing nails of the fingers and toes [63,67]. Small oral ulcers are rarely described [63,67].

Table 1
Epidermal growth factor receptor inhibitors: potential indications and cutaneous reactions

Drug	Class	Potential indications	Skin reactions
Gefitinib (Iressa, ZD1839)	Small-molecule EGFR-TK inhibitor	NSCLC, prostate cancer, head and neck tumors, colorectal cancer	Acneiform rashes, dry skin, pruritus, hair changes, paronychia
Erlotinib (Tarceva, OSI-774)	Small-molecule EGFR-TK inhibitor	NSCLC, head and neck tumors, pancreatic carcinoma	As above
Cetuximab (Erbitux, C225)	Chimeric monoclonal anti-EGFR antibody	Metastatic colorectal cancer, head and neck tumors, lung cancer	As above

Abbreviation: NSCLC, non–small cell lung cancer.

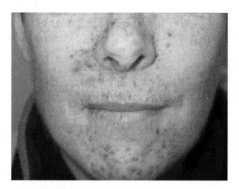

Fig. 2. Acneiform facial rash after treatment with cetuximab, an EGFR inhibitor.

Histopathology

Histopathologic effects of gefitinib on the skin have been reported [70]. Skin biopsy specimens taken after 28 days of gefitinib treatment showed thinner, more compact stratum corneum, with loss of basket-weave pattern, as compared with pretreatment specimens. Lichenoid reactions (with mononuclear infiltrates, vacuolar degeneration of the basal cell layer, and apoptotic keratinocytes) in follicular and interfollicular areas were seen in some cases. Comedo-like structures with keratin plugs and microorganisms in dilated infundibula were noted. In addition, acute folliculitis was seen in a few patients. The authors suggested that EGFR-TK inhibition may cause these skin changes by affecting terminal maturation of suprabasal keratinocytes.

Mechanism

The exact mechanism by which EGFR inhibition causes cutaneous reactions is not known. Effects on terminal differentiation of keratinocytes and effects on hair cycle control are proposed mechanisms [63–68]. Studies in EGFR-null mice have shown that EGFR has an important role in hair follicle cycling and differentiation and may protect the hair follicle from immunologic reactions [71].

Treatment

Patients should be advised at initiation of EGFR inhibitor therapy to expect some degree of skin dryness or acnelike rash [66]. This advice may help patients better tolerate the rash when it appears. Dry skin and pruritus are managed with emollients and topical corticosteroids. Sedative antihistamines, such as hydroxyzine, may be useful for severe pruritus.

Acneiform eruptions respond partially to topical antibiotics (eg, clindamycin), topical corticosteroids, and topical retinoids. One study reported that topical tretinoin 0.025% cream reduced follicular lesions in one patient but aggravated skin scaling in another [65]. These local treatments tend to control the follicular rash, but typically, patients may continue to have some signs of skin involvement until the EGFR inhibitors are discontinued. A response to 100-mg/day dosages of oral minocycline has been described [65].

Paronychial inflammation partially improved with the use of topical mupirocin ointment and with soaking and cushioning of the affected areas [63,67].

Summary

Adverse drug interactions and reactions continue to be significant and challenging areas in clinical medicine. This article has highlighted some current issues of clinical relevance to the practicing dermatologist. Absorption interactions between drugs and compounds containing polyvalent cations should be avoidable with appropriate advice. Herbal remedies are increasingly used and potentially interact with conventional medicines. A history of adverse reaction to sulfonamide antimicrobial agents should not exclude patients from receiving sulfonamide non-antimicrobial medications. Cutaneous reactions from EGFR inhibitors will become more prevalent as development of these agents proceeds.

References

[1] Shapiro LE, Knowles SR, Shear NH. Drug interactions of clinical significance for the dermatologist. Am J Clin Dermatol 2003;4(9):623–39.

[2] Aria N, Kauffman L. Important drug interactions and reactions in dermatology. Dermatol Clin 2003;21: 207–15.

[3] Roos TC, Merk HF. Important drug interactions in dermatology. Drugs 2000;59(2):181–92.

[4] Lebwohl M, Gelfand JM, Tan MH. Clinically significant therapeutic interactions for the practicing dermatologist. Adv Dermatol 1999;14:1–26.

[5] Sadowski D. Drug interactions with antacids. Drug Saf 1994;11:395–407.

[6] Carrasco DA, Vander Straten M, Tyring SK. A review of antibiotics in dermatology. J Cutan Med Surg 2002; 6(2):128–50.

[7] Neuvonen PJ. Interactions with the absorption of tetracyclines. Drugs 1976;11:45–54.

[8] Leyden JJ. Absorption of minocycline hydrochloride and tetracycline hydrochloride. Effect of food, milk, and iron. J Am Acad Dermatol 1985;12:308–12.

[9] Sable D, Murukawa GJ. Quinolones in dermatology. Clin Dermatol 2003;21:56–63.

[10] Lomaestro BM, Bailie GR. Absorption interactions with fluoroquinolones. Drug Saf 1995;12:314–33.

[11] Boling EP. Secondary osteoporosis: underlying disease and the risk for glucocorticoid-induced osteoporosis. Clin Ther 2004;26:1–14.

[12] Lin JH. Bisphosphonates: a review of their pharmacokinetic properties. Bone 1996;18:75–85.

[13] Liu V, Mackool BT. Mycophenolate in dermatology. J Dermatol Treat 2003;14:203–10.

[14] Kato R, Ooi K, Ikura-Morii M, Tsuchishita Y, Hashimoto H, Yoshimura H, et al. Impairment of mycophenolate mofetil absorption by calcium polycarbophil. J Clin Pharm 2002;42:1275–80.

[15] Morii M, Ueno K, Ogawa A, Kato R, Yoshimuro H, Wada K, et al. Impairment of mycophenolate mofetil absorption by iron ion. Clin Pharmacol Ther 2000; 68:613–6.

[16] Pirmohamed M. Herbal medicines. Postgrad Med J 2003;79:489.

[17] De Smet PAGM. Herbal remedies. N Engl J Med 2002; 347:2046–56.

[18] Williamson EM. Drug interactions between herbal and prescription medicines. Drug Saf 2003;26:1075–92.

[19] Fugh-Berman A, Ernst E. Herb-drug interactions: review and assessment of report reliability. Br J Clin Pharmacol 2001;52:587–95.

[20] Izzo AA, Ernst E. Interactions between herbal medicines and prescribed drugs. Drugs 2001;61:2163–75.

[21] Fugh-Berman A. Herb-drug interactions. Lancet 2000; 355:134–8.

[22] Brazier NC, Levine MAH. Drug-herb interaction among commonly used conventional medicines: a compendium for health care professionals. Am J Ther 2003;10:163–9.

[23] Henderson L, Yue QY, Bergquist C, Gerden B, Arlett P. St. John's wort (hypericum perforatum): drug interactions and clinical outcomes. Br J Clin Pharmacol 2002;54:349–56.

[24] Wang Z, Gorski C, Hamman MA, Huang SM, Lesko LJ, Hall SD. The effects of St. John's wort (Hypericum perforatum) on human cytochrome P450 activity. Clin Pharmacol Ther 2001;70:317–26.

[25] Markowitz JS, Donovan JL, DeVane CL, Taylor RM, Ruan Y, Wang JS, et al. Effect of St John's wort on drug metabolism by induction of cytochrome P450 3A4 enzyme. JAMA 2003;290:1500–4.

[26] Zhou S, Yihuai G, Jiang W, Huang M, Xu A, Paxton JW. Interactions of herbs with cytochrome P450. Drug Metab Rev 2003;35:35–98.

[27] Moore LB, Goodwin B, Jones SA, Wisely GB, Serabjit-Singh CJ, Willson TM, et al. St. John's wort induces hepatic drug metabolism through activation of the pregnane X receptor. Proc Natl Acad Sci U S A 2000;97:7500–2.

[28] Durr D, Stieger B, Kullak-Ublick GA, Rentsch KM, Steinert HC, Meier PJ, et al. St. John's wort induces intestinal P-glycoprotein/MDR1 and intestinal and hepatic CYP3A4. Clin Pharmacol Ther 2000;68: 598–604.

[29] Hennessy M, Kelleher D, Spiers JP, Barry M, Kavanagh P, Back D, et al. St. John's wort increases expression of P-glycoprotein: implications for drug interactions. Br J Clin Pharmacol 2002;53:75–82.

[30] Johne A, Schmider J, Brockmoller J, Stadelmann AM, Stormer E, Bauer S, et al. Decreased plasma levels of amitriptyline and its metabolites on comedication with an extract from St. John's wort (Hypericum perforatum). J Clin Psychopharmacol 2002;22: 46–54.

[31] Ernst E. St. John's wort supplements endanger the success of organ transplantation. Arch Surg 2002; 137:316–9.

[32] Johne A, Brockmoller J, Bauer S, Maurer A, Langheinrich M, Roots I. Pharmacokinetic interaction of digoxin with an herbal extract from St. John's wort (Hypericum perforatum). Clin Pharmacol Ther 1999; 66:338–45.

[33] Wang Z, Hamman MA, Huang SM, Lesko LJ, Hall SD. Effect of St. John's wort on the pharmacokinetics of fexofenadine. Clin Pharmacol Ther 2002;71: 414–20.

[34] Piscitelli SC, Burstein AH, Chaitt D, Alfaro RM, Falloon J. Indinavir concentrations and St. John's wort. Lancet 2000;355(9203):547–8.

[35] de Maat MMR, Hoetelmans RMW, Mathot RAA, van Gorp ECM, Meenhorst PL, Mulder JW, et al. Drug interaction between St. John's wort and nevirapine. AIDS 2001;15:420–1.

[36] Wang LS, Zhou G, Zhu B, Wu J, Wang JG, Abd El-aty AM, et al. St John's wort induces both cytochrome P450 3A4-catalyzed sulfoxidation and 2C19-dependent hydroxylation of omeprazole. Clin Pharmacol Ther 2004;75:191–7.

[37] Maurer A, Johne A, Bauer S, Brockmoller F, Donath F, Roots I, et al. Interaction of St. John's wort extract with phenprocoumon. Eur J Clin Pharmacol 1999;55:A22.

[38] Sugimoto K, Ohmori M, Tsuruoka S, Nishiki K, Kawaguchi A, Harada K, et al. Different effects of St. John's Wort on the pharmacokinetics of simvastatin and pravastatin. Clin Pharmacol Ther 2001;70: 518–24.

[39] Mai I, Stormer E, Bauer S, Kruger H, Budde K, Roots I. Impact of St. John's wort treatment on the pharmacokinetics of tacrolimus and mycophenolic acid in renal transplant patients. Nephrol Dial Transplant 2003;18: 819–22.

[40] Nebel A, Schneider BJ, Baker RK, Kroll DJ. Potential metabolic interaction between St. John's wort and theophylline. Ann Pharmacother 1999;33:502.

[41] Yue QY, Bergquist C, Gerden B. Safety of St. John's wort (Hypericum perforatum). Lancet 2000;355:576–7.

[42] Schwarz UI, Buschel B, Kirch W. Unwanted pregnancy on self-medication with St. John's wort despite hormonal contraception. Br J Clin Pharmacol 2003; 55:112–3.

[43] Hall SD, Wang Z, Huang SM, Hamman MA, Vasavada

N, Adigun AQ, et al. The interaction between St. John's wort and an oral contraceptive. Clin Pharmacol Ther 2003;74:525–35.

[44] Pfrunder A, Schiesser M, Gerber S, Haschke M, Bitzer J, Drewe J. Interaction of St. John's wort with low-dose oral contraceptive therapy: a randomized controlled trial. Br J Clin Pharmacol 2003;56:683–90.

[45] Knowles S, Shapiro L, Shear NH. Should celecoxib be contraindicated in patients who are allergic to sulfonamides. Revisiting the meaning of "sulfa" allergy. Drug Saf 2001;24:239–47.

[46] Cribb AE, Lee BL, Trepanier LA, Spielberg SP. Adverse reactions to sulphonamide and sulphonamide-trimethoprim antimicrobials: clinical syndromes and pathogenesis. Adverse Drug React Toxicol Rev 1996; 15:9–50.

[47] Naisbitt DJ, Hough SJ, Gill HJ, Pirmohamed M, Kitteringham N, Park BK. Cellular disposition of sulphamethoxazole and its metabolites: implications for hypersensitivity. Br J Pharmacol 1999;126:1393–407.

[48] Harle DG, Baldo BA, Wells JV. Drugs as allergens: detection and combining site specificities of IgE antibodies to sulfamethoxazole. Mol Immunol 1988; 25:1347–54.

[49] Wiholm BE. Should celecoxib be contraindicated in patients who are allergic to sulfonamides? Drug Saf 2002;25:297–300.

[50] Strom BL, Schinnar R, Apter AJ, Margolis DJ, Lautenbach E, Hennessy S, et al. Absence of cross-reactivity between sulfonamide antibiotics and sulfonamide nonantibiotics. N Engl J Med 2003;349: 1628–35.

[51] Saxon AS, Macy E. Cross-reactivity and sulfonamide antibiotics. N Engl J Med 2004;350(3):302–3.

[52] Pichler WJ. Pharmacological interaction of drugs with antigen-specific immune receptors: the p-i concept. Curr Opin Allergy Clin Immunol 2002;2:301–5.

[53] Depta JPH, Pichler WJ. Cross-reactivity with drugs at the T cell level. Curr Opin Allergy Clin Immunol 2003;3:261–7.

[54] Shapiro LE, Knowles SR, Weber E, Neuman MG, Shear NH. Safety of celecoxib in individuals allergic to sulfonamide. A pilot study. Drug Saf 2003;26:187–95.

[55] Yano S, Kondo K, Yamaguchi M, Richmond G, Hutchison M, Wakeling A, et al. Distribution and function of EGFR in human tissue and the effect of EGFR tyrosine kinase inhibition. Anticancer Res 2003;23:3639–50.

[56] Nanney LB, Magid M, Stoscheck CM, King LE. Comparison of epidermal growth factor binding and receptor distribution in normal human epidermis and epidermal appendages. J Invest Dermatol 1984;83: 385–93.

[57] Jost M, Kari C, Rodeck U. The EGF receptor: an essential regulator of multiple epidermal functions. Eur J Dermatol 2000;10:505–10.

[58] Ritter CA, Arteaga CL. The epidermal growth factor receptor-tyrosine kinase: a promising therapeutic target in solid tumors. Semin Oncol 2003;30(Suppl 1):3–11.

[59] Liu CY, Seen S. Gefitinib therapy for advanced non-small cell lung cancer. Ann Pharmacother 2003; 37:1644–53.

[60] Bonomi P. Clinical studies with non-iressa EGFR tyrosine kinase inhibitors. Lung Cancer 2003;41(Suppl 1): S43–8.

[61] Reynolds NA, Wagstaff AJ. Cetuximab in the treatment of metastatic colorectal cancer. Drugs 2004; 64:109–18.

[62] Lage A, Crombet T, Gonzalez G. Targeting epidermal growth factor receptor signaling: early results and future trends in oncology. Ann Med 2003;35:327–36.

[63] Busam KJ, Capodieci P, Motzer R, Kiehn T, Phelan D, Halpern AC. Cutaneous side-effects in cancer patients treated with the antiepidermal growth factor receptor antibody C225. Br J Dermatol 2001;144:1169–76.

[64] Kimyai-Asadi A, Jih MH. Follicular toxic effects of chimeric anti-epidermal growth factor receptor antibody cetuximab used to treat human solid tumors. Arch Dermatol 2002;138:129–31.

[65] van Doorn R, Kirtschig G, Scheffer E, Stoof TJ, Giaccone G. Follicular and epidermal alterations in patients treated with ZD1839 (Iressa), an inhibitor of the epidermal growth factor receptor. Br J Dermatol 2002;147:598–601.

[66] Herbst RS, LoRusso PM, Purdom M, Ward D. Dermatologic side effects associated with gefitinib therapy: clinical experience and management. Clin Lung Cancer 2003;4:366–9.

[67] Lee MW, Seo CW, Kim SW, Yang HJ, Lee HW, Choi JH, et al. Cutaneous side effects in non-small cell lung cancer patients treated with Iressa (ZD1839), an inhibitor of epidermal growth factor. Acta Derm Venereol 2004;84:23–6.

[68] Wong GA, Nigen S, Walsh S, Shear NH. Acneiform eruptions caused by an epidermal growth factor receptor-tyrosine kinase inhibitor ZD1839 [abstract]. J Am Acad Dermatol 2004;50(3 Suppl):39.

[69] van Zandwijk N. Tolerability of gefitinib in patients receiving treatment in everyday clinical practice. Br J Cancer 2003;89(Suppl 2):S9–14.

[70] Albanell J, Rojo F, Averbuch S, Feyereislova A, Mascaro JM, Herbst R, et al. Pharmacodynamic studies of the epidermal growth factor receptor inhibitor ZD1839 in skin from cancer patients: histopathologic and molecular consequences of receptor inhibition. J Clin Oncol 2001;20:110–24.

[71] Hansen LA, Alexander N, Hogan ME, Sundberg JP, Dlugosz A, Threadgill DW, et al. Genetically null mice reveal a central role for epidermal growth factor receptor in the differentiation of the hair follicle and normal hair development. Am J Pathol 1997;150: 1959–75.

DERMATOLOGIC
CLINICS

ELSEVIER
SAUNDERS

Dermatol Clin 23 (2005) 343 – 363

The Evolution of Soft Tissue Fillers in Clinical Practice

Christian A. Murray, BSc, MD, FRCPC[a],*, David Zloty, BSc, MD, FRCPC[b],
Laurence Warshawski, BSc, MD, FRCPC[b]

[a]Division of Dermatology, Department of Medicine, Sunnybrook and Women's College Health Sciences Centre,
University of Toronto, 76 Grenville Street, Toronto, ON M5S 1B2, Canada
[b]Division of Dermatology, Department of Medicine, The Skin Care Centre, 835 West 10th Avenue Vancouver,
BC V5Z 4E8, Canada

The recent movement toward a healthier society has encouraged practices that not only eradicate disease but also diminish perceived imperfections in individuals' appearance that are associated with being unwell or aged. As facial skin ages, it develops dynamic and static rhytids while losing the soft tissue fullness associated with youth. Traditional approaches to achieving a youthful appearance have focused on tightening of the skin through resection and remodeling of the superficial skin with resurfacing. These procedures generally meant significant downtime for patients and a substantial financial commitment. The softening of facial lines and augmentation of tissue volume using fillers allow physicians and patients an opportunity to re-create a natural appearance of youthfulness. Furthermore, soft tissue fillers are minimally invasive, have good safety records, and can be used conveniently in the office setting.

Physicians should understand all factors impacting on a patient's appearance and how best to manage his or her aesthetic concerns. A thorough knowledge of the properties (benefits, limitations, and complications) of the ever-expanding array of fillers is essential for any physician treating patients with cosmetic complaints. This article describes soft tissue fillers, industry recommendations, literature evidence, and the authors' experience.

Historical overview

Physicians have been searching for the ideal filler for more than a century (Box 1) [1–3]. The use of injected paraffin more than 100 years ago for cosmetic purposes resulted in paraffinomas. Autologous fat transfer was first described by Neuber in 1893 [4], but more recent modifications in technique have renewed the use of fat as a viable filling substance. Medical-grade liquid silicone was used successfully in thousands of patients in the United States and elsewhere since the 1960s for off-label cosmetic purposes. Silicone has never been approved by the US Food and Drug Administration (FDA) for cosmetic use, however. In 1981, a new era in soft tissue fillers emerged with the FDA approval of bovine collagen. To date, however, the ideal filler does not exist (see Box 1). The most widely used, legal products available worldwide today are the collagens, hyaluronic acids (HAs), polymethylmethacrylate (PMMA), and autologous fat. Fillers may be derived from autogenic (the patient), allogenic (another human), xenogenic (animal or bioengineered from bacteria), or synthetic sources (Box 2).

Preoperative preparation

Soft tissue augmentation is generally a minor procedure that can be performed in an office setting. The most important component of preoperative preparation is the full understanding and informed consent of the patient. A thorough discussion should take place to discuss the indications, advantages, and

---

* Corresponding author.

derm.theclinics.com

Box 1. The ideal filler

Safety: nonimmunogenic, noncarcino-
   genic, nonteratogenic, noninfectious,
   physiologic, low abuse potential
Efficacy: long-term benefit, nonmigratory,
   natural feeling, reproducible results
Practical: cost-effective, easy to use,
   approved, removable if required,
   long shelf life

disadvantages of the proposed filler agents. Alternative therapies, such as botulinum toxin (BTX) or
resurfacing, should be discussed and, in some cases,
recommended for certain indications (Table 1). Special attention should focus on ensuring the patient's
expectations are realistic in terms of side effects,
efficacy, and duration of correction. A mirror is
helpful for the patient to outline specific sites of
concern. Preoperative photographs or detailed dia-
grams are useful when documenting the status of the
patient before treatment begins.

It is important to remember that patients who are
interested in cosmetic procedures are often anxious
or embarrassed about their aesthetic concerns. The
consultant must be attentive, considerate, and non-
judgmental. Patients frequently have spent considerable time researching their options on the Internet
or in the lay press. Physicians should have a thorough
knowledge of the latest products available and at least
a cursory understanding of the most common concerns addressed in popular fashion magazines.

Minimizing risk

Techniques used to lower the risk of complications are similar to those of any minor surgical procedure. Cosmetic patients require careful attention
and tolerate adverse events poorly. Consequently, it is
important that consideration be paid to each element
of the process (Table 2).

Technique

The proper placement of soft tissue fillers requires
appropriate needle selection and method of insertion
(angle, depth, volume, needle positioning, method
of delivery). Each of these factors is addressed in general later, and filler-specific modifications are discussed in the relevant sections.

Needle selection

Most injectable fillers are supplied with a syringe
and needle. The choice of needle is determined by
the filler viscosity, and some viscous products cannot
be delivered effectively with smaller gauge needles.
Many experienced physicians will replace the supplied needles with an alternate choice, based on what
works best in their practice. As a general rule, it is
ideal to use the smallest needle that can deliver the
filler appropriately, without compromising control
(Table 3).

Superficial defects require shallow injection, with
the needle inserted almost parallel to the skin. The
needle is often beveled up, and the needle tip barely
enters the skin. Blanching and a small bleb should
be seen with correct placement. Gentle massage of
the product after insertion results in even correction.
Care should be taken to avoid displacing the product
entirely with aggressive kneading. Viscous products
should not be placed superficially, because they will
cause lumps, nodules, or unpleasant palpability.

Needle placement in the mid-dermis is best performed with an angle of 30° to 45°. Blanching should
occur, but the volume change is less apparent. Careful
attention to the evolving correction and volume of
filler deposited is required. The filler should not be
highly viscous because of the possibility of nodule
formation. Products with low viscosity may not
adequately correct mid-dermal defects, or they may
require excessive volume.

Delivery into the deep dermis, dermal-fat junction
or directly into the subcutaneous fat is reserved for
the most viscous products. Less viscous fillers will be
lost into the fat and not augment significantly at this
depth. The needle should be angled between 45° and
90° for the serial puncture technique, or between 30°
and 45° if threaded.

Box 2. Filler sources

Autogenic: dermis, fat, plasma,
   cultured fibroblasts, collagen
Allogenic: cultured collagen, cadaveric
   collagen, cadaveric fascia
Xenogenic: bovine collagen,
   avian-derived hyaluronan,
   bacterial-derived hyaluronan
Synthetic: hydrogels, calcium hydroxylapatite, PMMA, dextran, silicone, expanded polytetrafluoroethylene

Table 1
Problems that may be best managed with other methods

Problem	Description	Plan
Solar elastosis	Furrows between areas of elastosis often do not do well with fillers	Remove elastotic material with ablative resurfacing
Superficial contour defects	Fine defects may be too shallow for dermal fillers	Ablative resurfacing
Significant laxity	Excessive fillers in these areas may result in lumpiness	Correct surgically (rhytidectomy, liposuction) or perform nonablative tightening
Deep dynamic folds	Fillers may dislodge easily in dynamic areas	Should use BTX first or at the same time as fillers[a]

[a] Fillers do better in areas also treated with BTX.

Methods of delivery

The serial puncture technique is commonly used for superficial placement of fillers along a rhytid or to augment the lip. The skin is held taut, and the needle is placed at the appropriate depth and angle. The product is delivered in a small bolus to full correction, and then the needle is removed. Repeated injections are used until the entire length of the defect is corrected.

The threading technique is used to deliver the filler through a single insertion point. The needle

Table 2
Minimizing complications of soft tissue fillers

Complication	Common causes	Practical approach
Bleeding	1. Medications: ASA, NSAIDs, ticlopidine, clopidogrel, anticoagulants, vitamin E, various herbals 2. Large bore needle, vascular site, thin skin	1. Hold for 1 wk prior to procedure (and 24–48 h after) if not medically necessary 2. Use caution in high-risk areas (around eyes, lips), use the smallest bore needle possible
Infection	Colonized with pathogenic bacteria, herpes simplex	Remove makeup, careful antisepsis (alcohol or chlorhexidine), consider antivirals for those with a history of recurrent herpes
Anxiety	Anxious personality, new environment, new to the procedure	Explanations of all necessary steps, comfortable positioning, consider light sedation in some cases Beware of lying the patient down, which may alter the effects of gravity and prevent ideal correction
Immunologic reaction	Allergy to component of filler, latex allergy	Patient history of allergies, allergy testing as per product recommendations
Pain	No anesthetic used, large bore needle	Use the smallest needle possible Anesthesia as needed: topical for superficial injections, nerve or field blocks for lips Beware of excessive local anesthesia that may distort contours and obscure effective correction Postoperative cold packs
Postoperative unreal, expectations	Unreasonable patient, inadequate preoperative communication	Ensure patient has a full understanding of expectations, side effects Always consider a trial of a temporary filler first Be available to address concerns at all times

Abbreviations: ASA, acetylsalicyclic acid; NSAID, nonsteroidal anti-inflammatory drug.

Table 3
The choice of angle, depth, and product depends on the indication

Indication	Depth	Angle	Product viscosity (examples)
Fine lines and thin rhytids	Superficial (papillary) dermis	$10°-30°$	Low (Cosmoderm 1, Restylane Finelines)
Moderate to deep rhytids	Mid (reticular) dermis	$30°-45°$	Mid (Restylane, Zyderm 2)
Deeper rhytids or folds	Deep dermal-fat junction or below	$45°-90°$	High (Artecoll, Cosmoplast)

tunnels through the defect at the appropriate depth. As the needle is withdrawn, the product is delivered into the tunnel created.

Certain situations lend themselves best to a particular choice of equipment, technique, and product. Variations are the rule rather than the exception, however. Once the fundamental aspects of soft tissue augmentation are understood, every physician must decide which combination of variables to select for each patient. Ultimately, the right choices will be those that yield the consistently best results.

Optimizing outcomes

The most important factor determining outcome is proper patient selection. Those patients who cannot tolerate complications or who have unrealistic expectations are not suitable candidates. The layering of fillers allows fine-tuning and may provide for more complete correction. For example, more viscous products may be placed deeply and form a scaffold for less viscous fillers to be placed superficially. For melolabial and marionette lines, it is preferable to direct injections medial to the fold to avoid further pronouncement of the rhytid. Consider temporary fillers before permanent options. Most patients feel more secure in their choice to have permanent fillers placed if they have tolerated temporary correction. This method not only demonstrates the benefits of augmentation but allows the physician the opportu-

nity to avoid placing unforgiving, permanent fillers in patients who will not accept minor adverse events (Box 3).

Adverse events

Most side effects of injectable fillers are transient and minor. Attention to detail will reduce the rate of complications and ensure the best result. Despite expert technique, however, adverse events will occur (Box 4). It is important to discuss rare occurrences as a component of informed consent.

Xenogenic products

Nonhuman sources of dermal molecules, such as bovine collagen, have been used successfully as filling agents for decades. They are readily available from protected animal or bioengineered bacterial sources, and consequently mass production is possible. The main concern is that although xenogenic molecules are similar to human, they are not identical

---

Box 3. Postoperative care

Consider cold compresses regularly for first 24 to 48 hours
Courses of antivirals or antibiotics should be completed, if deemed necessary
Minimize aggressive movement or manipulation of the area (consider soft foods for lips)
Resume blood thinners after 24 to 48 hours
Consider follow-up examination at 2 to 4 weeks (touch-ups, evaluation)

Box 4. Adverse events of fillers

Minor local (temporary and present within days)

Discomfort, bruising, swelling, needle marks, incomplete correction

Problematic local

Hematoma, asymmetry, hypersensitivity, palpability in the skin, scarring, acneiform or milia reaction, hyperpigmentation, infection, extrusion or migration of the implant, neuropraxia, glabellar or perioral skin necrosis

Systemic

Vasovagal, blindness, systemic infection

and thus carry a risk of immunogenicity. Despite efforts to reduce the rate of antigenicity of bovine collagen with biochemical processing, there remains hypersensitivity potential, and allergy testing is required before use. HA is not species dependent and carries a much lower immunogenic potential. HA is currently derived from rooster combs or bacterial cultures. Xenogenic products remain the most popular fillers because of their high-use potential, years of successful experience, and forgiving side-effect profile. Analogous to autogenic and allogenic molecules, xenogenic fillers are resorbed over a period of months. This transient nature means repeated treatments are necessary, but problems are equally short-lived (Table 4).

Collagens

Collagen is a fibrous, extracellular, insoluble protein comprising a major component of connective tissues throughout the animal kingdom (Fig. 1). Injectable collagen consists of varying concentrations of highly purified bovine or human collagen. Bovine collagen is obtained from the skins of cattle. The herds are isolated and carefully controlled against contact with other animals, thus reducing the risk of viral or prion contamination [5]. Human-based collagens are obtained from cadavers or human fibroblastic cell culture grown in a controlled laboratory environment. Biochemical processing or cross-linking may reduce the antigenicity or the rate of proteolytic cleavage of the collagen molecule. An estimated 3% to 10% of patients develop an immunologic reaction to bovine collagen; however, a much smaller number actually manifests a clinically relevant response. Accordingly, two negative collagen test injections over a 4-week period are required prior to the use of bovine collagen. Approximately 3% of all patients tested will have a positive result [6], manifesting as a delayed-type hypersensitivity response. Bovine collagen still represents the "gold standard" injectable filler, against which all other implantable fillers are measured.

Zyderm and Zyplast are sterile, purified fibrillar suspensions of bovine collagen. The natural molecule is processed to remove most antigenic components while retaining the helical structure of the collagen fiber. The implant is injected into the dermis and, as the saline is lost, it forms a soft, cohesive network of fibers. Over months, host connective tissue cells grow into the network, giving it the texture and appearance of normal host tissue. There is also some suggestion that the inflammatory edematous response to the

foreign material may account for much of the augmentation noted with collagen implantation [7]. Over a period of weeks to months, the injected collagen material is detected as a foreign substance and degraded by collagenases and inflammatory cells. Studies have shown undetectable levels of collagen in the dermis of injected sites 3 months after delivery [8]. Accordingly, most patients require frequent reinjection to maintain clinical benefit.

Zyderm 1 contains 35 mg/mL of purified bovine dermal collagen, 3.5% collagen by weight. It is used to treat fine lines, wrinkles, and shallow scars. It should be injected to overcorrect by approximately 100%. Zyderm 2 contains 65 mg/mL of collagen, 6.5% collagen by weight. Having almost twice the collagen concentration, it is used to treat moderate lines, wrinkles, and scars. It should be injected to overcorrect by approximately 50%. Zyplast collagen is cross-linked with glutaraldehyde. It is 3.5% collagen by weight, but its latticework arrangement makes it more viscous than Zyderm 1 or 2, less immunogenic, and more resistant to proteolytic degradation. It is useful in treating deeper lines and scars. It should be injected without any overcorrection. Zyderm is often layered over Zyplast for longer lasting results.

Zyplast should be used with caution in the glabellar region because of the risk of local tissue necrosis and rare occurrence of blindness or arterial occlusion [9]. Zyplast or significant overcorrection with Zyderm should be avoided in areas of thin skin, such as the eyelids, because of the increased risk of beading. Bruising and overfilling are common complaints in the crow's-feet region; therefore, the needle should be just barely buried, and lots of massage should be provided in this site. A yellowish hue may be detected after treatment of fine perioral or periorbital lines. In most cases, this is not cosmetically bothersome.

Sensitivity reactions (1%–3%) and granulomatous (0.5%) responses have occurred in patients, even following a negative "double pretest" [6]. In the current authors' experience, time, reassurance, and 2.5 to 5 mg/mL of intralesional triamcinolone are usually successful in eliminating the reaction by 6 months. Other less common reactions include abscess formation and local tissue necrosis [10]. There has been no proven association between bovine collagen and autoimmune disease [11].

Patients receive an immediate, visible difference after the first treatment. Implants reportedly may last between 1 to 18 months, but in the authors' experience, reimplantation is usually required in approximately 3 to 6 months, especially in the most dynamic

Table 4
Xenogenic products

Molecule	Trade name[a]	Use	Durability	Technique	Advantages	Disadvantages	Approved
Bovine collagen	Zyderm 1: 3.5% dermal collagen	Superficial defects	3–4 mo	Papillary dermal injection, overcorrect 100%	Safe, reliable, user friendly, contains lidocaine	Allergic reaction rate of 1%–3%, short-lived correction, requires two prior skin tests	Yes: FDA and HPB for cosmetic use
	Zyderm 2: 6.5% collagen	Moderate depth defects, lip augmentation	3–6 mo	Mid-dermal delivery, 50% overcorrection	Safe, reliable, user friendly, contains lidocaine	Allergic reaction rate of 1–3%, short-lived correction, requires two prior skin tests	Yes: FDA and HPB for cosmetic use
	Zyplast: 3.5% cross-linked collagen	Deeper defects, lip augmentation	3–6 mo	Deep reticular dermis, no overcorrection, augmentation	Safe, reliable, user friendly, more viscous than Zyderm and more resistant to degradation, contains lidocaine	Can cause arterial occlusion if used in glabella, allergic reactions less than 3%, requires two prior skin tests	Yes: FDA and HPB for cosmetic use
Avian-derived hylan B gels	Hylaform (6 mg/mL), Hylaform gel (5.5 mg/mL)	Moderate depth defects, lip augmentation	4–6 mo	Mid-dermal delivery with 30-gauge needle, no overcorrection	Safe, reliable, user friendly, predictable results, no need for allergy testing	Temporary, rare immunologic reactions, contraindicated if allergic to avian products	Yes: FDA and HPB for cosmetic use
	Hylaform Fine Line	Superficial defects	3–6 mo	Superficial delivery with 30–32-gauge needle, no overcorrection	Safe, reliable, user friendly, predictable results, no need for allergy testing	Temporary, rare immunologic reactions, contraindicated if allergic to avian products	Yes: HPB cosmetic, not FDA approved
	Hylaform Plus	Deeper defects, lip augmentation	4–6 mo	Deep dermal delivery with 27-gauge needle, no overcorrection	Safe, reliable, user friendly, predictable results, no need for allergy testing	Temporary, rare immunologic reactions, contraindicated if allergic to avian products	Yes: HPB and FDA for cosmetic use

Bacterial cultured and stabilized hyaluronans	Restylane (20 mg/mL)	Moderate depth defects, lip augmentation	4–6 mo	Mid-dermal delivery with 30-gauge needle, no overcorrection	Safe, reliable, user friendly, predictable results, no need for allergy testing, evidence that it is longer lasting and safer than bovine collagen	Temporary, rare immunologic reactions	Yes: FDA and HPB for cosmetic use
	Restylane Finelines, Restylane Touch	Superficial defects	3–6 mo	Superficial delivery with 30-gauge needle, no overcorrection	Safe, reliable, user friendly, predictable results, no need for allergy testing	Temporary, rare immunologic reactions	Yes: HPB cosmetic, not FDA approved
	Perlane	Deeper defects, lip augmentation	4–6 mo	Deep dermal delivery with 27-gauge needle, no overcorrection	Safe, reliable, user friendly, predictable results, no need for allergy testing	Temporary, rare immunologic reactions	Yes: HPB cosmetic, not FDA approved
	Rofilan (Rofil)	Superficial defects, lip augmentation	4–6 mo	Superficial delivery with 30-gauge needle, no overcorrection	Safe, user friendly, predictable results, no need for allergy testing	Temporary, rare immunologic reactions, few studies done	Yes: HPB cosmetic, not FDA approved
	Juvederm 18, 24, and 30	18 (superficial), 24 (moderate), 30 (deeper defects)	3–6 mo	Deliver according to product viscosity	Safe, user friendly, predictable results, no need for allergy testing	Temporary, rare immunologic reactions, few studies done	Yes: HPB cosmetic, not FDA approved
Elastin and collagen	Endoplast 50	Deeper defects, lip augmentation	Up to 1 y	Mid-deep dermal injection	Longevity	Two allergy tests required, limited North American experience	No

[a] For a complete listing of fillers and manufacturers/distributors, see Table 9.

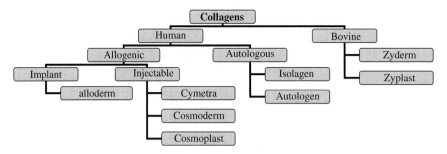

Fig. 1. Collagens.

regions. Two or more implant sessions, at intervals of at least 2 weeks, may be required to achieve the desired correction. The reproducible results combined with the extensive clinical experience with these products make them a comfortable and reliable choice for most soft tissue defects. The inconvenience associated with sensitivity testing and the short duration of correction limit their overall efficacy, however. More recently, bovine prion disease identification in North America has not helped reduce the anxiety associated with the use of animal products for surgical implantation.

Hyaluronic acid

Hyaluronan, also called hyaluronic acid (HA), is a component of all connective tissues and is abundant within the human dermis. It is a naturally occurring glycosaminoglycan biopolymer, which provides a fluid matrix or lattice on which collagen and elastic fibers may develop. The hydrophilic nature of HA attracts and maintains water within the extracellular space. It hydrates, lubricates, and stabilizes connective tissue, thus allowing cell movement and tissue remodeling [2]. The chemical structure is uniform throughout all living species, thus there is minimal chance of immunogenicity. HA is a large molecule, which forms a hydrated chain arrangement. The chains entangle and bind together at a relatively low concentration, imparting a highly elastoviscous quality.

As individuals age, the amount of HA decreases in their skin, with resultant loss of tissue hydration. Filling the skin with this molecule seems ideal, but it lasts only 1 to 2 days in the natural form because it is locally degraded and eventually metabolized to CO_2 and water in the liver. The challenge was to create a product with longevity, while maintaining low antigenicity and the natural beneficial properties of this matrix component.

Hylan B gels were developed in the mid-1980s, borne of the concept that the nonimmunologic, highly elastoviscous, hydrating, and space-occupying properties of hyaluronan would create the ideal filler. The material is extracted from rooster combs, and cross-links between the hydroxyl groups of the HA molecule are introduced to render the molecule more stable (less biodegradable) following injection [12]. The resultant polymer is insoluble, resistant to migration, and has greater elasticity than hyaluronan. Results from preclinical and human clinical studies found the product to be safe and efficacious for soft tissue augmentation. The isovolemic pattern of degradation occurs because of the increasing ability of the hyaluronan network to bind water over time. This enables HA products to retain greater volume for longer periods, as compared with bovine collagen products. Hylan B gels, such as Hylaform (Inamed), are manufactured in varying viscosities and are currently approved and distributed in Canada, Europe, and the United States.

Stabilized HA molecules are similar to hylan B gels but differ in their processing and product concentrations. Restylane (Q-Med) is more viscous and less elastic than Hylaform. In addition, Restylane has 20 mg/mL of HA, whereas Hylaform contains 5.5 mg/mL but is of higher molecular weight. Hylaform is extracted from rooster combs, whereas the Restylane product line is manufactured through bacterial fermentation. Restylane therefore has been called a non–animal-sourced HA.

Hyalform Fineline and Restylane Finelines are used in the treatment of superficial rhytids, whereas Hylaform and Restylane are useful for moderate to deep wrinkles. The greater viscosity of Hylaform Plus and Perlane allow their use for deeper lines and grooves, such as nasolabial folds and deep oral commissures. In general, compared with bovine collagen, the clinical effects and longevity of hyaluronan correction are similar. Restylane was compared with bovine collagen (Zyplast) in a recent randomized, double-blind study of 138 patients with prominent nasolabial folds and was shown to perform better than bovine collagen [13].

Hylaform and Restylane are supplied in preloaded syringes. One syringe of either is usually adequate for one treatment of moderately deep nasolabial folds or initial treatment of two lips. Skin testing is not required. HA gels have low viscosity at high shear rates, such as when forced through a needle, which make them favorable for injection. Warming the syringe in the hands before use has been reported to improve product flow [12]; however, the authors have not found this step to be clinically relevant. A 30-gauge, 1.2-cm needle is used with a threading technique in the dermis, with constant pressure on the syringe plunger as the needle is withdrawn. The more viscous hyaluronan products, if placed too superficially, can impart a bluish tinge to the treated area. The needle may be directed bevel-up for superficial delivery, but this is not essential to success. A plumping of the treatment area will be seen, and this should be followed by gentle massage of the area to smooth the implant and ensure that it is uniform. Successive threads are then laid down, until the entire area is treated. No overcorrection is required, which allows more accurate delivery of the desired augmentation. The current authors' approach is to have patients return for evaluation in 2 to 4 weeks after injection to assess if further product is required to achieve adequate results. The typical longevity of satisfactory correction is 4 to 6 months [14]; however, it is not unusual for patients to exhibit 7 to 9 months of augmentation.

HAs and particularly Restylane are especially useful in lip enhancement procedures. Before the procedure, a nerve or ring block is typically required. The lip margin is defined by injection just inside the vermillion border, in successive threadlike aliquots. Each lip margin may require five or six such threads. If placed properly, the needle will find a potential space allowing the product to flow smoothly. Personal preference will dictate whether the physician works from the commissure toward the philtrum, or the reverse. The lip must be stabilized firmly and uniformly to enable accurate placement. Approximately half the syringe is used for the lip margin. The other half is injected using the threading technique along the long axis of the "wet line" (the junction of the dry outer mucosa and the wet inner mucosa) of the lip. This step is followed by gentle massage. Postoperative swelling and bruising is a complication of lip enhancement that may be exacerbated by excessive tunneling. In some cases, edema may cause an immediate asymmetry between the right and left vermillion border. Correcting this asymmetry should be avoided because it tends to resolve on its own within a few hours. The triangular isthmus of the lip should be treated with a fan-shaped threading technique to uniformly fill the site.

Significant adverse events are uncommon and were recently reported to be less than 0.1% [15]. Unusual hypersensitivity [16] and granulomatous foreign body reactions [17] have been reported and observed by the authors. These reactions are characterized by recurrent erythematous nodules, which resolve spontaneously over several months. One case of arterial occlusion following glabellar injection was also reported [18]. In summary, immunologic reactions are rare and have not been associated with systemic adverse events.

Hyaluronic derivatives are safe and practical and eliminate the need for allergy testing. Both the Hylaform and Restylane product lines impart a natural texture and appearance to the skin. Overcorrection is not required, and the products are relatively straightforward to use by a trained physician. These products last longer than collagen products but are not permanent. Restylane has the advantage of containing no animal components and has been subjected to more extensive clinical evaluation than has Hylaform. HA derivatives fulfill many criteria of the ideal injectable filler and, when experience within the United States grows, may replace collagen as the gold-standard filler.

Autogenic products

The concept of using the patient's own tissue was introduced for several reasons. First, immunogenic reactions could be avoided. Second, the risk of microbial disease transmission could be reduced. Third, the injectable material is often available from the patient in ample supply. These factors were hoped to contribute to longer lasting and consistent results with limited adverse events. Their fundamental shortcoming is that they are impractical, requiring donor tissue harvesting and processing before the reimplantation stage. If the patient is considering liposuction or rhytidectomy, the harvesting is not a problem. Processing requires a series of steps that must ensure sterility and viability of the material. By and large, the results from autogenic fillers have not lived up to expectations. Fat transfer and dermal grafting have efficacy comparable to bovine collagen in the best hands but have unpredictable efficacy and complications. Similarly, cultured fibroblasts and collagens have great potential, but the lengthy

Table 5
Autologous products

Molecule	Use	Durability	Technique	Advantages	Disadvantages	Approved
Dermal graft	Moderate to deep defects	Months to years	Deep dermis is excised and implanted into pocket created at defect site	Safe, the concept makes sense	Limited supply, donor morbidity, unpredictable efficacy	No formal approval required
Viable fat	Deeper defects	Variable, several months, may last years with newer techniques	Harvested, washed and "microlipoinjection" with 14–25-gauge needle into subcutis or muscle, overcorrect 50%–100%	Abundant supply, safe, inexpensive, may last years	Donor site morbidity, variable results, processing required, viscous product	No formal approval required
Lipocyte dermal augmentation	Superficial to moderate defects	Several months	Harvested, processed, injected with 25–30-gauge needle into mid-dermis	Abundant supply, safe, inexpensive	Donor site morbidity, variable results, complex processing required	No formal approval required
Plasma (Fibrel)[a]	Moderate defects	Months to years	Pretest injection required, 30-gauge needle into mid-dermis	Potential for longevity	Not currently available from company	Yes
Cultured fibroblasts (Isolagen)[a]	Superficial to moderate defects	Months (up to 20 mo with 2–3 treatments)	3-mm punch taken from patient and processed (6 wk), test dose, injected mid to deep dermis 2 weeks after test	Safe, may be stored for future use	Costly, inconvenient, inconsistent results	No: FDA has asked for further testing because of the use of growth factors during culture
Collagen (Autolagen)[a]	Moderate to deep defects	Months to years	Processed (3–4 wk) from surgically excised skin, injected into mid-dermis	Can be stored up to 6 mo in fridge	Donor morbidity, painful, costly process, not currently available from company	Yes

[a] For a complete listing of fillers and manufacturers/distributors, see Table 9.

processing time and high cost make them less appealing for most applications (Table 5).

The term *autologous collagen* has been used to describe in vitro culture of autologous fibroblasts (Isolagen) [19], intact collagen fibers isolated from excised skin (Autologen) [7], or the process of separating extracted adipose tissue for reinjection of the fibrous components.

Autologous fat

Neuber [4] introduced the use of autologous fat for tissue augmentation in 1893. Cosmetic soft tissue augmentation occurred in 1910 by Lexer [20], but most surgeons were unable to duplicate these results, and its use declined until the late 1970s, paralleling the advent of liposuction. Over the years, this method's popularity has grown and the techniques have been refined, but there still remains no gold-standard method that ensures consistently successful outcomes. Various harvesting, processing, and delivery techniques have been described. Some propose to graft fat into a recipient site with the expectation of

long-term graft take. As such, little manipulation of the donor tissue would be anticipated to generate optimal long-term results [21]. Another approach is to aggressively process the fat to use only those components that trigger a local healing response and ultimate collagen production. In this method, the fat cells are nonviable, but rather, sources of an inflammatory response (Box 5).

The longest lasting results are seen when used for atrophic conditions, such as in scleroderma, postsurgical or traumatic atrophy, and depressed scars. Results when used for changes associated with aging are initially good, but there is a higher rate of resorption. Overall correction and duration approximate bovine collagen, although cases have been reported with viable augmentation of more than 7 years [22]. The nasolabial folds and nondynamic sites seem to do better than the lips or glabella. Adverse events, such as fat necrosis and clumping, are temporary but not uncommon. Rare side effects, such as local tissue necrosis and blindness, have been reported with glabellar injection [23].

Allogenic products

Similar to autologous tissue, human-based products have the advantage of high biocompatibility with low antigenicity. In comparison, allogenic sources provide a generous supply without donor site morbidity for the patient. Allogenic material is obtained from cadaveric dermis or fascia, or engineered using human cell lines. Donors have been screened with tests licensed by the FDA or Health Protection Branch of Health Canada (HPB) to rule out microbial disease. Cell lines used for tissue production are also tested for microbes, cell morphology, karyology, isoenzymes, and tumorigenicity. Each lot produced then undergoes further testing to ensure the product meets required specifications. In general, products harvested from cadaveric sources have been limited by their cost, practicality, and variable efficacy (Table 6).

Cosmoderm (1 and 2; Inamed) and Cosmoplast (Inamed) are tissue-engineered collagen implants derived from human fibroblastic cell culture. Cosmoderm 2 has almost twice the collagen concentration as Cosmoderm 1. Cosmoplast is cross-linked with glutaraldehyde to increase viscosity and longevity. These products are similar in indication and technique to the bovine collagens; however, no skin testing is required. In the authors' experience, although the flow characteristics are excellent, the longevity is less than with bovine collagens or HA products.

Box 5. Factors affecting fat cell viability

Epinephrine in local anesthesia has not been shown to decrease viability.

Blood in the transplanted fat accelerates degradation.

Harvesting method (syringe, liposuction, surgical harvest) does not influence results.

The donor site probably does not influence outcome.

If freezing fat, slow freezing to $-20°C$ is preferable to obtain viable adipocytes.

Centrifugation before separating fat fractions has not shown increased viability.

There is no known correlation between injection needle size and longevity.

The major factor that determines fat cell viability is the vascularity of the recipient site.

Data from Sommer B, Sattler G. Current concepts of fat graft survival: histology of aspirated adipose tissue and review of the literature. Dermatol Surg 2000;26: 1159–66.

Table 6
Allogenic products

Molecule	Trade name[a]	Use	Durability	Technique	Advantages	Disadvantages	Approved
Collagen derived from fibroblasts	Cosmoderm 1, 35 mg/mL collagen	Superficial defects, lip augmentation	3–4 mo	Papillary dermal injection, overcorrect 100%	No skin tests required, safety	Short-lived correction	Yes: FDA and HPB for cosmetic use
Collagen derived from fibroblasts	Cosmoplast, 35 mg/mL cross-linked collagen	Deeper defects, significant lip augmentation	3–4 mo	Deep reticular dermis or fat, no overcorrection	No skin tests required, safety	Short-lived correction	Yes: FDA and HPB for cosmetic use
Cadaveric collagen sheets	Alloderm	Deep rhytids or scars, lip augmentation	3–12 mo	Surgically implanted deeply using full sterile technique	No allergy testing, semi-invasive procedure	Swelling for a week, costly, palpability, shrinkage	Yes: FDA for cosmetic use
Cadaveric injectable collagen	Cymetra	Deep rhytids or scars, lip augmentation	3–4 mo	Injected into deep dermis or fat, overcorrect 25%	No allergy testing	Glabellar necrosis reported, clumps in needle, costly	Yes: FDA for cosmetic use
Cadaveric injectable collagen	Dermalogen	Moderate to deep defects	Months	Injected into mid-deep dermis	No allergy testing required, but many suggest one test	Costly, painful	Not available from manufacturer
Cadaveric implantable collagen	Dermaplant	Deep defects	Months	Injected deep dermis	No allergy testing	Inflammatory reactions, painful injection, costly	Not available from manufacturer
Cadaveric fascia lata	Fascian particulate	Deep rhytids or scars, lip augmentation	3–6 mo	Available in various sizes, rehydrate before use, anesthesia needed	Viscosity can be adjusted, no allergy testing	Tends to clump in needle, impractical, painful, limited evidence available	Yes: FDA for cosmetic use

[a] For a complete listing of fillers and manufacturers/distributors, see Table 9.

Synthetic products

Biologic products require a complex development process, generally provide transient correction, and contain a risk of antigenicity. Inert synthetic (alloplastic) agents may be identically mass-produced at a much lower cost and have the potential for permanent implantation. One of the first synthetic fillers was silicone. Reports of migration and granulomatous responses have prevented FDA approval of silicone as a filler and currently its use is off-label for cosmetic purposes. Other synthetic microsphere products have been approved, however, and are listed in Table 7. Hydrogels are polymers that draw water into the area. Polylactic acid, polyalkylamide, and polyacrylamide have been used as semipermanent dermal hydrogel fillers. Polytetrafluoroethylene (PTFE; Teflon) and expanded PTFE (e-PTFE; Goretex) have been used for permanent tissue augmentation.

Synthetic fillers offer the advantages of lower cost, consistent formulation, longevity, and limited hypersensitivity. Conversely, adverse events can be serious and enduring when they occur. Generally, synthetics are delivered into the deep dermis or below and require injection with larger bore needles or surgical implantation. The demand for a permanent means of correcting soft tissue defects has compelled the production of many synthetic options. Safer and more practical choices have become available recently, and the pipeline is rich with substitutes in the development stage of production (Table 7).

Polymethylmethacrylate

PMMA has been used for medical applications for more than 60 years. For example, as bone cement, PMMA has been used for 30 years in millions of patients without proven immunologic reaction or carcinogenicity. It is also used in ocular lenses, dental work, artificial joints, and pacemakers, and has been shown to be biocompatible and nondegradable. Lemperle [24] developed PMMA for cosmetic use. After reformulation to reduce inflammatory nodules, the product was named Artecoll. Artecoll received approval as the first permanent injectable dermal filler in Canada in 1998. In the United States, the FDA granted marketing approval in February 2003 for the product, which will be marketed under the trade name Artefill.

Artecoll consists of 25% PMMA microspheres suspended in a 3.5% bovine collagen solution (75%) containing lidocaine. The microspheres are characterized by surface smoothness and homogenicity

[24]. Their diameter of 30 of 40 μm is small enough to allow subdermal implantation using a 26-gauge needle. Phagocytosis and dislocation of the implant is theoretically limited by encapsulation with connective tissue. The atelocollagen, which serves as a delivery system for the PMMA, has been chemically modified to reduce antigenicity. The collagen is biodegraded over several weeks, whereas the PMMA remains in place. The microspheres induce tissue fibroblasts to encapsulate the foreign material, which results in a fixed fibrous stroma.

Artecoll is user-dependent, and the learning curve should be respected. The depth and volume of product administered is crucial for gradual and nodule-free augmentation with Artecoll to occur. Because of its high viscosity, a 26- to 27-gauge needle is used to deliver the product into the deep dermis-subcutaneous fat junction. It is important to avoid superficial placement, which will result in a beaded appearance. If blanching is noted, an aggressive and immediate kneading of the area to disperse the spheres is suggested. Deposition into muscle may cause nodule development [24]. Artecoll is administered using the tunneling technique. This approach uses the needle to create a space for injection with two to three small liposuction-styled movements, before approximately 0.1 mL of the filler is deposited on final withdrawal. Success may also be achieved with a single tunnel and withdrawal method [2]. This method is the authors' preferred technique. Overcorrection should be avoided. During treatment, if excessive pressure is required to inject the material, withdraw the needle, check to ensure the product is flowing freely, then reinsert along the same tunnel. Do not force the injection, because inadvertent placement of excessive product could result. Ensure accurate depth and direction of the tunnel is maintained along the entire length of the needle. This result is achieved by maintaining good skin fixation with the noninjecting hand. Some physicians describe immobilizing the site post injection to prevent nodule formation and product migration. In the authors' experience, this has not proved necessary or practical. Patients are asked to avoid excessive facial movements for 1 day and not manipulate the treated area. One 0.5-mL syringe will treat one deep melolabial fold, one lip for augmentation, or several mild to moderate rhytids. Second treatments generally use lesser volumes within the site, and the third or fourth visits should be an opportunity to fine-tune the correction.

The initial correction provided by the product slowly decreases as the collagen vehicle is degraded. Typically, 50% to 75% of immediate correction is

Table 7
Injectable synthetics

Molecule	Trade name[a]	Use	Durability	Technique	Advantages	Disadvantages	Approved
PLA	Sculptra (previously New-Fill)	HIV lipodystrophy, deep defects	Months to years	Deep injection	Longevity, PLA has long safety record as implant and suture material	Granulomas have been reported	Yes: FDA for HIV lipodystrophy, not HPV approved
Polyalkylamide	Bio-Alcamid	Deep defects, including lipodystrophy	Months to years	Deep injection	Potential for permanence	Untested in North America	No
Polyacrylamide	Argifom (Bioform)	Deep defects	Years	Deep injection	Potential for permanence	Untested in North America	No
Polyethylene beads	Profill	Deep defects	Months to years	Deep injection	Potential for permanence	Untested in North America	No
Acrylic hydrogel (40–65 μm) in HA carrier	Dermalive	Moderate defects	Months to years	Injected into deep dermis or superficial subcutis	Longevity, no allergy testing required	Granulomas have been reported	Yes: HPB, not FDA approved
Acrylic hydrogel (80–110 μm) in HA carrier	Dermadeep	Deep defects	Months to years	Injected into subcutis	Longevity, no allergy testing required	Granulomas have been reported	Yes: HPB, not FDA approved
Calcium hydroxlapatite microspheres	Radiesse, (previously Radiance FN)	Deep defects, lipodystrophy	2–5 y	Deep injection of small volumes	No allergy testing, shelf life 2 y, longevity	Nodules common, especially in lips	Off-label cosmetic, FDA for vocal cord surgery, oral/maxillofacial defects and radiographic marking

PMMA spheres in 3.5% bovine collagen carrier and 0.3% lidocaine	Artecoll Artefill	Deep defects, lip augmentation	Permanent, but 50% of initial correction resorbs	Deep placement of small volumes using serial puncture or threading	Permanence, long-term experience in Europe and Canada, safe, most problems are self-limited	Problems if placed superficially or in excess, FDA requires allergy testing (HPB does not), learning curve for injectors	Yes: HPD and preliminary FDA for cosmetic use
Dextran beads suspended in hylan gel	Reviderm Intra	Deep defects and lip augmentation	Months to 2 y	Deep injection of small volumes with a 30-gauge needle, no overcorrection	Longevity, safe, effective, practical	Limited North American experience, swelling for 4 d	Yes: HPB for cosmetic
Liquid silicone (1000 cs)	Silikon-1000	Deep defects and lip augmentation	Permanent	Deep injection of small volumes	Permanence, safe, effective, practical, years of clinical experience	Migration and inflammatory reactions, difficult to remove, hostile public opinion	Off-label cosmetic, FDA for retinal tamponade, not HPB approved
Silicone microparticles in a carrier gel	Bioplastique	Deep defects and lip augmentation	Permanent	Deep injection of small volumes	Permanence	Unproven in North America, migration reported	No

All products are problematic if delivered in excessive doses or superficially, and all are difficult to remove.

Abbreviation: PLA, polylactic acid.

[a] For a complete listing of fillers and manufacturers/distributors, see Table 9.

maintained long-term because of the permanence of the PMMA microspheres. Accordingly, patients should be advised that complete correction will require two to four treatment sessions, at intervals of 3 to 4 months. This time period allows resorption of the collagen and a more accurate assessment of the degree of permanent correction before retreatment. In addition, dynamic and gravity-dependent sites will continue to deepen naturally over time; therefore, patients should understand that touch-ups will be necessary to maintain optimal correction.

The most common side effects are related to the injection technique. The reported allergy rate with Artecoll collagen is 0.78% [2]. Although skin testing is not required by Health Canada, allergy testing to the collagen component is recommended by the manufacturer, and required by the FDA, 1 month before treatment. Although granuloma formation is a rare event, reported in less than 0.01% of patients, it is the most significant complication associated with Artecoll and may be delayed by several years. Nodules, hypertrophic scarring, and granulomas generally respond to intralesional corticosteroids [25]. In the authors' experience, multiple monthly treatments are required. More extensive cases of Artecoll granulomas also have been treated effectively with oral allopurinol [26]. Superficial ridging or beading is difficult to correct with steroid treatment, and excision may be required in these cases. Nodules can recur if excision of the product is incomplete.

Artecoll or Artefill offers the opportunity for long-lasting results for patients but is unforgiving of treatment errors. Complications are uncommon, but significant, and can happen to the most experienced injector. Slow correction over several sessions is the philosophy suggested by these authors.

Radiance

Calcium hydroxylapatite is the major mineral constituent of bone and has been used safely and effectively for more than a decade in reconstructive surgery and dentistry. More recently, its successful use in urologic surgery and vocal cord paralysis has sparked interest in this molecule for soft tissue augmentation. Radiance fine needle (FN) is composed of calcium hydroxylapatite microspheres (25–45 μm) suspended in an aqueous gel formulation. It has been FDA-approved for vocal cord surgery and is used off-label for soft tissue augmentation. It is packaged within a 1-cc syringe and can be used effectively with a 27-gauge needle. It does not require refrigeration or prior allergy testing.

The product is highly viscous, thus subdermal or intramuscular placement is recommended. Intradermal placement will predispose to nodule formation. Avoid delivery of the product as the needle is withdrawn to prevent intradermal placement. No overcorrection is required. The threading technique is effective for delivery. Patients often notice a throbbing sensation after injection, which resolves spontaneously. Conservative molding of the filler is suggested immediately after placement to even the correction. Side effects, such as granuloma and nodule formation, have been reported, especially with superficial placement or in the lips. In addition, Radiance is radiopaque and thus shows up on radiographs, but this situation has never been shown to be problematic.

Radiance shows promise, with early results suggesting that it may last years without migrating. The rate of nodule formation in the lips is 20%; therefore, its use in this site is not recommended [27]. Radiance FN seems to be most effective for the nasolabial folds, glabella, and tear trough. Like all new and more permanent fillers, the learning curve is steep and the adverse events unforgiving. This product should be approached with caution until longer term studies are available.

Silicone

Medical-grade silicone is an inert, clear, oily liquid derived from silica and composd of polymerized dimethylsiloxane [28]. Viscosity is graded in centistokes (cs); water viscosity is 1 cs, whereas Silikon-1000 (1000 cs; Alcon Laboratories) and Adatosil-5000 (5000 cs, Bausch and Lomb) are much more resistant to flow. Webster and Orentreich established the microdroplet technique in the 1980s. Minuscule volumes (0.01 cc) are injected with a 27- to 30-gauge needle into the deep dermis and fat with serial puncture. The silicone locally disperses in the tissue and becomes individually encapsulated by fibrous tissue over weeks. Undercorrection is imperative and repeat treatments at 4- to 12-week intervals will offer a steady correction to desired effect. The best outcomes are noted to feel more natural, compared with most permanent implants. In addition, the injection of silicone is user-friendly for the physician and an inexpensive alternative for patients. It also provides permanent augmentation and is associated with few adverse outcomes despite years of product use. Rarely, serious granulomatous reactions occur.

Table 8
Permanent (but reversible) expanded polytetrafluoroethylene implants

Formulation of e-PTFE	Trade name[a]	Advantages	Disadvantages	Approved
Low-porosity tubes	SoftForm	Long clinical experience. Easier to remove	Palpability, extrusions, unnatural feel	Yes: FDA and HPB for cosmetic
Higher porosity tubes	UltraSoft and UltraSoft-RC	Softer than low-porous products. UltraSoft-RC used for larger defects	Palpable and unnatural feel can occur. More difficult to remove?	Yes: FDA and HPB for cosmetic
Low-porosity sheets, strands, strings	Gore S.A.M.	Longest history of safety. Easier to remove. Available in various sizes	Palpability, extrusions, unnatural feel	Yes: FDA and HPB for cosmetic
Dual-porosity tubes	Advanta	Softer feel, less migration or extrusion? Available in various sizes	Difficult to remove? Limited long-term experience	Yes: FDA and HPB for cosmetic

All products are implanted deeply to correct deep defects and lip augmentation.
  [a] For a complete listing of fillers and manufacturers/distributors, see Table 9.

Most, but not all, result from misuse or adulteration of the product. Inflammatory reactions typically resolve spontaneously but may be unpredictable and result in considerable local and systemic morbidity [29,30]. In addition, its removal is often problematic, leading to further complications. Silicone is currently approved only for ophthalmic indications, and its off-label use remains at best controversial and at worst illegal in some states.

Expanded polytetrafluoroethylene

In 1971, William and Robert Gore created e-PTFE from PTFE (Teflon). The product was named Goretex, and its inert, strong, and flexible nature allowed it to be used safely in millions of vascular surgery procedures since the 1970s [31]. It was subsequently used off-label for cosmetic purposes and later approved for subdermal augmentation. The extent of tissue in-growth is determined by the pore size of the e-PTFE product. Less porous implants promote fixation through encapsulation but limit in-growth. This characteristic provides stability in mobile areas, while permitting removal if required. Products with higher porosity offer more integration with the tissue, less migration, and theoretically a softer feel. Goretex is solid and supplied as sheets, strips, strings, or tubes, which are surgically implanted. Gore Technologies manufactures Gore S.A.M. (subcutaneous augmentation material) for this purpose. Injectable forms are being developed, but none is available at this time.

Tubular forms of e-PTFE implants include Soft-form (Tissue Technologies.), Ultrasoft (Tissue Technologies), and Advanta (Atrium Medical). These products are used to augment lips, melolabial folds, and deep contour deficiencies. Further details regarding their application can be found elsewhere (Table 8) [32–35].

Summary

Options for soft tissue augmentation have increased substantially in the last few years. Despite new products entering the marketplace routinely, well-done clinical trials remain sparse. Although the quest for the perfect filler continues, the available assortment offers many satisfactory choices for each indication. Patients frequently have spent considerable time researching their options on the Internet or in the lay press; physicians therefore should have a thorough knowledge of the latest products available. Ideally, elective procedures should bear little risk of morbidity, and the outcomes should be predictably efficacious. These features should not be sacrificed for longevity.

It is prudent to gain experience with user-friendly and approved temporary products before performing less forgiving procedures. Products will have a different efficacy and side-effect profile in another physician's hands. It is therefore wise to acquire confidence with the use of a select number of fillers before widespread product usage. Most complications are secondary to the misuse of products. Slow and

Table 9
Filler companies

Company	Contact	Fillers
Alcon Laboratories	6201 South Freeway Fort Worth, Texas 76134, USA Tel.: (817) 551-8430 http://www.alconlabs.com	Silikon-1000
Artes Medical	4660 La Jolla Village Drive Suite 825 San Diego, California 92122, USA Tel.: (858) 550-9999 Fax: (858) 550-9997 http://www.artecoll-usa.com	Artecoll (USA) Artefill
Atrium Medical	5 Wentworth Drive Hudson, New Hampshire 03051, USA Tel.: (603) 880-1433 Fax: (603) 880-6718 http://www.atriummed.com	Advanta
Bausch & Lomb	One Bausch & Lomb Place Rochester, New York 14604-2701, USA Tel.: (585) 338-6000 Fax: (585) 338-6007 http://www.bausch.com	Adatosil-5000
Bioform	Krasnobogatyrskay Street 42/1103 Moscow, Russia Tel./fax: +7-(095)-161-0524/161-0537 http://www.bioform.ru	Argiform Farmacryl
Bioform Medical	4133 Courtney Road Suite 10 Franksville, Wisconsin 53126, USA Tel.: (262) 835.9800 Fax: (262) 835.9311 http://www.bioforminc.com	Radiesse
Canderm Pharma	5353 Thimens St-Laurent, QC H4R 2H4, Canada Tel.: (514) 334-3835 Fax: (514) 334-7078 http://www.canderm.com	Artecoll (Canada)
Collagenesis	500 Cummings centre Suite 464-C Beverly, Massachusetts 01915, USA Tel: (508) 232-0333 Fax: (978) 232-9601	Autologen Dermalogen
Dermatech S.A.R.L	10 rue Saint Claude 75003 Paris, France	Dermadeep (international) Dermalive
Dermik (A Division of Aventis Pharmaceuticals)	1050 Westlakes Drive Berwyn, Pennsylvania 19312, USA Toll-free: (800) 981-2491 http://www.aventis.com	Sculptra

(continued on next page)

Table 9 (*continued*)

Company	Contact	Fillers
Fascia Biosystems	9663 Santa Monica Boulevard PMB 840 Beverly Hills, California 90210, USA Tel.: (888) 332-7242 http://www.fascian.com	Fascian
Inamed	5540 Ekwill Street Santa Barbara, California, USA 93111 Tel.: (805) 683-6761 Fax: (805) 692-5432 http://www.inamedaesthetics.com	Cosmoderm 1 Cosmoplast Hylaform Hylaform Fine Line Hylaform Plus Juvederm (Canada) Zyderm 1 Zyderm 2
Intradermal Distribution	P.O. Box 1071 Hudson, QC J0P 1H0, Canada Toll-free: (888) 458-8673 Tel.: (450) 455-9779 http://www.intradermaldistribution.com/index.htm	Dermadeep (Canada) Dermalive
Isolagen Technologies	2500 Wilcrest 5th Floor Houston, Texas 77042, USA Tel.: (713) 780-4754 Fax: (713) 781-9396 http://www.isolagen.com	Isolagen
Laboratories Filorgra	Paris, France	Endoplast 50
L.E.A. Derm	28, rue Caumartin 75009 Paris, France Tel.: +1-49240686 http://www.leaderm.com	Juvederm (international)
Lifecell	One Millennium Way Branchburg, New Jersey 08876-3876, USA Tel.: (908) 947-1100 http://www.lifecell.com	Alloderm Cymetra
Medicis Aesthetics Canada	355 McCaffrey Montreal, QC H4T 1Z7, Canada Tel.: (866) 551-5567	Perlane (Canada) Restylane Restylane Finelines Restylane Touch
Medicis Aesthetics USA	8125 North Hayden Road Scottsdale, Arizona 85258-2463, USA http://www.q-medesthetics.com	Restylane (USA)
Mentor	600 Pine Avenue Goleta, California 93117, USA Toll-free: (800) 235-5731	Fibrel
Polymekon Research	Via Savona 19/a 20144 Milano, Italy http://www.polymekonresearch.com	Bio-Alcamid

(continued on next page)

Table 9 (*continued*)

Company	Contact	Fillers
Q-Med	Seminariegatan 21 SA 75228 Uppsala, Sweden Tel: +46-18-504-210 http://www.q-medesthetics.com	Perlane Restylane Restylane Finelines Restylane Touch
Rofil Medical International	Heusing 16 4817 ZB Breda, The Netherlands Tel.: +31-(0)-76 5315670 Fax: +31-(0)-76 5315660 http://www.rofil.com	Artecoll (international) Resoplast Reviderm Intra Rofilan
Tissue Technologies	1612 Union Street San Francisco, California 94123, USA Toll-free: (866) 349-3223 Tel.: (415) 771-7960 Fax: (415) 771-1387 http://www.tissuetechnologies.com	SoftForm UltraSoft UltraSoft-RC
Uroplasty BV	Hofkamp 2 6161 DC, Geleen, The Netherlands Tel.: +31-(0)-464237920 Fax: +31-(0)-464237922	Bioplastique
W.L. Gore & Associates	Medical Products Division Flagstaff, Arizona 86003-2400, USA Toll-free: (800) 437-8181 Tel.: (928) 779-2771 http://www.goremedical.com	GORE S.A.M.

steady correction provides the safest means of achieving the best results. Reporting complications in peer-reviewed journals and informal meetings will lead to a safer environment for patients and physicians (Table 9).

References

[1] Dzubow LM, Goldman G. Introduction to soft tissue augmentation: a historical perspective. In: Klein AW, editor. Tissue augmentation in clinical practice: procedures and techniques. New York: Marcel Dekker; 1998. p. 1–22.

[2] Pollack SV. Some new injectable dermal filler materials: Hylaform, Restylane, and Artecoll. J Cutan Med Surg 1999;3:S4–27.

[3] Klein AW, Elson ML. The history of substances for soft tissue augmentation. Dermatol Surg 2000;26: 1096–105.

[4] Neuber F. Fettransplantation [in German]. Chir Kongr Verhandl Dsch Gesellch Chir 1893;22:66.

[5] Carruthers J, Carruthers A. Mad cows, prions, and wrinkles. Arch Dermatol 2002;138:667–70.

[6] Cooperman LS, Mackinnon V, Bechler G, Pharriss BB. Injectable collagen: a six-year clinical investigation. Aesthetic Plast Surg 1985;9:145–51.

[7] Fagien S. Facial soft tissue augmentation with autologous and homologous injectable collagen (Autologen and Dermalogen). In: Klein AW, editor. Tissue augmentation in clinical practice: procedures and techniques. New York: Marcel Dekker; 1998. p. 97–124.

[8] Robinson JK, Hanke CW. Injectable collagen implant: histopathologic identification and longevity of correction. J Dermatol Surg Oncol 1985;11:124–30.

[9] Cucin RL, Barek D. Complications of injectable collagen implants. Plast Reconstr Surg 1983;71:731.

[10] Hanke CW, Hingley HR, Jolivette DM, et al. Abscess formation and local necrosis after treatment with Zyderm or Zyplast collagen implant. J Am Acad Dermatol 1991;25:319–26.

[11] Elson ML. Injectable collagen and autoimmune disease. J Dermatol Surg Oncol 1993;19:165–8.

[12] Duranti F, Salti G, Bovani B, Calandra M, Rosati ML. Injectable hyaluronic acid gel for soft tissue augmentation: a clinical and histological study. Dermatol Surg 1998;24:1317–25.

[13] Narins RS, Brandt F, Leydon J, Lorenc ZP, Rubin M, Smith S. A randomized, double-blind, multicenter comparison of the efficacy and tolerability of Resty-

lane versus Zyplast for the correction of nasolabial folds. Dermatol Surg 2003;29:588–95.

[14] Olenius M. The first clinical study using a new biodegradable implant for the treatment of lips, wrinkles, and folds. Aesthetic Plast Surg 1998;22:97–101.

[15] Friedman PM, Mafong EA, Kauvar AN, Geronemus RG. Safety data of injectable nonanimal stabilized hyaluronic acid gel for soft tissue augmentation. Dermatol Surg 2002;28:491–4.

[16] Lowe NJ, Maxwell CA, Lowe P, Duick MG, Shah K. Hyaluronic acid skin fillers: adverse reactions and skin testing. J Am Acad Dermatol 2001;45:930–3.

[17] Lupton JR, Alster TS. Cutaneous hypersensitivity to injectable hyaluronic acid gel. Dermatol Surg 2000; 26:135–7.

[18] Schanz S, Schippert W, Ulmer A, Rassner G, Fierlbeck G. Arterial embolization caused by injection of hyaluronic acid (Restylane). Br J Dermatol 2002;146: 928–9.

[19] Boss WK, Marko O. Isolagen. In: Klein AW, editor. Tissue augmentation in clinical practice: procedures and techniques. New York: Marcel Dekker; 1998. p. 335–47.

[20] Lexer E. Euber freie fettransplantation [in German]. Klin Ther Wehnscher 1911;18:53.

[21] Niechajev I, Sevcuk O. Long-term results of fat transplantation. Plast Reconstr Surg 1994;94:496–506.

[22] Sommer B, Sattler G. Current concepts of fat graft survival: histology of aspirated adipose tissue and review of the literature. Dermatol Surg 2000;26:1159–66.

[23] Teimourian B. Blindness following fat injections [letter]. Plast Reconstr Surg 1988;82:361.

[24] Lemperle G, Gauthier-Hazan N, Lemperle M. PMMA-microspheres for long-lasting correction of wrinkles: refinements and statistical results. Aesthetic Plast Surg 1998;22:356–65.

[25] Kim KJ, Lee HW, Lee MW, Choi JH, Moon KC, Koh JK. Artecoll granuloma: a rare reaction induced by microimplant in the treatment of neck wrinkles. Dermatol Surg 2004;30:545–7.

[26] Reisberger EM, Landthaler M, Wiest L, Schroder J, Stolz W. Foreign body granulomas caused by polymethylmethacrylate microspheres: successful treatment with allopurinol. Arch Dermatol 2003;139:17–20.

[27] Sklar JA, White SM, Radiance FN. A new soft tissue filler. Dermatol Surg 2004;30:764–8.

[28] Duffy DM. Injectable liquid silicone: new perspectives. In: Klein AW, editor. Tissue augmentation in clinical practice: procedures and techniques. New York: Marcel Dekker; 1998. p. 237–67.

[29] Ellenbogen R, Rubin L. Injectable fluid silicone therapy: human morbidity and mortality. JAMA 1975; 234:308–9.

[30] Rapaport MJ, Vinnik C, Zarem H. Injectable silicone: cause of facial nodules, cellulites, ulceration and migration. Aesthetic Plast Surg 1996;20:267–76.

[31] Soyer T, Lempinen M, Cooper P, Norton L, Eiseman B. A new venous prosthesis. Surgery 1972;72(6):864–72.

[32] Wall SJ, Adamson PA, Bailey D, van Nostrand AW. Patient satisfaction with expanded polytetrafluoroethylene (Softform) implants to the perioral region. Arch Facial Plast Surg 2003;5:320–4.

[33] Truswell WH. Dual-porosity expanded polytetrafluoroethylene soft tissue implant: a new implant for facial soft tissue augmentation. Arch Facial Plast Surg 2002;4:92–7.

[34] Hanke CW. A new ePTFE soft tissue implant for natural-looking augmentation of lips and wrinkles. Dermatol Surg 2002;28:901–8.

[35] Maas CS, Spiegel J, Greene D. ePTFE (Softform) augmentation of folds and wrinkles. In: Klein AW, editor. Tissue augmentation in clinical practice: procedures and techniques. New York: Marcel Dekker; 1998. p. 191–205.

ELSEVIER
SAUNDERS

Dermatol Clin 23 (2005) 365 – 371

DERMATOLOGIC
CLINICS

Current Therapy

A Conservative Approach to the Nonsurgical Rejuvenation of the Face

Marsha L. Gordon, MD

Department of Dermatology, Mount Sinai School of Medicine, 5 East 98th Street, 5th Floor, Box 1048,
New York, NY 10029, USA

With ever-increasing frequency, dermatology patients are requesting information and treatments that improve the appearance of their skin. Corresponding to this trend, there is an ever-increasing number of products and procedures available that claim to aid in this pursuit. Finding a suitable regimen is a challenge for patients and physicians alike. Patients desire prompt improvement, whereas clinicians require safety and efficacy. Is there a right or a wrong way? In fact, there are nearly as many approaches as there are physicians in this field. Many different approaches may be helpful. This article outlines one general approach to choosing effective and safe treatments and procedures.

In broad terms, treatment may be divided into two categories: topical care and procedures. Topical care includes a cleansing-exfoliating, moisturizing, and sun protection regimen, and the use of therapeutic creams or gels. *Procedures* refers to office-based treatments, such as the injection of tissue-augmenting fillers and botulinum toxin, and peels. This article is limited to the discussion of Food and Drug Administration (FDA)–approved procedures (along with off-label uses) and does not discuss surgical procedure options or device-driven procedures, such as laser treatments.

Before embarking on any treatment plan, it is essential to understand the needs and wishes of the patient. Although the physician often sees where the obvious problems are and which therapeutic options are most helpful, the initial conversation about cosmetic issues must be guided by the patient. Begin

the consultation with a simple open-ended question that elicits which concerns have prompted the office visit, such as "What can we do for you today?" Offering the patient a mirror in which he or she can point out problem areas is another useful technique. If the patient points to a specific area or problem, that is the jumping-off point of the consultation. If the patient expresses general dissatisfaction, the physician is being invited to proceed as he or she sees fit. First-time patients often feel nervous or awkward and want to start slowly with one problem at a time. If the problem is correctible, starting slowly can nurture trust and comfort on the part of the patient such that, in time, the physician may be able to expand the breadth of the treatment appropriately. Very often a consultation that begins with a specific issue, such as one disturbing facial line or area, may progress to a complete discussion of all problems during the first or second office visit. In all cases, at some point it is necessary to discuss both topical care and available procedures.

Topical care

Cleansing

Proper cleansing of the face is essential. This means gentle, but effective cleansing. Patients often express the concern that cleansing is drying and irritating and should be avoided. Some *cleanse* with water alone.

Harsh surfactants and the high pH of some cleansers can lead to damage of skin proteins and

E-mail address: marsha.gordon@mssm.edu

lipids [1] causing the tight, dry, and uncomfortable postwash feeling patients describe. Patients must understand that foundation makeup [2] and airborne pollutants [3] may be irritating to the skin and that cleansers have been formulated to be gentle and compatible with almost every skin type.

For most people, the nonsoap synthetic detergent cleansers are effective and nonirritating. These formulations, available from most cosmetic companies, are soap free, contain *mild* surfactants, and are engineered to have a pH near that of the skin so they do not feel as drying or irritating as soap. Both foaming and nonfoaming varieties exist. The foaming formulations tend to be slightly more astringent (able to lift more dirt, debris, and oil). The nonfoaming formulations are milder and useful for sensitive skin types. Some formulations actually contain emollients, which are delivered to the skin during washing.

For those with extremely dry or sensitive skin, wipe-off cleansers and cold creams are available. At the other end of the spectrum, those with oilier skin may prefer an exfoliating cleanser, formulated with salicylic acid or an alpha hydroxy acid. One must remember that an exfoliating topical therapeutic preparation will most likely be added. Because the goal is to rejuvenate, not to irritate, a good general rule for cleansers is to go as mild and as gentle as possible.

Many patients wish to use a toner or astringent. These can be useful in moderation and damaging when used to excess. Toner does not need to be used daily. The frequency of use is determined by the dryness or oiliness of the skin and the ambient humidity. Again, gentle care must be stressed. Some patients think that if they can just exfoliate enough of the top layer away, they will reveal the younger skin underneath. They forget that aggressive exfoliation only irritates their skin. In the author's opinion, after application, toner should be splashed off with water to further remove oil and debris that the toner has dislodged, and to remove the toner fluid itself from the face. Granular scrubs, which have the potential to be irritating, should be used with great care.

Moisturizing

The topic of moisturizing is one that is fraught with confusion. Many people believe that moisturizing is the key to the fountain of youth. Properly moisturized skin feels good to most people and looks better than dry skin. Additionally, the daily application of a moisturizing cream is effective in improving mild subclinical inflammation of the face in winter [4]. There is disagreement in the literature, however, about the long-term effects of moisturizing the skin. Some authors have found that moisturizers prevent irritant skin reactions and improve barrier function [5]. Others have suggested that long treatment with moisturizers on normal skin may increase susceptibility to irritants. [6]. Specifics of the moisturizing formulations may account for these disparate reports. Emulsifiers in some formulations may weaken the skin barrier function, whereas other ingredients, such as petrolatum, have a barrier-repairing effect [7]. Ceramide and urea ingredients may also be helpful.

Therapeutic ingredients in over-the-counter moisturizers may improve the appearance of the skin, but none of these ingredients have been unequivocally proved to do so in good scientific studies. Sun protection, avoidance of cigarette smoke, certain retinoid creams (discussed later), good nutrition, and the procedures described later help prevent and treat aging changes of the skin. I give patients free reign on their choice of moisturizers, as long as they are not irritating and do not discourage the patient from using a great sunscreen every day.

Sun protection

Excellent sun protection is essential. Ultraviolet irradiation reduces production of type I procollagen, the major structural protein in human skin [8]. Patients must understand that chronic low-dose irradiation by the sun adds up. A surprising number of patients do not understand that daily exposure to sun as they go to work and run their errands is damaging. Patients arrive at the dermatologist's office without sunscreen, explaining that they had not been in the sun that day. (I ask them how they got to the office.) In fact, evidence suggests that chronic low-dose ultraviolet (UV) exposure is likely to cause wrinkles [9]. People who are interested in turning back the clock of photoaging must use excellent sun protection every day.

It is essential to protect against both UV rays B and A (UVB and UVA) radiation. The sun protection factor (SPF) is more a measure of UVB protection than UVA protection. There is not a good standardized numerical measurement of UVA radiation in the United States. Patients are advised to choose a sunscreen with a high SPF number (SPF 15 is adequate, but higher is better) and, additionally, they are instructed to read the active ingredient list to be sure that the product contains one of the better UVA-shielding ingredients. At the moment, there is not a perfect UVA-protecting sunscreen ingredient available. For this reason, sunscreen alone is imperfect sun protection and an adequate sun protection program also requires the use of protective clothing, hats, and sun avoidance when possible. Titanium dioxide, micronized zinc, and avobenzone are good UVA-protecting ingredients to look for. Newer UVA protecting ingredients may be approved by the FDA in upcoming years.

Therapeutic creams

Many creams and cream ingredients purport to be therapeutic and antiaging. Only tretinoin and tazarotene, however, have been FDA approved for this purpose. Although it is quite possible that some, if not many, of the non-FDA products have antiaging properties, it is impossible to really know what is being recommended in this area. For this reason, I always start by recommending one of the FDA-approved ingredients and only move on to over-the-counter products if effectiveness or tolerability becomes a problem.

Both tretinoin (Retin-A, Renova, and others) and tazarotene (Tazarac, Avage) significantly improve mottled hyperpigmentation and fine wrinkles [10,11]. Concern about facial irritation is an important deterrent to use among both patients and physicians. To minimize this problem, patients may be started on a relatively mild formulation, such as tretinoin 0.02% cream (Renova 0.02% cream). If this concentration is irritating, patients may reduce application frequency to every other evening or twice weekly. With regular use, many patients become *used to* the retinoids and can tolerated increased frequency of application and stronger preparations over time. The patient who starts with tretinoin 0.02% cream nightly might expect to tolerate tretinoin 0.05% cream by the time they are ready for another prescription. Some patients, however, are not able to progress in strength. For these patients, I use the highest concentration that can be tolerated without significant irritation.

Procedures

Temporary augmenting and filling agents

Beginning in the early to mid-1980s, bovine collagen became widely available for the temporary filling of facial wrinkles. This relatively simple and quick office procedure heralded the age of the *lunchtime* procedure trend.

Bovine collagen is available in several formulations (Box 1). Zyderm 1 and Zyderm 2 (Zyderm 2

Box 1. Partial list of temporary dermal fillers

Collagen

   Bovine collagen
     Zyderm 1
     Zyderm 2
     Zyplast

   Human-based collagen
     Cosmoderm
     Cosmoplast

Hyaluronic acid

     Restylane
     Hylaform
     Hylaform Plus

Others

     Poly-L-lactic acid
     Calcium hydroxylapatite

---

contains almost twice the collagen concentration of Zyderm 1) are useful for fine lines. Zyplast, a glutaraldehyde cross-linked preparation, is best for improving the contour of deeper lines and folds. Both contain 0.3% lidocaine. These preparations are still used successfully today. Because of rare allergic reactions, however, patients must be allergy tested to these materials. Test collagen tubes are provided for this purpose. It is recommended that two tests be performed, approximately 3 weeks apart, and that treatment with a bovine product not begin until 3 to 4 weeks after the second allergy test has been placed, to minimize the occurrence of allergic reaction once the material has been placed in the facial skin.

An additional drawback to the use of these products is their bovine derivation. Although the manufacturer has gone to great lengths to ensure the safety and sterility of the product and there is every reason to believe that these materials are free from infectious diseases or prions, there is a lingering doubt in the mind of some patients.

Because it eliminated the time consuming nuisance of allergy testing and because it is not a bovine product, human-based collagen (Cosmoderm and Cosmoplast) has been well received. As with the bovine products, both a cross-linked formulation

(Cosmplast) for deeper folds and a non–cross-linked preparation (Cosmoderm) are available. These products became a favorite among first-time patients who wanted immediate improvement without the 4- to 6-week wait for allergy testing.

Although human collagen largely eliminated the problem of allergic reaction, the collagen fillers in general have two other clinically relevant issues. One is the concern about autoimmune disease [12,13]. Although the collagen products ultimately have not been linked to the development or exacerbation of autoimmune diseases, such as lupus or dermatomyositis and polymyositis [14], concern in this regard limits their use in patients with these conditions. Autoimmune diseases tend to wax and wane over time. As a result, most physicians hesitate to inject these products into patients with such autoimmune diseases for fear that injection might be blamed for an unrelated disease flare.

The other major drawback is the lifespan in terms of clinical improvement. In the author's experience, most patients need to return in about 3 months for follow-up treatment. Although some fortunate individuals have longer time intervals between treatments, others must return as often as monthly for touch-ups to maintain the appearance that they want. The relatively minor side effects of bruising, redness, and swelling, seen after injection of the collagen products, tend to resolve in several days and are rarely of clinical significance.

Injectable hyaluronic acid products are an answer to several of the problems and concerns listed previously. They have not been linked to autoimmune disease. Although there is always the possibility of allergy, the incidence of allergic reactions to the FDA-approved hyaluronic acid products is so low that no allergy testing is required. It seems that correction using these products lasts longer in many individuals than correction with the collagen products.

Three hyaluronic acid products have been approved by the FDA for the correction of moderate to severe facial wrinkles and folds, such as nasolabial folds. Restlyane, which was approved in December 2003, is not animal derived (it is generated by *Streptococcus* species of bacteria). Hylaform, approved in April 2004, is derived from rooster combs and so the patient must not have an allergy to avian products. Hylaform Plus was approved in October 2004. None of these products contain lidocaine. Although they were not approved for this purpose, the hyaluronic acid products are often used for augmenting thin lips and for restoring the natural convex contour of the chin, which often looses subcutaneous tissue over time. Of note, when the chin has lost some of the

substance of its subcutaneous tissue, it is no longer able to bolster up the corners of the mouth. This is partially responsible for the down-turned appearance of the lateral lips and for the formation of marionette lines. These cosmetic problems can be improved with the approved hyaluronic acid product. Hyaluronic acid can also be used to restore the fullness of the cheek when the buccal fat pad has been displaced and may even enhance the appearance of the malar prominence to make a higher or more dramatic *cheek bone*.

Formulations of hyaluronic acid available elsewhere but not yet approved by the FDA include Perlane, which is a more robust product that is especially useful for restoring contour defects and is reported to last 8 to 18 months [15], and Fine Line Restlyane, which is expected to fill some of the finer superficial lines not addressed with the currently approved hyaluronic acid products.

As with collagen, temporary local bruising, erythema, and edema may be expected after treatment. These reactions may be more pronounced with hyaluronic acid than with collagen. Although they usually resolve in a day or two, they may persist for up to a week. Rare allergic reactions have also been reported. Lumpiness, which has been described as a problem with these products, largely has to do with product placement. If the material is carefully placed, lumps may be kept to a minimum. Additionally, small lumps may be massaged smooth by the physician immediately after injection.

The decision to use a collagen or a hyaluronic acid product is a complex one. It is the author's experience that the hyaluronic acid products provide a soft, natural, and longer-lasting improvement. At the moment, however, one of the collagen products (Zyderm or Cosmoderm) is necessary for fine lines and the collagen products may be preferred overall in selected patients. Some patients with more deeply lined faces and *crepe paper*–type skin do better with collagen implants. Others request collagen because of the incorporated lidocaine. With regard to lip augmentation, collagen may be preferable in certain patients, both because of the lidocaine and because some patients report longer-lasting results with collagen in this area. In fact, there are subsets of patients who clearly prefer the result they obtain with the collagen products and only trial and error can determine which patient falls into which category.

The FDA recently approved poly-L-lactic acid (Sculptra) for the correction of HIV-related facial lipoatrophy. Outside of the United States, poly-L-lactic acid has been used as a cosmetic filling agent for years and it can be expected that physicians will use this product for similar off-label uses in the United States. Although correction may last for 1 to 2 years, the development of granulomas, especially in the perioral area, has been reported [16] and is of concern. Further experience with this product is necessary before determining if and how poly-L-lactic acid might be incorporated into the cosmetic dermatology armamentarium.

Calcium hydroxylapatite-based implants have been used for noncosmetic purposes for years and are now being used as a cosmetic tissue augmenting agent (Radiesse). Again, further studies and experience are needed to determine the safely and efficacy of this product for cosmetic use [17].

Botulinum neurotoxin

Botulinum neurotoxin is a paralyzing agent. It has been approved by the FDA for weakening or paralyzing the corrugator supercilii and procerus muscles, which cause the glabellar frown lines. Its cosmetic functions, however, also include off-label use for softening of the horizontal forehead lines, crow's feet, and perioral *smile lines*; elevation of the eyebrows and lateral corners of the mouth; smoothing the *peau d'orange* appearance of the chin; and softening of the platysmal bands of the neck.

Botulinum toxin type A (Botox Cosmetic) comes available as a vacuum-dried complex of the neurotoxin and several accessory proteins, and human albumin and sodium chloride. It is reconstituted by the physician. The package insert instructs reconstitution with 0.9% sterile, nonpreserved saline (100 units in 2.5 mL saline). A wide range of dilutions, however, have been used. The author reconstitutes with 2 mL. Some physicians have suggested that bacteriostatic water is less painful than nonpreserved saline because of the partial numbing effect of the benzyl alcohol preservative [18]. It has also been said that vigorous turbulence during reconstitution may decrease the effectiveness of the material. The diluent should be injected somewhat slowly into the vial, which should be gently swirled to dissolve the toxin. Before injecting botulinum toxin, a careful history should be taken to rule out possible complicating neurologic problems or the ingestion of medications that may potentiate the effect of the toxin.

Many techniques have been described and are still being developed for the administration of Botox. In terms of treating the glabellar frown complex, it is important to weaken both the procerus and the corrugator muscles. To begin with, between 4 and 10 U (usually 5 to 7.5 U) can be given in one or two injection sites to the procerus. Weakening this muscle has the double effect of partially improving the frown line and allowing for a small elevation of the medial brow. As for the corrugator, the base should be injected with 3 to 5 U. The belly may also be injected with an additional 2 to 4 U. Asking the patient to make a frown allows the physician to place the injection at the site of maximal muscle contraction. As the patient frowns, it becomes obvious that fibers of the corrugator stretch upward and laterally in a diagonal across the forehead. These fibers can also be weakened by injecting small quantities (approximately 2 U) in three to four sites (each approximately 1.5 cm apart) in a diagonal upward and outward across the forehead. These injections also partially treat the frontalis muscle and the horizontal forehead lines. If the angle of injections is approximately 45 degrees upward and outward from the center of the brow toward the upper temple, and small quantities are used, this should not depress the brow in most cases. Botox diffuses between 1 and 1.5 cm from the site of injection. For this reason, injections should be kept 1 to 2 cm above the mid-lateral brow to reduce the risk of brow ptosis.

Diffusion from a full frown treatment allows partial treatment of the frontalis muscle, softening the horizontal forehead lines. (Note that treating only the frontalis and not the glabellar frown complex somewhat increases the risk of eyebrow ptosis.) The number of additional units injected into the upper frontalis after full treatment of the frown lines is less than expected. Often 7.5 to 15 U given in small aliquots over the upper frontalis is sufficient. Be sure to ask the patient to raise their brows so that injections can be given into the areas of maximal contracture. Watch where the patient engages the lateral aspect of the frontalis and inject 1 to 2 U there (at least 2 cm above the eyebrow) to prevent the so-called *quizzical look* of an overly raised or arched lateral brow.

Weakening the depressor aspect of the orbicularis oculi muscle provides the double improvement of softening the crow's feet and raising the lateral brow. Between 7.5 and 15 U may be injected just outside the orbital rim in three to five injection sites. Sometimes, treating the crow's feet results in a new line forming just below the treated area. This is a tricky problem, because injecting too low on the cheek may cause diffusion into the zygomaticus muscles. Asking the patient to smile deeply and injecting just 1 U into the most inferior lateral line, however, may partially soften this line.

Injecting botulinum toxin into the lower aspect of the face must be done with great caution. Softening of the perioral lines may be achieved by injecting 1 to 2 U in two to four sites just outside (onto the cutaneous surface) of the upper and lower vermilion borders. Be sure not to inject into the Cupid's bow, because this may flatten that area. Also, be sure to undertreat initially because overtreatment may cause functional difficulties.

The depressor anguli oris muscle may be injected with 2.5 to 5 U of botulinum neurotoxin to induce an upturn of the lateral lips in some patients. Platysmal bands of the neck may also be improved with botulinum neurotoxin. Because of concern for functional problems here, start with a modest dose of 2 to 2.5 U injected into three to five sites vertically along each of the two major bands. If the platysma is particularly contracted in one area, an extra injection may be placed there. The dose may be increased in subsequent visits if improvement without any functional difficulties is reported. One may also inject 2 U horizontally in three to five sites along the horizontal lines of the neck, although that is not always helpful.

A good rule of thumb for first time botulinum toxin patients is to slightly undertreat. This allows the patient to get used to the new look and feel. Additionally, because rare patients are exquisitely sensitive to the toxin, it reduces the risk of functional and cosmetic problems. At the follow-up appointment, more toxin can be given if and where needed. Keep precise notes of injection sites and dosages so that future treatments may be fully accomplished in one visit.

The author recommends that the patient remain upright and does not physically manipulate the treated area for 4 hours after treatment. This may reduce the risk of the toxin *flowing* to adjacent sites and causing such side effects as eyelid ptosis. Contracting the treated muscles several times per hour during these 4 hours may increase uptake of the toxin and increase the effectiveness of the treatment. Finally, remember that the goal is the softening of facial lines, not paralysis.

Peels

In general terms, the topic of peels may be divided into three categories: (1) deep peels (eg, phenol peels); (2) medium peels (eg, 30% trichloroacetic acid peels); and (3) superficial peels (eg, alpha-hydroxy and salicylic acid peels [microdermabrasion also *peels* at approximately this level]). Although

space limitations preclude an extensive discussion of peels, suffice it to say that as lunchtime procedures go, the superficial peels may be helpful when incorporated into a complete regimen, including excellent sun protection. Removal of the topmost stratum corneum allows for a smoother skin surface and, possibly, enhanced penetration of therapeutic topical preparations, such as tretinoin or tazarotene.

Summary

A great many products and procedures exist for nonsurgical improvement of the facial skin. Safety and effectiveness must be considered when embarking on a treatment plan. First, a topical regimen that includes a cleanser, moisturizer, and sunscreen must be chosen. Second, relatively simple lunchtime procedures, such as the injection of augmenting fillers and botulinum toxin, may be used to smooth surface lines and shadows. With just these relatively simple techniques, physicians may achieve remarkable improvements in the facial skin of their patients.

References

[1] Ananthapadmanabhan KP, Moore DJ, Subramanyan K, et al. Cleansing without compromise: the impact of cleansers on the skin barrier and the technology of mild cleansing. Dermatol Ther 2004;17(Suppl 1): 16–25.

[2] Draelos ZD. Degradation and migration of facial foundations. J Am Acad Dermatol 2001;45:542–3.

[3] Fischer T, Bjarnason B. Sensitizing and irritant properties of 3 environmental classes of oil and their indicator dyes. Contact Dermatitis 1996;34:309–15.

[4] Kikuchi K, Kobayashi H, Hirao T, et al. Improvement of mild inflammatory changes of the facial skin induced by winter environment with daily applications of a moisturizing cream. Dermatology 2003;207:269–75.

[5] Ramsing DW, Agner T. Preventive and therapeutic effects of a moisturizer: an experimental study of human skin. Acta Derm Venereol 1997;77:335–7.

[6] Held E, Sveinsdottir S, Agner T. Effect of long-term use of moisturizer on skin hydration, barrier function and susceptibility to irritants. Acta Derm Venereol 1999;79:49–51.

[7] Loden M. Role of topical emollients and moisturizers in the treatment of dry skin barrier disorders. Am J Clin Dermatol 2003;4:771–88.

[8] Quan T, He T, Kang S, et al. Solar ultraviolet irradiation reduces collagen in photoaged human skin by blocking transforming growth factor-beta type II receptor/Smad signaling. Am J Pathol 2004;165: 741–51.

[9] Kambayashi H, Yamashita M, Odake Y, et al. Epidermal changes caused by chronic low-dose UV irradiation induce wrinkle formation in hairless mouse. J Dermatol Sci 2001;27:19–25.

[10] Kligman AM, Grove GL, Hirose R, et al. Topical tretinoin for photoaged skin. J Am Acad Dermatol 1986; 15(4 Pt 2):836–59.

[11] Kang S, Leyden JJ, Lowe NJ, et al. Tazarotene cream for the treatment of facial photodamage: a multicenter, investigator-masked, randomized, vehicle-controlled parallel comparison of 0.01%, 0.025%, 0.05% and 0.1% tazarotene creams with 0.05% tretinoin emollient cream applied once daily for 24 weeks. Arch Dermatol 2001;137:1597–604.

[12] Cukier J, Beauchamp R, Spindler J, et al. Association between bovine collagen dermal implants and a dermatomyositis polymyositis-like syndrome. Ann Intern Med 1993;118:920–8.

[13] Rosenberg M, Reichlin M. Is there an association between injectable collagen and polymyositis/dermatomyositis? Arthritis Rheum 1994;37:747–53.

[14] Zyderm Collagen Implant [Inamed]. Physician package insert.

[15] Lowe N. New filler agents: what can we learn from Europe? Practical Dermatology 2004;1:29–33.

[16] Lombardi T, Samsom J, Plantier F, et al. Orofacial granulomas after injection of cosmetic fillers: histopathologic and clinical study of 11 cases. J Oral Pathol Med 2004;33:115–20.

[17] Tzikas TL. Evaluation of the radiance FN soft tissue filler for facial soft tissue augmentation. Arch Facial Plast Surg 2004;6:234–9.

[18] Bartfield JM, May-Wheeling HE, Raccio-Robak N, et al. Benzyl alcohol with epinephrine as an alternative to lidocaine with epinephrine. J Emerg Med 2001;21:375–9.

ELSEVIER
SAUNDERS

Dermatol Clin 23 (2005) 373–381

DERMATOLOGIC
CLINICS

Index

Note: Page numbers of article titles are in **boldface** type.

A

Acne, photodynamic therapy for, 204–205

Actinic keratoses, imiquimod for, 249–250

Acyclovir, indications for, 314–315

Aldara. *See* Topical immunotherapy, imiquimod.

Alefacept. *See* Systemic immune modulators.

Allogenic fillers, in facial rejuvenation, 367–368
in soft tissue augmentation, 353

Alopecia areata. *See* Hair loss.

Alopecia totalis. *See* Hair loss.

Alopecia universalis. *See* Hair loss.

Aminolevulinic acid, in photodynamic therapy, 204

Anesthetics, topical, in pediatric dermatology, 174

Anthralin, for alopecia areata, 237

Antiandrogen therapy, for female pattern hair
loss, 232

Antibiotics, **301–312**
dalbavancin and oritavancin, 309
daptomycin, 301–303
adverse effects of, 302–303
clinical data on, 301–302
historical aspects of, 301
indications for, 301
interactions with, 302
mechanism of action of, 301
pharmacokinetics and dosing of, 302
gatifloxacin and moxifloxacin, 307–309
adverse effects of, 308–309
clinical data on, 308
historical aspects of, 307
indications for, 307–308
interactions with, 308
mechanism of action of, 307
pharmacokinetics and dosing of, 308
in wound healing, 185, 188
interactions with, 335–336

linezolid, 303–306
adverse effects of, 305–306
clinical data on, 304
for diabetic foot ulcers, 189
historical aspects of, 303
indications for, 303–304
interactions with, 304–305
mechanism of action of, 303
pharmacokinetics and dosing of, 304
spectrum of activity of, 303
quinupristin-dalfopristin, 306–307
adverse effects of, 307
clinical data on, 306
historical aspects of, 306
indications for, 306
interactions with, 307
mechanism of action of, 306
pharmacokinetics and dosing of, 306–307

Antimicrobial dressings, in wound healing, 189–190

Antioxidant therapy, for hypomelanosis, 216

Antiviral therapy, **313–322**
acyclovir in, 314–315
cidofovir in, 316, 318, 319
experimental vaccines in, 319–320
for herpesvirus infections, 319
for human papillomavirus, 319–320
famciclovir in, 315
fomivirsen in, 316
for cytomegalovirus, 314
for Epstein–Barr virus, 314
for herpes simplex–1, 313
for herpes simplex–2, 313–314
for herpes zoster, 314
for human papillomavirus, 317–318
for molluscum contagiosum, 318–319
foscarnet in, 316–317
ganciclovir/valganciclovir in, 315–316
helicase primase inhibitors in, 317
highly active antiretroviral therapy in, 319
immunomodulators in, 317–318
nucleoside agents in, 314

penciclovir in, 315
valacyclovir in, 315

Apligraf, for diabetic foot ulcers, 189

Artecoll, in soft tissue augmentation, 355, 358

Artefill, in soft tissue augmentation, 355, 358

Arterial ulcers, healing of, 188

Ascorbic acid, for hypermelanosis, 217

Autogenic fillers, in soft tissue augmentation, 351, 353

Autologous fat, in soft tissue augmentation, 353

Avelox. *See* Antibiotics, gatifloxacin and moxifloxacin.

Azathioprine. *See* Systemic immune modulators.

Azelaic acid, for hypermelanosis, 217, 219

B

Basal cell carcinoma, imiquimod for, 250

Betamethasone, for alopecia areata, 234

Biochemotherapy, for melanoma, 325, 328

Bleaching products, for hypermelanosis, 219

Blister grafts, for hypomelanosis, 215

Botulinum neurotoxin, in facial rejuvenation, 369–370

Burn wounds, autologous cultured keratinocytes for, 185

Butyl cyanoacrylate, in skin closure, 193

4-N-Butylresorcinol, for hypermelanosis, 217

C

Cadexomer iodine, in wound healing, 190

Calcineurin inhibitors, indications for, 251

Calcipotriol, for hypomelanosis, 213–214

Camouflaging, for melanotic pigmentary disorders, 222

Chemical peels, for hypermelanosis, 219–221
in facial rejuvenation, 370

Chemotherapy, for melanoma, 325

Cidofovir, indications for, 316, 318, 319

Cilostazol, for arterial ulcers, 188

Collagens, in facial rejuvenation, 367–368
in soft tissue augmentation, 347, 350

Condylomata acuminata, imiquimod for, 248

Congestive heart failure, infliximab and, 285

Conscious sedation, in pediatric dermatology, 175

Cosmoderm, in facial rejuvenation, 367–368
in soft tissue augmentation, 353

Cosmoplast, in facial rejuvenation, 367–368
in soft tissue augmentation, 353

Cryotherapy, for hypermelanosis, 221

Cubicin. *See* Antibiotics, daptomycin.

Cultured epidermal cell transplantation, for hypomelanosis, 215

Cyanoacrylates, in skin closure, **193–198**
and wound hemostasis, 196
as drug delivery device, 196
as wound dressings, 195–196
butyl cyanoacrylate, 193
indications for, 196
octyl cyanoacrylate, 193–195
and infections, 194
cosmetic outcome of, 194
cost of, 194–195

Cyclophosphamide. *See* Systemic immune modulators.

Cyclosporine, systemic. *See* Systemic immune modulators.
topical, indications for, 251

Cyproterone acetate, for female pattern hair loss, 232

Cytokines, in wound healing, 182

Cytomegalovirus infections, antiviral therapy for, 314
mycophenolate mofetil and, 273

D

Dalbavancin, indications for, 309

Daptomycin. *See* Antibiotics.

Demyelinating diseases, etanercept and, 281
infliximab and, 285

Depigmentation therapy, for hypermelanosis. *See* Hypermelanosis.
for hypomelanosis, 215–216

Dermabrasion, for hypermelanosis, 221

Dermagraft, for diabetic foot ulcers, 189

Diabetic foot ulcers, healing of, 188–189

Dimethyl triazino imidazole carboxamide, for melanoma, 325

Diphenylcyclopropenone, for alopecia areata, 236–237

Drug delivery, cyanoacrylates in, 196

Drug interactions, **335–342**
    adverse binding interactions between drugs and polyvalent cations, 335–336
        bisphosphonates, 336
        mycophenolate mofetil, 336
        quinolone antibiotics, 336
        tetracyclines, 335–336
    adverse interactions between herbal and conventional drugs, 336–337
        St. John's wort, 336–337
    epidermal growth factor receptor inhibitors, 339–340
        clinical features of, 339
        histopathology of, 340
        management of, 340
        mechanism of, 340
    sulfa allergy, 337–339
        definition of, 337
        patient advice on, 338–339
        versus other antibiotics, 337
    with antibiotics. *See* Antibiotics.
    with systemic immune modulators. *See* Systemic immune modulators.

Duke boot, for venous ulcers, 188

E

Efalizumab. *See* Systemic immune modulators.

Elidel, indications for, 252

Epidermal cell transplantation, for hypomelanosis, 215

Epidermal growth factor receptor inhibitors, interactions with. *See* Drug interactions.

Epstein-Barr virus, antiviral therapy for, 314

Erbium:YAG laser therapy, indications for, 202

Etanercept. *See* Systemic immune modulators.

Eutectic mixture of local anesthetics, in pediatric dermatology, 174

Excimer laser therapy, for hypomelanosis, 212–213, 214

Expanded polytetrafluoroethylene, in soft tissue augmentation, 359

Extracellular matrix, in wound healing, 183

F

Facial rejuvenation, nonsurgical, **365–371**
    botulinum neurotoxin in, 369–370
    chemical peels in, 370
    temporary augmenting and filling agents in, 367–369. *See also* Soft tissue fillers.
        collagens, 347, 350, 367–368
        hyaluronic acid, 350–351, 368
        poly-L-lactic acid, 368–369
        Radiance, 358, 369
    topical care, 365–367
        cleansing in, 365–366
        moisturizing, 366
        sun protection, 366–367
        therapeutic creams, 367

Famciclovir, indications for, 315

Fatty acids, unsaturated, for hypermelanosis, 218

Female pattern hair loss. *See* Hair loss.

Finasteride, for female pattern hair loss, 232
    for male pattern hair loss, 228–229

FK-506, indications for, 213–214, 251–252

Flip-top transplantation, for hypomelanosis, 215

Fluocinolone, for alopecia areata, 235

Flutamide, for female pattern hair loss, 232

Fomivirsen, indications for, 316

Foot ulcers, diabetic, healing of, 188–189

Foscarnet, indications for, 316–317

Fusion protein vaccines, for human papillomavirus, 320

G

Ganciclovir/valganciclovir, indications for, 315–316

Gastrointestinal complications, of azathioprine, 260, 262
    of cyclophosphamide, 265
    of methotrexate, 267–268
    of mycophenolate mofetil, 272

Gatifloxacin. *See* Antibiotics.

Glabridin, for hypermelanosis, 218

Glycolic acid, for hypermelanosis, 219–220

Gore-Tex, in soft tissue augmentation, 359

Grafts, blister, for hypomelanosis, 215
    punch, for hypomelanosis, 214
    split-thickness, for hypomelanosis, 215

Growth factors, in wound healing, 182–183

H

Hair loss, **227–243**
    alopecia areata, 234–240
        management of, 239–240
            anthralin in, 237
            combination therapy in, 239
            diphenylcyclopropenone in, 236–237
            intralesional steroids in, 235
            minoxidil in, 238–239
            psoralen plus ultraviolet light therapy in,
                237–238
            squaric acid dibutylester in, 236–237
            systemic steroids in, 235–236
            topical steroids in, 234–235
    female pattern, 231–235
        management of, 232–233
            antiandrogen therapy in, 232
            cyproterone acetate in, 232
            finasteride in, 232
            flutamide in, 232
            hair transplantation in, 233
            minoxidil in, 231–232
            spironolactone in, 232
    male pattern, 227–231
        management of, 230–231
            combination therapy in, 229
            finasteride in, 228–229
            hair transplantation in, 230–231
            minoxidil in, 227–228, 229
    telogen effluvium, 233–234

Hair removal, light therapy in, 202

Hair transplantation, for female pattern hair loss, 233
    for male pattern hair loss, 230–231

Helicase primase inhibitors, indications for, 317

Hematologic complications, of azathioprine, 260
    of cyclophosphamide, 265
    of methotrexate, 267
    of mycophenolate mofetil, 272

Hemostasis, wound, cyanoacrylates and, 196

Herbal medications, versus conventional
    medications, interactions with, 336–337

Herpesvirus infections, antiviral therapy for,
    313–314
    experimental vaccines for, 319

Highly active antiretroviral therapy, indications
    for, 319

Histoplasmosis, infliximab and, 284

Human papillomavirus, antiviral therapy for,
    317–318
    experimental vaccines for, 319–320
    imiquimod for, 248

Hyaluronic acid, in facial rejuvenation, 368
    in soft tissue augmentation, 350–351

Hydroquinones, for hypermelanosis, 216–217, 219,
    220–221

Hylaform, in facial rejuvenation, 368
    in soft tissue augmentation, 350–351

Hypermelanosis, management of, 216–222
        chemical peels in, 219–221
        depigmenting agents in, 216–219
            ascorbic acid, 217
            azelaic acid, 217
            bleaching products, 219
            4-N-butylresorcinol, 217
            combination therapies, 218–219
            hydroquinone, 216–217
            kojic acid, 217
            licorice extracts, 218
            monobenzylether of hydroquinone, 217
            monomethyl ether of hydroquinone, 217
            retinoids, 218
            thioctic acid, 218
            unsaturated fatty acids, 218
        dermabrasion in, 221
        future directions in, 223
        lasers in, 221–222
        liquid nitrogen cryotherapy in, 221
    Wood's light examination in, 209–210

Hypersensitivity reactions, azathioprine and, 262

Hypertension, cyclosporine and, 270

Hypomelanosis, management of, 210–216
        camouflaging in, 222
        combination phototherapies in, 213–214
        depigmentation in, 215–216
        future directions in, 223
        immunomodulators in, 213
            steroids in, 213
        melagenin in, 216
        micropigmentation in, 215
        photoprotection in, 222
        phototherapy in, 210–213
            excimer lasers, 212–213
            focused microphototherapy, 212

psoralens with, 211–212
ultraviolet A, 211–212
ultraviolet B, 212
psychologic support in, 222–223
surgical, 214–215
blister grafts, 215
cultured epidermal cell transplantation, 215
flip-top transplantation, 215
melanocyte suspension transplantation, 215
punch grafts, 214
split-thickness grafts, 215
systemic antioxidant therapy in, 216
tacrolimus in, 213
Wood's light examination in, 209–210

I

Imiquimod. *See* Topical immunotherapy.

Immune modulators, for hypomelanosis, 213
systemic. *See* Systemic immune modulators.

Immune response modifiers, topical.
See Topical immunotherapy.

Immunotherapy, topical. *See* Topical immunotherapy.

Infections, alefacept and, 276
azathioprine and, 262
cyclophosphamide and, 266
efalizumab and, 279
etanercept and, 281
infliximab and, 284
methotrexate and, 268
mycophenolate mofetil and, 273
octyl cyanoacrylate and, 194

Infliximab. *See* Systemic immune modulators.

Intense pulsed light therapy. *See* Light therapy.

Interferons, for melanoma, 323–324

Interleukins, for melanoma, 325, 328

K

Kenalog, for alopecia areata, 235

Keratinocytes, in wound healing, 182–183, 185

Kligman formula, for hypermelanosis, 218

Kojic acid, for hypermelanosis, 217, 219

L

Laser therapy. *See* Light therapy.

Leukopenia, cyclophosphamide and, 265
mycophenolate mofetil and, 272

Licorice extracts, for hypermelanosis, 218

Lidocaine, in pediatric dermatology, 174–175

Light therapy, **199–207**
lasers and intense pulsed light in, 200–203
extending therapeutic range of, 201
for hair removal, 202
for hypermelanosis, 221–222
for hypomelanosis, 212–213, 214
for nonablative dermal remodeling, 202
for skin resurfacing, 202
need for trials in, 202–203
photodynamic therapy in, 204–205
for acne, 204–205
for hypomelanosis. *See* Hypomelanosis.
tissue optics and photobiologic reactions in, 199–200
ultraviolet light in, 203–204
for alopecia areata, 237–238
for hypomelanosis, 211–212
narrow-band UVB, 203
novel sources of, 203–204

Linezolid. *See* Antibiotics.

α-Lipoic acid, for hypermelanosis, 218

Liquid nitrogen cryotherapy, for hypermelanosis, 221

Liquiritin, for hypermelanosis, 218

L-M-X anesthetic, in pediatric dermatology, 174

M

Male pattern hair loss. *See* Hair loss.

Melagenina, for hypomelanosis, 216

Melanin pigmentary disorders.
See Hypermelanosis; Hypomelanosis.

Melanocyte suspension transplantation, for hypomelanosis, 215

Melanoma, management of, **323–333**
advanced disease, 325–328
biochemotherapy for, 325, 328
chemotherapy for, 325
combination chemotherapy for, 325
interleukins for, 325, 328
radiation therapy in, 330
stage III, adjuvant therapy for, 323–325
vaccines in, 328–330
multipolyvalent, 329
univalent, 329–330

Methotrexate. *See* Systemic immune modulators.

8-Methoxypsoralen, for hypomelanosis, 211

Methylprednisolone, for alopecia areata, 235

Microphototherapy, focused, for hypomelanosis, 212

Micropigmentation, for hypomelanosis, 215

Minoxidil, for alopecia areata, 238–239
    for female pattern hair loss, 231–232
    for male pattern hair loss, 227–228, 229

Molluscum contagiosum, antiviral therapy for, 319–320

Monobenzylether of hydroquinone, for
    hypermelanosis, 217
    for hypomelanosis, 215–216

Monomethyl ether of hydroquinone, for
    hypermelanosis, 217, 218–219

Moxifloxacin. *See* Antibiotics.

Mycophenolate mofetil, systemic. *See* Systemic
    immune modulators.
    topical, indications for, 252, 254

Myelosuppression, azathioprine and, 260
    cyclophosphamide and, 265

N

Nd:YAG laser therapy, indications for, 201

Nongenital cutaneous warts, imiquimod for,
    248–249

O

Octyl cyanoacrylate, in skin closure.
    See Cyanoacrylates.

Oritavancin, indications for, 309

Oxygen tension, in wound healing, 184

P

Pediatric dermatology, **171–180**
    adherence to treatment programs in, 175–179
        age factors in, 176
        cognitive factors in, 176
        developmental factors in, 175–176
        family's role in, 177–178
        physician's role in, 178–179
        psychologic factors in, 177
        social and emotional factors in, 176–177
    office visit in, 171–173
        for adolescents, 172–173
        for infants, 171–172

    for school–aged children, 172
    for toddlers and preschool–aged children, 172
    pain and intrusive procedures in, 173–175
        nonpharmacologic approaches to, 173–174
            in adolescents, 174
            in infants, 173
            in school-aged children, 174
            in toddlers and preschool–aged children,
                173–174
        pharmacologic approaches to, 174–175
            conscious sedation, 175
            lidocaine, 174–175
            topical anesthetics, 174

Penciclovir, indications for, 315

Pentoxifylline, for arterial ulcers, 188

Peptide-based vaccines, for human
    papillomavirus, 320

Pexiganan, for diabetic foot ulcers, 189

Phenol compounds, for hypermelanosis, 216–217

Phenolic-thioether, for hypermelanosis, 217

Photodynamic therapy, for hypomelanosis.
    See Hypomelanosis.
    indications for, 204–205

Photoprotection, against hypomelanosis, 222

Pigmentary disorders, melanin.
    See Hypermelanosis; Hypomelanosis.

Pigmented lesion dye laser therapy, for
    hypermelanosis, 221–222

Pimecrolimus, indications for, 252

Poly-L-lactic acid, in facial rejuvenation, 368–369

Polymethylmethacrylate, in soft tissue augmentation,
    355, 358

Prednisone, for alopecia areata, 235

Psoralens, for alopecia areata, 237–238
    for hypomelanosis, 211–212

Psoriasis, efalizumab for, 279–280
    mycophenolate mofetil for, 273
    ultraviolet light therapy for, 203

Punch grafts, for hypomelanosis, 214

Q

Q-switched alexandrite laser therapy, for
    hypermelanosis, 221–222

Q-switched Nd:YAG laser therapy, for
    hypermelanosis, 221–222

Q-switched ruby laser therapy, for hypermelanosis, 221–222

Quinolone antibiotics, interactions with, 336

Quinupristin-dalfopristin. *See* Antibiotics.

R

Radiance, in facial rejuvenation, 369
  in soft tissue augmentation, 358

Radiation therapy, for melanoma, 330

Renal complications, of cyclosporine, 270

Renova, in facial rejuvenation, 367

Reproductive complications, of
  cyclophosphamide, 265
  of methotrexate, 268

Resiquimod, indications for, 318

Restylane, in soft tissue augmentation, 350–351

Retin-A, in facial rejuvenation, 367

Retinoids, for hypermelanosis, 218–219
  in facial rejuvenation, 367

S

Sculptra, in facial rejuvenation, 368–369

Sedation, conscious, in pediatric dermatology, 175

Silicone fillers, in soft tissue augmentation, 358–359

Silver-based antimicrobial dressings, in wound
  healing, 189

Skin closure, cyanoacrylates in. *See* Cyanoacrylates.

Skin equivalents, in wound healing, 185

Skin resurfacing, lasers in, 202

Soft tissue fillers, **343–363**. *See also*
  Facial rejuvenation.
  adverse effects of, 346
  allogenic, 353, 367–368
  autogenic, 351, 353
  autologous fat, 353
  collagens, 347, 350, 367–368
  expanded polytetrafluoroethylene, 359
  historical aspects of, 343
  hyaluronic acid, 350–351, 368
  manufacturers of, 360–362
  minimizing risks of, 344
  optimizing outcome of, 346
  polymethylmethacrylate, 355, 358
  preoperative preparation for, 343–344

Radiance, 358, 369
  silicone, 358–359
  synthetic, 355
  techniques for, 344–346
    methods of delivery, 345–346
    needle selection, 344
  xenogenic, 346–347

Spironolactone, for female pattern hair loss, 232

Split-thickness grafts, for hypomelanosis, 215

Squamous cell carcinoma, imiquimod for, 249–250

Squaric acid dibutylester, for alopecia areata,
  236–237

St. John's wort, versus conventional medications,
  interactions with, 336–337

Stem cells, in wound healing, 184

Steroids, for alopecia areata. *See* Hair loss.
  for hypomelanosis, 213
  in immunosuppressive therapy, 251

Sulfonamides, interactions with.
  See Drug interactions.

Synercid. *See* Antibiotics, quinupristin–dalfopristin.

Systemic immune modulators, **259–300**
  alefacept, 275–278
    adverse effects of, 276
      immune system, 276
      infections, 276
      injection site reactions, 276
      oncogenic potential, 276
    dosage and monitoring of, 278
    efficacy of, 276–277
    indications for, 277
    mechanism of action of, 275–276
    pharmacology of, 275–276
    usage guidelines for, 277–278
  azathioprine, 259–260, 262–263
    adverse effects of, 260, 262
      gastrointestinal, 260, 262
      hematologic, 260
      hypersensitivity reactions, 262
      oncogenic potential, 262
      opportunistic infections, 262
    dosage and monitoring of, 263
    indications for, 262–263
    interactions with, 263
    pharmacology of, 260
    usage guidelines for, 263
  cyclophosphamide, 263, 265–266
    adverse effects of, 265–266
      gastrointestinal, 265

hematologic, 265
    oncogenic potential, 265
    opportunistic infections, 266
    reproductive toxicity, 265
    urologic, 265
  dosage and monitoring of, 266
  indications for, 266
  interactions with, 266
  pharmacology of, 263, 265
  usage guidelines for, 266
cyclosporine, 269–272
  adverse effects of, 270
    nephrotoxicity and hypertension, 270
    oncogenic potential, 270
  dosage and monitoring of, 271–272
  indications for, 251, 270–271
  interactions with, 271
  pharmacology of, 269–270
  usage guidelines for, 271
efalizumab, 278–280
  adverse effects of, 278–279
    immune system, 279
    infections, 279
    oncogenic potential, 278–279
    thrombocytopenia, 279
  dosage and monitoring of, 280
  efficacy of, 279
  indications for, 279–280
  interactions with, 280
  mechanism of action of, 278
  pharmacology of, 278
  usage guidelines for, 280
etanercept, 280–283
  adverse effects of, 280–282
    demyelinating disease, 281
    immune system, 281
    infections, 281
    injection site reactions, 281–282
    oncogenic potential, 280–281
  dosage and monitoring of, 283
  efficacy of, 282
  indications for, 282
  interactions with, 283
  mechanism of action of, 280
  pharmacology of, 280
  usage guidelines for, 282–283
infliximab, 283–287
  adverse effects of, 283–285
    congestive heart failure, 285
    demyelinating disease, 285
    immune system, 284–285
    infections, 284
    infusion reactions, 285
    oncogenic potential, 283–284

  dosage and monitoring of, 287
  efficacy of, 285–286
  indications for, 286
  interactions with, 287
  mechanism of action of, 283
  pharmacology of, 283
  usage guidelines for, 286–287
methotrexate, 267–269
  adverse effects of, 267–268
    gastrointestinal, 267–268
    hematologic, 267
    oncogenic potential, 268
    opportunistic infections, 268
    reproductive toxicity, 268
  dosage and monitoring of, 269
  indications for, 268–269
  interactions with, 269
  pharmacology of, 267
  usage guidelines for, 269
mycophenolate mofetil, 272–275
  adverse effects of, 272–273
    gastrointestinal, 272
    hematologic, 272
    infections, 273
    oncogenic potential, 272–273
  dosage and monitoring of, 274
  indications for, 252, 254, 273–274
  interactions with, 274
  pharmacology of, 272
  usage guidelines for, 274

T

Tacrolimus, for hypomelanosis, 213, 214
  indications for, 251–252

Tazarotene, for hypermelanosis, 218

Telogen effluvium, management of, 233–234

Tequin. *See* Antibiotics, gatifloxacin
  and moxifloxacin.

Tetracyclines, interactions with, 335–336

Thioctic acid, for hypermelanosis, 218

Thrombocytopenia, efalizumab and, 279

Tissue-engineered skin products, for diabetic foot
  ulcers, 189

Topical immunotherapy, **245–258**
  for alopecia areata, 236–237
  immunosuppressive agents in, 251–252, 254
    calcineurin inhibitors, 251
    cyclosporine, 251
    mycophenolate mofetil, 252, 254

pimecrolimus, 252
steroids, 251
tacrolimus, 213, 214, 251–252
Toll-like receptor agonists in, 246–248
imiquimod, 246–251, 317–318
as antineoplastic agent, 249–250
for human papillomavirus, 248
for nongenital cutaneous warts, 248–249
future directions in, 250–251
Toll-like receptors in, 245–246

Tretinoin, for hypermelanosis, 218–219
in facial rejuvenation, 367

Triamcinolone acetonide, for alopecia areata, 235

Tuberculosis, reactivation of, infliximab and, 284

U

Ulcers, healing of. *See* Wound healing.

Ultraviolet light therapy, for hypomelanosis, 211–212
indications for, 203–204

Urologic complications, of cyclophosphamide, 265

V

Vaccines, experimental, for herpesviruses, 319
for human papillomavirus, 319–320
for melanoma. *See* Melanoma.

Valacyclovir, indications for, 315

Venous ulcers, healing of, 188

Viruslike particles, for human papillomavirus, 319–320

Vitiligo. *See* Hypomelanosis.

W

Westerhof formula, for hypermelanosis, 219

Wood's light examination, of melanin pigmentary disorders, 209–210

Wound dressings, cyanoacrylates as, 195–196

Wound healing, **181–192**
antibiotics in, 185, 188
antimicrobial dressings in, 189–190
cytokines in, 182
extracellular matrix in, 183
growth factors in, 182, 183
keratinocytes in, 182–183, 185
of arterial ulcers, 188
of diabetic foot ulcers, 188–189
of venous ulcers, 188
oxygen tension in, 184
prohealing elements in skin and, 181–182
serum versus plasma in, 182–183
skin equivalents in, 185
stem cells in, 184

Wound hemostasis, cyanoacrylates and, 196

Z

Zyderm, in facial rejuvenation, 367
in soft tissue augmentation, 347

Zyplast, in facial rejuvenation, 367
in soft tissue augmentation, 347

Zyvox. *See* Antibiotics, linezolid.

Changing Your Address?

Make sure your subscription changes too! When you notify us of your new address, you can help make our job easier by including an exact copy of your Clinics label number with your old address (see illustration below.) This number identifies you to our computer system and will speed the processing of your address change. Please be sure this label number accompanies your old address and your corrected address—you can send an old Clinics label with your number on it or just copy it exactly and send it to the address listed below.

We appreciate your help in our attempt to give you continuous coverage. Thank you.

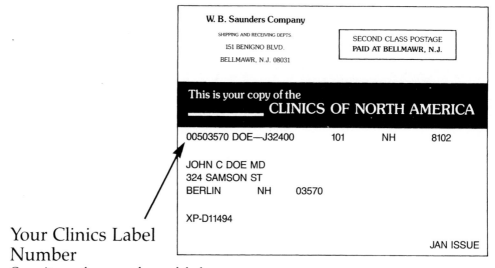

W. B. Saunders Company

SHIPPING AND RECEIVING DEPTS.
151 BENIGNO BLVD.
BELLMAWR, N.J. 08031

SECOND CLASS POSTAGE
PAID AT BELLMAWR, N.J.

This is your copy of the
_____ **CLINICS OF NORTH AMERICA**

00503570 DOE—J32400   101   NH   8102

JOHN C DOE MD
324 SAMSON ST
BERLIN   NH   03570

XP-D11494

JAN ISSUE

Your Clinics Label
Number
Copy it exactly or send your label
along with your address to:
W.B. Saunders Company, Customer Service
Orlando, FL 32887-4800
Call Toll Free 1-800-654-2452

Please allow four to six weeks for delivery of new subscriptions and for processing address changes.

Practice, Current, Hardbound:
SATISFACTION GUARANTEED

Please Print:

Name _____

Address_____

City_____ State _____ ZIP _____

Method of Payment

❑ Check (payable to **Elsevier**; add the applicable sales tax for your area)

❑ VISA　　❑ MasterCard　　❑ AmEx　　❑ Bill me

Card number _____ Exp. date _____

Signature _____

Staple this to your purchase order to expedite delivery

Adolescent Medicine Clinics
- ❑ Individual $95
- ❑ Institutions $133
- ❑ *In-training $48

Anesthesiology
- ❑ Individual $175
- ❑ Institutions $270
- ❑ *In-training $88

Cardiology
- ❑ Individual $170
- ❑ Institutions $266
- ❑ *In-training $85

Chest Medicine
- ❑ Individual $185
- ❑ Institutions $285

Child and Adolescent Psychiatry
- ❑ Individual $175
- ❑ Institutions $265
- ❑ *In-training $88

Critical Care
- ❑ Individual $165
- ❑ Institutions $266
- ❑ *In-training $83

Dental
- ❑ Individual $150
- ❑ Institutions $242

Emergency Medicine
- ❑ Individual $170
- ❑ Institutions $263
- ❑ *In-training $85
- ❑ Send CME info

Facial Plastic Surgery
- ❑ Individual $199
- ❑ Institutions $300

Foot and Ankle
- Individual $160
- Institutions $232

Gastroenterology
- ❑ Individual $190
- ❑ Institutions $276

Gastrointestinal Endoscopy
- ❑ Individual $190
- ❑ Institutions $276

Hand
- ❑ Individual $205
- ❑ Institutions $319

Heart Failure (NEW in 2005!)
- ❑ Individual $99
- ❑ Institutions $149
- ❑ *In-training $49

Hematology/Oncology
- ❑ Individual $210
- ❑ Institutions $315

Immunology & Allergy
- ❑ Individual $165
- ❑ Institutions $266

Infectious Disease
- ❑ Individual $165
- ❑ Institutions $272

Clinics in Liver Disease
- ❑ Individual $165
- ❑ Institutions $234

Medical
- ❑ Individual $140
- ❑ Institutions $244
- ❑ *In-training $70
- ❑ Send CME info

MRI
- ❑ Individual $190
- ❑ Institutions $290
- ❑ *In-training $95
- ❑ Send CME info

Neuroimaging
- ❑ Individual $190
- ❑ Institutions $290
- ❑ *In-training $95
- ❑ Send CME inf0

Neurologic
- ❑ Individual $175
- ❑ Institutions $275

Obstetrics & Gynecology
- ❑ Individual $175
- ❑ Institutions $288

Occupational and Environmental Medicine
- ❑ Individual $120
- ❑ Institutions $166
- ❑ *In-training $60

Ophthalmology
- ❑ Individual $190
- ❑ Institutions $325

Oral & Maxillofacial Surgery
- ❑ Individual $180
- ❑ Institutions $280
- ❑ *In-training $90

Orthopedic
- ❑ Individual $180
- ❑ Institutions $295
- ❑ *In-training $90

Otolaryngologic
- ❑ Individual $199
- ❑ Institutions $350

Pediatric
- ❑ Individual $135
- ❑ Institutions $246
- ❑ *In-training $68
- ❑ Send CME info

Perinatology
- ❑ Individual $155
- ❑ Institutions $237
- ❑ *In-training $78
- ❑ Send CME inf0

Plastic Surgery
- ❑ Individual $245
- ❑ Institutions $370

Podiatric Medicine & Surgery
- ❑ Individual $170
- ❑ Institutions $266

Primary Care
- ❑ Individual $135
- ❑ Institutions $223

Psychiatric
- ❑ Individual $170
- ❑ Institutions $288

Radiologic
- ❑ Individual $220
- ❑ Institutions $331
- ❑ *In-training $110
- ❑ Send CME info

Sports Medicine
- ❑ Individual $180
- ❑ Institutions $277

Surgical
- ❑ Individual $190
- ❑ Institutions $299
- ❑ *In-training $95

Thoracic Surgery (formerly Chest Surgery)
- ❑ Individual $175
- ❑ Institutions $255
- ❑ *In-training $88

Urologic
- ❑ Individual $195
- ❑ Institutions $307
- ❑ *In-training $98
- ❑ Send CME info

Order your subscription today. Simply complete and detach this card and drop it in the mail to receive the best clinical information in your field.

BUSINESS REPLY MAIL

FIRST-CLASS MAIL   PERMIT NO 7135   ORLANDO FL

POSTAGE WILL BE PAID BY ADDRESSEE

PERIODICALS ORDER FULFILLMENT DEPT
ELSEVIER
6277 SEA HARBOR DR
ORLANDO FL 32821-9816